DETECTION AND TREATMENT OF BREAST CANCER

Second Edition

DETECTION AND TREATMENT OF BREAST CANCER

Second Edition

IAN S FENTIMAN, MD FRCS

Professor of Surgical Oncology

Hedley Atkins Breast Unit

Guy's Hospital

London, UK

MARTIN DUNITZ

© Ian S Fentiman 1990, 1998

First published in the UK in 1990 by
Martin Dunitz Ltd
The Livery House
7–9 Pratt Street
London NW1 0AE

Second edition 1998

A CIP catalogue record for this book is available
from the British Library.

ISBN 1-85317-223-5

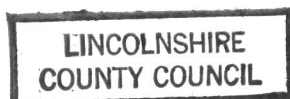

Composition by Scribe Design, Gillingham, Kent
Printed and bound in Great Britain by Biddles Ltd,
Guildford and King's Lynn

Contents

Preface to the second edition

A book that furnishes no quotations is, me judice, *no book – it is a plaything.*

Thomas Love Peacock

It is now seven years since the first edition of this book was published and the field of breast cancer has made substantial progress. Mortality from the disease is falling, and should fall further as screening makes its impact. Breast conservation is no longer regarded as experimental by surgeons, more of whom are specializing in looking after women with breast problems. As a result of clinical research, great improvements have been achieved.

Rather than being slightly modified, this book has been completely re-written and given a new title. It has expanded as a result of new topics being covered. Of necessity, this is one person's view of aspects of early breast cancer, but I hope that it achieves a more united synthesis than is possible with multi-author books.

I owe a great debt to my colleagues who have kindly advised me on the text, particularly Murid Chaudhury, Hisham Hamed, Andy Hanby, Elisabeth Heap, David Miles, Rosemary Millis, Tony Rowsell, Robert Rubens, David Tong, Dennis Wang, and Phil Wilson. Without their help, this book would not have been completed. Finally, I thank Pam Evans for her IT tuition and support.

Ian S Fentiman

I would like to dedicate this book to my
patients whose unfailing courage and
determination have been an inexhaustible
source of inspiration

ISF

1

The causes

If a man will begin with certainties he shall end in doubts, but if he will be content to begin with doubts he shall end in certainties.
                                                    Francis Bacon

Age and incidence • Carcinogenesis

The molecular jigsaw of breast cancer is still in fragments. It is likely that more than one mutagenic hit causes permanent alterations to mammary epithelium as a result of a failure of DNA repair mechanisms. The result, many years later, is the appearance of a breast cancer. So much of this is as yet conjectural but the pieces are being put together gradually, and a picture is emerging at molecular, cellular and clinical levels. The manifold causes are uncharacterized and the biological behaviour can be unpredictable but, despite this, the diagnosis and treatment of this capricious disease are the subjects of continual, modest, yet significant, improvements. A guaranteed cure and a totally effective prevention scheme require a greater understanding of basic events, together with a different viewpoint on the epidemiology of the disease.

Present knowledge of risk factors gives powerful pointers to the aetiology of breast cancer: the disease affects between one in nine and one in twelve women, but fewer than one in a 1000 men. Hence the endocrine milieu associated with being female is a very powerful determinant of risk and most epidemiological studies have reiterated this truism. The other major risk factor is age. In the Western World, about half the cases of breast cancer occur in women aged over 65 years. The longer that an individual lives, the greater the cumulative exposure to carcinogens and the higher the probability of DNA damage remaining unrepaired.

AGE AND INCIDENCE

During a woman's lifetime, the cells of her body may undergo approximately 10^{16} divisions, associated with a spontaneous mutation rate of 10^{-6}/gene per cell division.[1] Almost all these cells undergo apoptosis with, it is thought, only the stem cells being programmed for survival, so that a mutation within this subset will lead to a robust malignant phenotype in daughter cells. Mammary epithelium is unusual in that there is cyclical proliferation during the reproductive years, together with surges of proliferation and differentiation during pregnancies.

Rather than carcinogenesis being a multistage process, it is likely that the first mutagenic hit gives rise to a transformed cell morphologically indistinguishable from the normal but, as a result of a second hit, manifesting as a malignant phenotype.[2] As support for this theory, Kodama et al compared age-specific incidence rates (ASIR) of breast cancers in British (high-risk) and Japanese (low-risk) women between

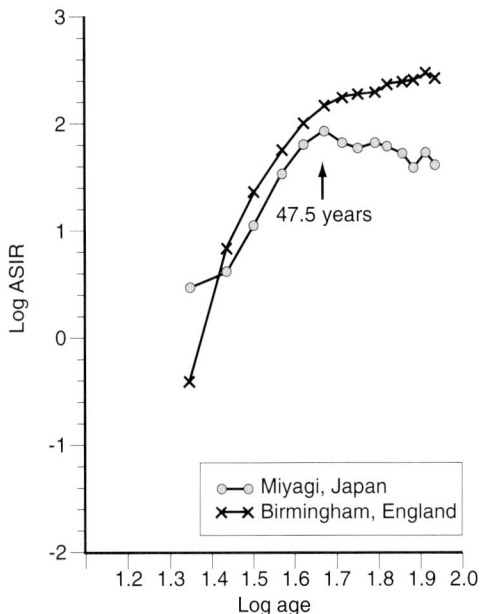

Fig. 1.1 Age-specific incidence rates for breast cancer in Japan and England. (From Kodama et al.[3])

1960 and 1980.[3] The two target populations were Birmingham, England and Miyagi, Japan. During these two decades there was a modest increase in incidence in Japan, but only a slight increase in Britain.

The log-transformed data are shown in Fig. 1.1, which indicates a similar ASIR in both populations up to the age of 47.5 years. At this breakpoint the two populations diverged, with a plateauing of incidence in the Japanese and a continued but slower rise among the British women. For cancers of the stomach and lung there was no perimenopausal breakpoint but instead an inflexion around age 70. This can be interpreted as showing that there was little change in epithelial turnover in stomach and lung until senescence, whereas mammary epithelial proliferation largely ceased at the time of the menopause in the Japanese but continued in the British women (possibly because of endogenous oestrogens derived from peripheral aromatization of adrenal androgens).

Taking into account the physiological breast changes at puberty, pregnancy and the menopause, Moolgavkar et al created a mathematical model based on a two-stage process of mammary carcinogenesis.[2] The assumptions upon which the model was based were the following: transformation of a single cell led on to clinical cancer; all cells were of similar susceptibility; and the time to clinical detection could be treated as a constant. When the model was applied to women from Iceland, Denmark, Slovenia, the USA, Finland and Japan, the predicted age-incidence curves were in close agreement with the observed data. In particular, the protective effect of early age at first full-term pregnancy predicted by the model was consistent with the available multinational epidemiological findings.

To quantify lifetime risks of developing breast cancer, Feuer reanalysed data from the National Cancer Institute's Surveillance, Epidemiology, and End Results (SEER) project.[4] In the group of women aged 80–89 years, the cumulative probability of developing breast cancer was 0.125 so that one in eight will have been diagnosed with the disease. The approximate incidence rates with age are given in Table 1.1 and these indicate that, by the age of 49, only one in 70 women will have developed

Table 1.1 Incidence of breast cancer with age

Age (years)	Incidence rate
< 20	1 in 170 000
20–29	1 in 5000
30–39	1 in 500
40–49	1 in 70
50–59	1 in 30
60–69	1 in 17
70–79	1 in 10
80–89	1 in 8

From Feuer et al.[4]

Table 1.2 Numbers of individuals with lymphocytes showing chromatid breaks after irradiation of cells from normal women and breast cancer patients with and without a family history

| | Chromatid breaks per 100 metaphase cells | | | | |
	20–60	61–100	101–140	141–160	>161
Normal	9	–	1	–	–
Normal + family history	1	–	1	–	1
Breast cancer	6	–	3	1	1
Breast cancer + family history	1	–	4	2	–

From Parshad et al.[7]

breast cancer, rising to one in 30 by age 59 and one in 10 at age 79. These figures indicate a higher incidence than often stated, in part because the data are derived from the high incidence in the USA, and also because they represent lifetime risks. The enormity of the problem of breast cancer is starkly illuminated by this calculation.

CARCINOGENESIS

Chemical carcinogens

Carcinogens are ubiquitous in nature, even in the absence of human industrial or recreational pollution. Although some have been identified that can therefore be avoided, the major protection against initiation of the process of carcinogenesis is the DNA repair mechanisms. Individuals with inherited deficiencies of DNA repair, such as Bloom's syndrome with anomalously heat labile ligase I, will develop early-onset malignancies.[5] It is likely that this arises from a missense mutation in the gene coding for ligase I. The rare condition of ataxia–telangiectasia, associated with an increased risk of breast cancer, is the result of an altered form of deoxyribose within DNA

leading to a failure to inhibit transcription from a damaged template.[6]

These rare conditions may hold the key to induction of some sporadic tumours. To investigate this, Parshad et al measured radiation-induced DNA repair in normal individuals and breast cancer patients with and without a family history.[7] Blood samples were taken from all individuals, lymphocytes were extracted and then transformed with phytohaemagglutinin (PHA), after which the cells were grown in vitro for 72 hours. At that time the cells were suspended and irradiated to a total dose of 0.48 Gy. Thereafter the cells were incubated and then treated with colcemid before examination for chromatid breaks. An outline of the results is given in Table 1.2, which shows the low incidence of chromatid breaks in lymphocytes from normal women (10% > 101). In contrast, there were over 101 chromatid breaks in 55% of those with breast cancer and in 86% of those with breast cancer and a family history. These data suggest that deficient DNA repair may predispose to both familial and sporadic breast cancer.

To examine the role of DNA repair capacity in neoplastic transformation of the breast, Sanford et al cultured normal human mammary epithelium extracted from a reduction mammoplasty specimen.[8] The normal mammary epithelium maintained a low level of chromatid breaks (<60 per 100 cells), after up to 12 passages in vitro. In contrast, those that had been transformed with benzo(a)pyrene had a threefold increase in chromatid breaks. When these cells became tumorigenic after treatment with HaMSV and SV40 T antigen there was a fivefold increase. This suggests that, at least in vitro, there is a link between DNA repair deficiency and tumorigenesis.

In a different approach, Shaw et al studied microsatellite instability in 78 screen-detected invasive breast cancers.[9] Microsatellite instability is a mutation in which there is tandem repetition of between one- and six-nucleotide motifs, probably as a result of deficiency in DNA-mismatch repair genes, with both copies being inactivated.[10] Shaw et al extracted DNA from representative malignant and non-malignant tissue and used the polymerase chain reaction (PCR) to determine microsatellite repeats. Microsatellite instability was found in tumours of four cases, but not in normal tissue from these individuals, suggesting that this was possibly an early event rather than a predisposing factor. Hence this particular DNA-repair deficiency is not an aetiological factor in breast cancer.

Radiation

The major source of human exposure to ionizing irradiation is the medical profession. As a result of both diagnostic and therapeutic interventions, there is a burgeoning of data indicating a link between radiation exposure and risk of malignancy, including breast cancers. Unfortunately, as radiotherapists tried to extend their role beyond malignancy many luckless individuals were irradiated for benign conditions such as ringworm, thymic enlargement, postpartum mastitis and fibroadenosis. Such practices have now been discontinued but follow-up results have provided us with important aetiological information.

A series of 10 384 Israeli children were treated with low-dose scalp irradiation for ringworm (tinea capitis), and were found to have a fourfold increase in risk of head and neck cancers.[11] In comparison with an age-matched non-irradiated group, after a longer follow-up of over 30 years, an excess of breast cancers (relative risk, RR = 2.9) was observed in the treated group.[12] The calculated dose to the breast was only 16 mGy. Increase in risk was confined to those who were aged 5–9 years at the time of irradiation, indicating the susceptibility of the prepubertal breast to ionizing radiation.

Hildreth et al studied a group of 1201 women who had radiotherapy to the anterior mediastinum because of thymic enlargement and their 2469 sisters who were not irradiated.[13] The estimated mean absorbed mammary dose was 0.69 Gy, and the two groups were followed for a mean of 36 years. There were 12 breast cancers diagnosed in the control group and 22 in the irradiated group (adjusted relative risk = 3.6), with the first breast cancer being diagnosed 28 years after irradiation.

Skin haemangioma was a further lapsed indication for radiotherapy and, between 1920 and 1959, 9675 women were treated for this condition in infancy at the Radiumhemmet, Stockholm.[14] The average age at irradiation was 6 months and the calculated mean breast exposure was 0.39 Gy. A total of 75 breast cancers were diagnosed whereas 61 would have been expected (RR = 1.24). There was a significant dose–response relationship but this did not become apparent until 40–50 years had elapsed.

Breast irradiation was used as treatment for women with acute postpartum mastitis and Shore et al conducted a mail survey of 571 women who had been treated at the University of Rochester, New York.[15] In years 10–34 after treatment the relative risk of breast cancer was 2.2 and, for years 20–34, it was 3.6. These data were reanalysed by Prince and Hildreth to determine whether there were biases.[16] These included selection bias, differential verification of diagnosis, differential diagnosis and confounding variables. Even after adjustment for these variables, there remained a significantly elevated risk of breast cancer (RR = 2.7)

Table 1.3 Follow-up studies of breast cancer incidence after radiotherapy for lymphoma

Number	Follow-up (years)	Observed	Expected	Relative risk	Reference
6171	15	41	46	0.89	Travis et al[18]
885	10	25	6	4	Hancock et al[19]

Table 1.4 Risk of breast cancer after multiple diagnostic X-rays

Number	Indication	Mean dose (Gy)	Follow-up (years)	Relative risk	Reference
1 742	Tuberculosis	0.96	30	1.86	Hrubec et al[20]
1 030	Scoliosis	0.12	26	1.82	Hoffman et al[21]
31 710	Tuberculosis	>0.1	30	1.6	Miller et al[22]

in those who had received radiotherapy. Mattsson et al reported the outcome of a group of 1216 women irradiated for postpartum mastitis, so-called chronic mastitis and fibroadenosis, who were followed for up to 60 years.[17] An increase in risk of breast cancer was first observed 25 years after irradiation and the overall relative risk was 3.6. Risk was greater in younger women but was seen in all age groups.

For patients with non-Hodgkin's (NHL) and Hodgkin's lymphoma, mantle irradiation has been an intrinsic part of therapy, which can result in a breast radiation dose of 14–40 Gy. In a cohort of patients from the Netherlands, the USA, Canada and Sweden the average age at diagnosis of NHL was 56 years and after 15 years of follow-up there were fewer breast cancers than expected in this group (RR = 0.89), as shown in Table 1.3.[18] In contrast a follow-up of 885 women with Hodgkin's lymphoma showed a fourfold increase in risk of breast cancer.[19] The probable explanation for the difference was that the average age of the

patients in the second study was 28 years. Indeed there was no increase in risk in those aged over 30 years, whereas for those aged 15–24 at the time of irradiation the relative risk was 19 and for those aged 24 to 29, it was 7.

As a result of chronic diseases such as pulmonary tuberculosis or scoliosis, many individuals were exposed to radiation because of the need for multiple X-rays to monitor the progress of their condition. Results of larger studies with long-term follow-up are summarized in Table 1.4.[20–22] In a study of 1742 women treated for tuberculosis at two sanatoria in the USA, there was a significantly increased risk of breast cancer in those who had repeated fluoroscopies as part of pneumothorax treatment.[20] There was a linear dose–response and risk diminished with increasing age. Hoffman followed 1030 women with scoliosis, who had a mean age at diagnosis of 12 years.[21] There was a significant elevated relative risk which was greater in those who had received more X-rays and increased with length of follow-up.

A Canadian cohort of women who had been treated for tuberculosis was examined, not for incidence of breast cancer but in terms of mortality from the disease.[22] There was a significant elevation of mortality (RR = 1.6), which showed a linear dose–response relationship and was greatest among those exposed to radiation between ages 10 and 14. There was a sharp diminution in risk with increasing age, which could be taken to indicate that carrying out X-rays such as mammograms in women over age 50 would not lead to any significant increase in radiation-induced breast cancers.

As an unexpected outcome of the atomic bombing of Hiroshima and Nagasaki in 1945, extensive information has accumulated in relation to age, radiation exposure and subsequent risk of cancer. In terms of breast cancer the populations had a low incidence. Between 1958 and 1987 the incidence of breast cancer doubled in both Hiroshima and Nagasaki.[23] Despite this, the age-specific incidence rate still shows a rise up to the age of 50 and a plateau thereafter, unlike that of women in Europe and North America.

The age of individuals at the time of the bombing had a major impact on risk of subsequent breast cancer. Among 63 275 female survivors of the bombing in both cities, 187 who had a quantifiable radiation exposure had been diagnosed with breast cancer.[24] There was a fourfold increase in risk for those who had been aged 10–19 at the time of the bombing, compared with a relative risk of 1.2 for those aged 20–34 and 0.9 in those who were 35–49. This indicates the increased sensitivity of the pubertal breast to irradiation and the possibly protective effect of irradiation in older women because of the induction of a premature menopause.

Land et al conducted a case-control interview study of 196 breast cancer cases diagnosed in both Hiroshima and Nagasaki and 566 controls based on age, city of residence, and whether or not exposed to radiation.[25] For those with a specific known dose estimate, four matched controls were selected. The aim of the study was to examine the interaction of known risk factors with radiation dose. There was a positive relationship between age at first full-term pregnancy. Negative (protective) effects were found with regard to number of births and duration of lactation. For postmenopausal women there was an increase in risk for those who were obese or had a history of either thyroid disease or uterine/ovarian surgery. Further analyses indicated that young age at first pregnancy, multiple births and prolonged lactation were protective, not only against breast cancer in those who had not been exposed to irradiation, but also in the exposed group.

Recently the Radiation Effects Research Foundation's extended Life Span Study (LSS) also reported non-radiation risk factors after 8 years of follow-up in a cohort of 22 000 women who participated in a mail questionnaire.[26] During the time of follow-up, 161 breast cancer cases had been diagnosed. Early age at first pregnancy was protective, but not the number of subsequent pregnancies. Obesity was associated with an increase in risk as was use of hormone replacement therapy and a history of diabetes. It was suggested that reproductive risk factors were acting independently of radiation exposure in this population.

Diet

There are several compelling reasons to believe that dietary intake has an important role in the genesis of breast cancer but the demonstration of specific cause and effect is lacking. Surgeons have been aware for many years that they are more likely to perform mastectomies on fat rather than thin women. More recently, this has been quantified using computed tomography at the level of the fourth lumbar vertebra.[27] In a case-control study of 40 breast cancer cases and 40 age-, weight- and height-matched controls, there was a significantly greater visceral fat area in the cases who also had significantly lower subcutaneous to visceral fat ratios. The breast cancer cases had about 45% more visceral fat than the controls.

Another pointer is the international difference in breast cancer incidence. In 1966, Lea

Table 1.5 Comparative incidence rates for breast cancer among Japanese, American, and Japanese–American women

Age (years)	Japanese (%)	Issei (%)	Nisei (%)	American (%)
35–64	18	52	65	100
65–74	7	56	–	100

From Buell.[30]

demonstrated that there was a highly signifi-cant relationship between national mortality rates from breast cancer and consumption of fats.[28] Subsequently, Armstrong and Doll examined incidence rates of breast cancer and diet in 37 countries and found that the compo-nent that gave the greatest correlation was fat. However, there was an even greater correlation between gross national product and incidence rates, suggesting that fat consumption was a wealth indicator and that other wealth-associ-ated variables might be responsible for mammary carcinogenesis.

It could be argued that international differ-ences in incidence rates of breast cancer are the result of different genetic susceptibilities rather than variations in diet. That this is not so is demonstrated by migrant studies of Japanese who moved from Japan to either Hawaii or San Francisco.[29,30] At the time of migration the incidence rate of breast cancer in Japan was one-fifth of that in the USA. Buell examined incidence rates in Japanese women aged 35–74 born in Japan but living in California (Issei).[30] These were compared with rates for second-generation Japanese, born in the USA (Nisei), aged 25–64, and Japanese women living in Okayama, Japan. Outline results are given in Table 1.5 and show that incidence in Japanese women living in Japan aged 65–74 was only 7% of that American women of the same age whereas the Issei had 56% of the US rate. For younger women aged 35–64, the Japanese rate

was 18% of the American but, for the Issei, 52% and for the Nisei, 56%. Thus there was a fairly rapid assimilation of the increased American risk by the migrating Japanese and this presum-ably has to be attributed to alterations in diet, water or air.

In the attempts that have been made to dissect out the dietary components that might increase the risk of breast cancer there is often a confusion as to whether diet is acting as an inducer or a promoter of tumorigenesis. Fats in particular are carriers of carcinogens, such as heterocyclic amines, which can be activated by cooking such as frying and barbecuing.[31] These mutagens can be identified using the in vitro Ames' mutation test and then be shown to be carcinogenic in rodent models.[32] However, there is the matter of quantum toxicology. As has been pointed out by Sugimara et al, the dose of carcinogen that can kill one rat in 250 may yet be able to activate one cell in a human (equivalent in weight to 250 rats), resulting in the death of that individual person.[33] Hence the search for cause and effect in mammary carcinogenesis is of herculean scale.

Although it is an easier task to establish links between diet and endocrine function, this is yet another way of rediscovering that sex hormones can promote the growth of both emerging and established breast cancers. As we are what we have eaten, an analysis of fatty acid composition of adipose tissue might well provide evidence of prior dietary solecisms.

Table 1.6 Case-control studies of fat consumption and breast cancer risk

Cases	Controls	Results	Reference
400	400	Saturated fat and oleic acid intake elevated	Miller et al[36]
2024	1463	No difference	Graham et al[37]
368	373	Milk and dairy product intake elevated	Talamini et al[38]
120	120	No difference	Katsouyanni et al[39]
1108	1281	Butter, margarine and oil intake elevated	La Vecchia et al[40]
344	688	No difference	Hirohata et al[41]
142	852	No difference	Mills et al[42]
451	451	No difference	Rohan et al[43]
120	120	No difference	Katsouyanni et al[44]
250	499	<28% of calories from fats reduced risk	Toniolo et al[45]
150	300	Increased intake of fats, sugars and proteins	Iscovitch et al[46]
186	186	Increased monounsaturated fat	Shun-Zhiang et al[47]
200	420	Red meat increased risk	Lee et al[48]
99	209	Red meat increased risk	Ingram et al[49]
265	431	No difference	Holmburg et al[50]

London et al carried out a case-control study of 380 women with breast cancer and 176 with benign breast conditions.[34] There was no consistent alteration in pattern of saturated, polyunsaturated or long-chain ω-3 fatty acids in those with breast cancer compared with benign controls. In a similar study conducted at the Memorial Sloane-Kettering Cancer Center, New York, the composition of breast and abdominal fat from 154 breast cancer patients and 125 benign controls was measured by gas chromatography.[35] The two groups had similar proportions of fats and fatty acids, indicating no difference between the fat consumption of women with and without breast cancer.

Results from case-control studies have yielded heterogeneous results with regard to fat intake. An outline of the results is given in Table 1.6.[36–50] Miller et al administered dietary questionnaires to women from four different areas of Canada and found that breast cancer cases had a higher total intake of all nutrients including fat.[36] Since the patients were questioned 3 months or more after treatment, it is possible that the findings could have been the result of 'comfort eating' during the period of recovery from the diagnosis.

The largest case-control study was that of Graham et al which found no difference in fat intake between 2024 breast cancer cases and 1463 controls.[37] A study from northern Italy reported higher consumption of dairy products by cases of borderline significance which disappeared after adjustment for other risk factors.[38] In a larger case-control study from Italy, La Vecchia et al found that there was a statistically significant trend in relation to dietary fat consumption and breast cancer risk which persisted in a multivariate analysis.[40]

Almost certainly, the reason for the many negative results was the narrow range of fat consumption in the population from which the cases were derived and this is exemplified by the lack of any observed difference between

Table 1.7 Relative risks of breast cancer and fat intake in pooled cohort studies

Nutrient increment per day	Relative risk	95% confidence interval	p value heterogeneity
Total fat (25 g)	1.02	0.94–1.11	0.24
Saturated (10 g)	1.03	0.95–1.11	0.27
Monounsaturated (10 g)	0.99	0.90–1.08	0.10
Polyunsaturated (10 g)	1.03	0.95–1.12	0.57
Animal fat (10 g)	1.00	0.96–1.03	0.27
Vegetable fat (10 g)	1.01	0.97–1.05	0.22

From Hunter et al.[51]

cases and controls who were Seventh-day Adventists.[42] An exception to this was the study from Singapore where there are still great individual differences in diet.[48] A quantitative food-frequency questionnaire was administered to determine probable diet during the year before interview and this revealed that high intakes of animal protein and red meat were significantly associated with an increased risk, whereas higher consumption of soya bean or polyunsaturated fatty acids led to a significant lowering of risk.

To investigate whether the lack of any association between fat consumption and breast cancer was the result of recall bias, Holmberg et al compared the results from a retrospective postdiagnostic questionnaire with a pre-diagnostic survey.[50] There were no significant differences between cases or controls in either the pre- or postdiagnostic questionnaires.

Not only were the case-control studies a source of confusion but so too were the very variable results of cohort studies. This may have arisen because of narrow ranges of consumption, difficulties in determining accurate intake and variation in statistical techniques. In an attempt to create order from this chaos, Hunter et al pooled the results from

eight major cohort studies.[51] The relative risks of breast cancer in relation to fat consumption are given in Table 1.7. This shows that there was no effect of fat intake on risk of breast cancer. Even those women whose intake of fat comprised less than 20% of their calorie intake did not have any reduction in risk. It was concluded that, for Western women, restriction of dietary fat intake would be unlikely to lead to any significant reduction in breast cancer incidence.

Weight

Although the relationship between fat intake and breast cancer remains the subject of heated debate, there is some agreement that the end-product, namely obesity, does influence risk. Although not all studies are in agreement, there is a trend towards a protective effect of obesity in the premenopausal and, conversely, an increase in risk for heavier postmenopausal women. In the Nurses' Health Study Cohort (NHSC), weight was sought from 115 534 women aged 30–55 years of whom 658 subsequently developed premenopausal breast cancer and 420 were diagnosed with postmenopausal disease.[52] When divided into quintiles on a basis

Table 1.8 Relative risks of breast cancer in relation to quintiles of weight, Quetelet's index and waist–hip ratio

Variable	Quintiles				
	1	2	3	4	5
Weight	1.00	1.00	1.31	1.33	1.63
Weight + family history	1.00	2.26	2.41	1.27	2.55
Quetelet's	1.00	1.02	1.00	1.32	1.50
Quetelet's + Family history	1.03	2.22	1.95	1.65	2.21
Waist–hip ratio	1.00	1.01	1.11	1.22	1.20
Waist–hip ratio + family history	0.85	2.19	1.25	1.24	3.24

From Sellers et al.[54]

of Quetelet's index (weight in kg/height in m^2), there was a highly significant relationship between relative weight and breast cancer risk in premenopausal women. Taking the relative risk of the lightest group as 1, this fell to 0.6 for the heaviest quintile. Obesity thus appears to be protective in the premenopausal women. In the NHSC there was no effect of obesity in the postmenopausal women, possibly because of the relatively few cases. In a case-control study of Asian–American women, Ziegler et al also found that obesity was protective in women aged 20–39, with the relative risk falling to 0.45 in the highest sextile.[53]

The Iowa Women's Health Study Cohort comprised 37 105 women aged 55–69 years.[54] Of these, 493 were subsequently diagnosed with breast cancer and the influences of weight and family history on risk were examined. Weight was expressed either in absolute terms, or as Quetelet's index or as the waist:hip ratio. As Table 1.8 shows, there was an elevation of relative risk with increasing weight or Quetelet's index. For those with a first-degree family history and obesity, there was an amplification of risk which rose from 1.2 in the highest quintile without a family history to 3.2 in those with a first-degree relative.

In a study of 16 355 postmenopausal women participating in the Utrecht screening project, den Tonkelaar et al measured both weight and fat distribution, using scapular and triceps skinfold thickness.[55] In terms of Quetelet's index the relative risk of breast cancer of the highest quintile was 1.6 times that of the lowest quintile, whereas for fat distribution there was no difference in relative risk for the highest and lowest quintile.

To determine whether the timing of weight gain had any impact on breast cancer risk, Kumar et al weighed 218 newly diagnosed cases and 436 age-matched controls, and asked for recollected weight at age <30, 30–40, 41–50, 51–60, 61–70 and 71–75, as appropriate.[56] The patients were more likely to have gained weight than the controls and this was true for each decade of adulthood. In a multivariate analysis, weight at age 30 was an independent variable with those who were heavier being at an increased lifetime risk of breast cancer. Van den Brandt et al carried out anthropometric measurements and collected recalled weights in 62 573 postmenopausal women in the Netherlands Cohort Study, of whom 626 were subsequently diagnosed with breast cancer.[57] Although weight and Quetelet's index at age 20

Table 1.9 Studies showing no relationship between height and breast cancer risk			
Type of study	**Numbers**	**Height measure**	**Reference**
Population	176:179	Self-recorded	Adami et al[61]
Hospital	777:2041	Self-recorded	Wynder et al[62]
Population	607:38 084	Self-recorded	Le Marchand et al[63]
Population	1486:1336	Self-recorded	Ewertz et al[64]
Population	229:1839	Self-recorded	Folsom et al[65]
Population/Hospital	213:213:213	Self-recorded	Kyogoku et al[66]
Hospital	2388:3600	Self-recorded	La Vecchia et al[67]
Population	422:527	Self-recorded	Lund et al[68]
Hospital	3247:3263	Self-recorded	Parazzini et al[69]
Hospital	5358:4555	Self-recorded	Zhang et al[70]

were associated with a reduction in risk, this effect disappeared on multivariate analysis whereas height remained a significant variable.

In a study of 6548 breast cancer cases and 9057 population-derived age-matched controls, premenopausal women in the heaviest quintile had a reduced risk of breast cancer (odds ratio, OR = 0.87).[58] In contrast, postmenopausal women in the highest quintile of weight had an increased risk (OR = 1.6). Postmenopausal women who had gained the most weight since the age of 18 were at the highest risk (OR = 1.5) and weight loss during that time reduced risk of breast cancer (OR = 0.89). That weight does influence breast cancer risk in the postmenopausal woman is to be expected. In this group of women the major source of endogenous oestrogens is from peripheral aromatization of adrenal androgens in fat. Women with more peripheral fat have higher levels of plasma oestrogens and so their weight could be acting as a promoter of breast cancer growth.[59]

Height

The adult height of a women is dependent upon several factors, partly genetic but mostly

as a consequence of nutrition, particularly food intake around the time of puberty. Thus, those who attain a greater height may have had a higher fat/carbohydrate intake, perhaps associated with increased exposure to carcinogens. In addition, high intake would lead to an earlier maturation of ovarian function as has been demonstrated in secular trends with regard to age at menarche. Conversely, starvation or nutritional deprivation will lead to a later menarche, with a protective effect in terms of breast cancer.[60]

There has been considerable inconsistency in the epidemiological literature with regard to the influence of height on breast cancer risk. The situation becomes clearer when account is taken of one variable not usually considered in scientific papers, namely vanity. It has been customary in epidemiological studies to ask the patient her height and weight, in order to simplify matters and improve compliance, rather than to add extra complexity and measure these variables. Those studies that have found no relationship between height and breast cancer risk are outlined in Table 1.9.[61–70] What emerges is that in all these studies the cases and controls were asked to record their height, without an objective measurement being performed.

Table 1.10 Studies finding a significant positive association between height and breast cancer risk

Type of study	Numbers	Height measure	Reference
Prospective	70:7259	Measured	De Waard et al[71]
Population	1006:4201	Measured	De Waard et al[72]
Prospective	1283:2154	Self-reported	Dubin et al[73]
Prospective	122:7413	Measured	Albanes et al[74]
Prospective	121:7028	Measured	Swanson et al[75]
Prospective	1182:46 570	Measured	Tornberg et al[76]
Population	2560:2679	Measured	Swanson et al[77]
Prospective	8427:570 000	Measured	Tretli[78]
Prospective	236:23 831	Measured	Vatten and Kvinnsland[79]
Hospital	3993:11 783	Self-recorded	Hseich et al[80]
Population	225:450	Measured	Bruning et al[81]
Hospital	200:420	Self-reported	Lee et al[82]
Prospective	168:6706	Measured	De Stavola et al[83]
Hospital	674:1155	Self-reported	Palmer et al[84]
Prospective	182:7622	Measured	Frenie et al[85]
Hospital	328:417	Measured	Mannisto et al[86]

Those studies that did find a significant positive association between height and breast cancer risk are outlined in Table 1.10.[71–86] Of these positive studies, 12 of 16 (75%) measured the height of participating individuals. Furthermore, 9 of 16 (56%) of those that showed a significant positive association were prospective whereas none of the negative studies was of this design. The effect of increased height leading to an elevated risk of breast cancer is predominantly found in postmenopausal women.

In the Guernsey project, the height of volunteers was self-reported in the first study but measured in the second, so that both could be compared for 2731 women.[87] Figure 1.2 shows the differences between self-reported and measured heights. Despite a high correlation between the two variables, it is apparent that here is significant divergence at both extremes.

Short women were more likely to report a greater height than measured and taller women more likely to report a decreased height. Hence a significant effect of height on breast cancer risk may be attenuated or obliterated if self-reported values are used.

Caffeine

Coffee and tea are almost universally consumed and so suspicions that the caffeine therein might increase the risk of breast cancer had to be taken very seriously. Circumstantial evidence came from the promotional effect of caffeine on mammary carcinomas induced in rats by dimethylbenzanthracene (DMBA).[88] In addition elevated levels of cyclic adenosine monophosphate (cAMP), which can be induced by caffeine, were found in human breast cancers.[89] However, in vitro studies of human

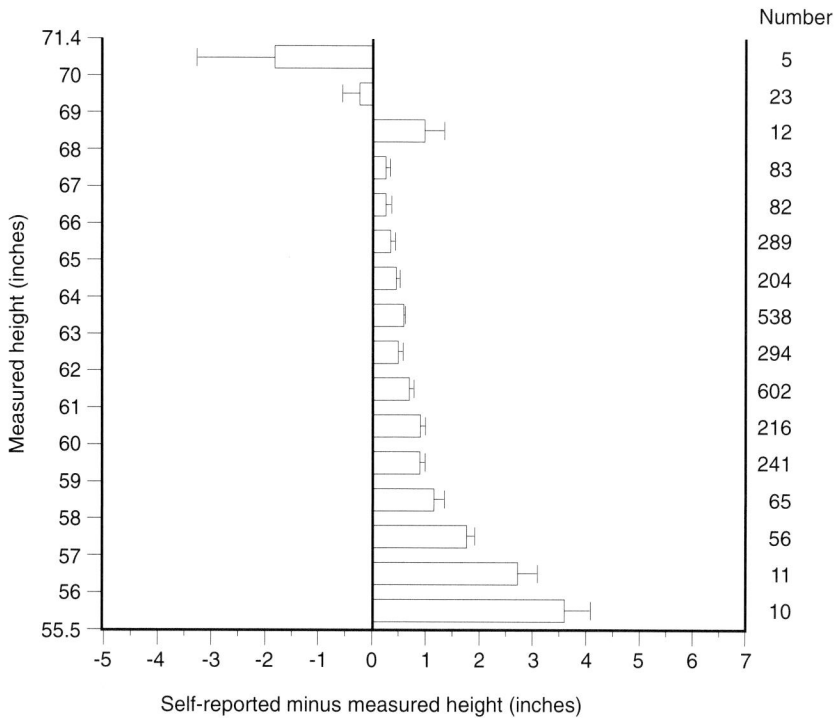

Fig. 1.2 Differences between reported and measured heights in Guernsey volunteers. (From Wang et al.[87])

breast cancer cell lines had shown consistently that elevation of cAMP was associated with an inhibition of cell proliferation.[90]

Most case-control studies that had examined the relationship between caffeine consumption in tea, coffee, and chocolate had shown either a weak association or no effect.[91–94] The UK National Case-Control Study Group examined a number of risk factors, including caffeine intake, in a comparison of 755 breast cancer cases aged less than 36 years and a similar number of age-matched population controls.[95] There were similar distributions of caffeine intake at age 16 and age 25 in both the cases and controls. Furthermore, there was no evidence of a significant association between consumption and risk or any trend in relation

to consumption at either 16 or 25. After adjustment for potentially confounding factors the relative risk approximated to unity. Thus reduction of caffeine intake is not a viable option for breast cancer prevention.

Alcohol

In 1977, as a result of the Third National Cancer Survey, which examined social habits, an association was reported between alcohol consumption and breast cancer.[96] This prompted over 50 investigations of which 10 were cohort studies and 28 of case-control design.[97] A series of meta-analyses has demonstrated a modest association between alcohol intake and breast cancer risk, with an evident dose–response rate.[98–100] This being so, it is important to establish whether this alcohol intake is an epiphenomenon or truly either an initiating or promoting agent in breast cancer. If our success in preventing lung cancer by dissuading individuals from smoking is taken as a model, however, this does not bode well for an enormous expenditure of resources to prove or disprove a link between alcohol and breast cancer.

As negative thoughts should not discourage us from trying to expand the bounds of knowledge, it is necessary to outline what are the potential mechanisms by which relatively low levels of alcohol might influence mammary neoplasia. In general these could be considered as initiating or promotional. Alcohol might act as a solvent for carcinogens, thereby allowing access of fat-soluble mutagens to mammary epithelium. Alternatively, congeners or congener metabolites might behave in a similar manner. Both in vitro and in vivo ethyl alcohol metabolism can lead to the generation of cytotoxic protein molecules which could facilitate entry of carcinogens to target cells.[101] These mechanisms remain speculative but all are susceptible to investigation.

An alternative possible action is that alcohol modulates oestrogen metabolism and thereby acts as a promoting agent. Evidence is available to show that administration of alcohol to non-alcoholic premenopausal women does lead to a modest rise in oestradiol (E2) levels, particularly at mid-cycle.[102,103] In addition long-term administration of alcohol leads to an increase in the percentage of biologically available oestradiol (free E2), so that the absolute amount of available E2 was increased.[103] In postmenopausal women alcohol consumption has also been shown to be associated with elevation of blood oestradiol levels, either as a direct effect on residual functioning ovarian tissue or as an indirect effect by causing obesity so that peripheral aromatization of adrenal androgens is increased.[104]

All of these effects could plausibly slightly increase risk, but it is difficult to equate these with an apparent risk consequent upon the consumption of one unit of alcohol per day. The possibility still exists that the apparent effect of alcohol may tell us more about the lifestyle and propensities of non-drinkers rather being a breast cancer risk factor. Moderate alcohol consumption can reduce the risk of coronary heart disease by increasing high-density-lipoprotein levels and for this reason alone, total abstinence could cause more harm than good.[105]

Smoking

As public health measures, such as clean water, uncontaminated air and availability of healthy food, have led to a prolongation of average life expectancy so the major current threat to human survival is from smoking. More premature deaths from vascular and pulmonary disease result from this cause than from any other identified agent. Without the unclaimed financial contribution of smokers to pension schemes, non-smokers would be paying substantially more to ensure their quality of life in old age. Curiously, it has been claimed that smoking could protect against breast cancer.[106] The putative mechanism was that smoking led to a reduction in urinary oestrogens in premenopausal women,[107] elevation of androgens in the postmenopausal woman,[108] and an earlier menopause which was advanced by an average of 1.5 years in smokers.[109,110]

The antioestrogenic action of smoking could lead to a theoretical benefit in terms of breast cancer, while of course greatly increasing the risk of heart disease and lung cancer. There is also evidence that smokers are less likely to develop endometrial cancer[111] and are at increased risk of osteoporosis,[112] both of which suggest that cigarettes exert an antioestrogenic effect. The case-control studies that have examined the relationship between cigarette smoking and breast cancer have used controls derived either from hospitals or from the community. As hospital controls were drawn from a group who were hospitalized because of diseases unrelated to cigarette smoking, this would immediately reduce the intake of those

Table 1.11 Relative risk of breast cancer and smoking in case-control studies using hospital-derived controls

Cases	Controls	Relative risk	Reference
799	2470	1.1	Valoaras et al[113]
340	340	1.0	MacMahon et al[114]
213	648	0.9	Lin et al[115]
536	1550	1.0	Mirra et al[116]
1167	2380	0.9	Williams and Horm et al[96]
1432	2650	0.8	Paffenbarger et al[117]
332	1353	0.8	Kelsey et al[118]
1176	1176	0.8	Vessey et al[119]
188	186	1.0	Porter and Jick et al[120]
2160	717	1.0	Rosenberg et al[121]

Table 1.12 Relative risk of breast cancer and smoking in case-control studies using population-derived controls

Cases	Controls	Relative risk	Reference
278	520	1.2	Janerich et al[122]
1473	1839	0.99	CDC et al[123]
173	246	1.0	Porter and Jick et al[120]
1547	1930	1.1	Brinton et al[124]
276	1519	0.8	O'Connell et al[125]
456	1693	1.4	Brownson et al[126]
451	451	1.3	Rohan and Baron et al[127]
254	762	1.0	Schecter et al[128]
317	951	1.2	Schecter et al[128]
1480	1332	0.93	Ewertz et al[129]

individuals and potentially bias the results. Those case-control studies that used hospital controls are summarized in Table 1.11.[96,113–121] Half of these studies show a relative risk equal or greater than unity, whereas the remainder showed a reduction of relative risk of breast cancer among smokers of between 0.8 and 0.9.

A different picture emerged from the studies which used population controls and results of these are given in Table 1.12.[120,122–129] Almost without exception, none of these studies showed any significant reduction in relative risk in smokers. In particular the Canadian Breast Cancer Screening Study showed no

Table 1.13 Case-control studies of organochlorines and breast cancer

Design	Cases	Controls	Odds ratio	Reference
Serum DDE	58	171	1.7	Wolff et al[139]
Serum DDE	150	150	1.0	Krieger et al[140]
Adipose DDE	265	3421	0.84	Van't Veer et al[141]

protective effect in terms of prevalent or incident breast cancers in either premenopausal or postmenopausal women.[128] A previous report had suggested an increased relative risk (1.4) in premenopausal smokers,[130] but this disappeared as the study became more mature. Other supportive evidence of the neutral status of smoking with regard to breast cancer risk has come from a large cohort study conducted in Norway.[131] Vatten and Kvinnsland studied a cohort of 24 329 Norwegian women of whom 242 developed breast cancer after 11–14 years of follow-up. Although there was a significant relationship between smoking and body mass index, with smokers being lighter than non-smokers, the age-adjusted incidence rate ratio was unity for both premenopausal and postmenopausal women.

Calle et al examined smoking and risk of fatal breast cancer in a cohort of 604 412 women of whom 880 died of breast cancer.[132] Smoking at the time of entry to the study was associated with a significantly increased risk of dying from breast cancer (RR = 1.3). The risk rose in relation to the number of cigarettes smoked so that smokers of more than 40 per day had a relative risk of 1.7. Almost certainly this tells us more about the personality of heavy smokers and their attitude towards health and screening. It is likely that such individuals may deny symptoms and present with more advanced breast cancers, or not attend when offered mammographic screening.

Taken together these results cannot be used as a source of comfort for cigarette smokers.

Their increased risk of premature death from vascular and pulmonary complications of smoking will not be offset by a reduced risk of breast cancer. Worse than this, their prognosis after diagnosis of breast cancer may be poorer than that of non-smokers for reasons that have yet to be fully elucidated but which probably result from their need for denial in order to persist with their sociopathic habit.

Organochlorines

In 1943, during the Second World War, dichloro-diphenyl-trichloroethane (DDT) was developed as an antimalarial agent, and in this role was responsible for saving large numbers of lives among both the military and civilians. Subsequently it was found that that DDT was present in animal milk[133] and also human fat and milk.[134] Levels of organochlorine residues in fat are up to 300 times greater than in serum and these are excreted during lactation.[135] DDT was found to produce a variety of cancers in animals, and possibly pancreatic cancer in humans.[136] In addition, DDT binds to oestrogen receptors and can stimulate the growth of rat mammary tumours in vitro.[137] Domestic use of DDT was banned in the USA in 1972 but the agent is still widely used in the developing world.

As a result of its excretory pathway and oestrogenic activity, DDT was a potential candidate as a mammary carcinogen with an early study showing higher levels of the metabolite dichloro-dichlorophenyl-ethylene (DDE) in patients with breast cancer.[138] Subsequently, three large studies (Table 1.13) have examined the relationship between DDT and breast cancer.[139–141] Wolff et al measured DDE levels in blood which had been taken as part of the New York University Women's Health Study.[139] There were 58 cases and 171 controls in a nested case-control study. Although DDE levels were 35% higher in the cases, the difference was only significant when adjustment was made for lactation. Furthermore, the blood had been taken within 6 months of diagnosis so that the disease itself might have had an influence on DDE levels.

Krieger et al used stored blood which had been taken during the 1960s as part of routine health testing in San Francisco.[140] As this was before the US ban on DDT use, mean serum levels of DDE were significantly elevated compared with those in the Wolff study (43 versus 8 parts per billion). A random sample was drawn of 50 women who had been subsequently diagnosed with breast cancer from three ethnic groups: white, black and Asian. There were 150 ethnically matched controls. Although serum DDE levels were significantly elevated in black and Asian women compared with whites, there were no differences between the cases and controls. Polychlorinated biphenyls (PCBs) were also measured and found to be no different in those with and those without breast cancer.

The European Study on Antioxidants, Myocardial Infarction and Cancer of the breast (EURAMIC) measured levels of DDE in subcutaneous buttock fat derived from 347 breast cancer patents and 374 hospital and population controls.[141] This was a multinational study with participants from the Netherlands, Germany, Britain, Switzerland and Spain. It emerged that breast cases had lower adipose levels of DDE compared with controls. The findings were essentially unchanged after adjustment for alcohol consumption, body weight and age at first birth. Although organochlorines are clearly toxic agents, they do not appear to have an aetiological role in breast cancer, either as carcinogens or as weak oestrogenic promoters.

SYNOPSIS

- The major risk factor for breast cancer is increasing age, possibly because of defective repair of DNA damage.
- Low level irradiation of the breast, particularly at the time of puberty, causes an increased risk of cancer.
- Japanese women have only one-fifth of the incidence of breast cancer compared with Americans but after migration this rises to 50% and 65% in second generation migrants.
- Case-control studies have not found a clear link between fat consumption and risk but most studies examined women who had a narrow range of fat intake.
- Heavier women are at decreased risk of premenopausal breast cancer but at increased risk of postmenopausal disease.
- When height has been measured rather than reported, studies show that taller women are at increased risk of breast cancer.
- Alcohol intake elevates breast cancer risk, possibly by increasing blood oestradiol levels in postmenopausal women, or as a result of unknown protective factors in non-drinkers.
- Neither smoking nor exposure to organochlorines has any impact on breast cancer risk.

REFERENCES

1. Cairns J. Mutation selection and the natural history of cancer. *Nature* 1975; **255:** 197–200.
2. Moolgavkar SH, Day NE, Stevens RG. Two-stage model for carcinogenesis: epidemiology of breast cancer in females. *J Natl Cancer Inst* 1980; **65:** 559–69.

3. Kodama M, Kodama T, Kodama M. The genesis of breast cancer is a two-step phenomenon. I. Differential effects of ageing on the cancer incidence in the United Kingdom and Japan. *Anticancer Res* 1992; **12**: 145–52.

4. Feuer EJ, Wun L-M, Boring CC et al. The lifetime risk of developing breast cancer. *J Natl Cancer Inst* 1993; **85**: 892–7.

5. Willis AE, Lindahl Y. DNA ligase I deficiency in Bloom's syndrome. *Nature* 1987; **325**: 355–6.

6. Shiloh Y, Tabor E, Becker Y. The response of ataxia–telangiectasia homozygous and heterozygous skin fibroblasts to neocarzinostatin. *Carcinogenesis* 1982; **3**: 815–18.

7. Parshad R, Price FM, Bohr VA et al. Deficient DNA repair capacity, a predisposing factor in breast cancer. *Br J Cancer* 1996; **74**: 1–5.

8. Sanford KK, Price FM, Rhim JS et al. Role of DNA repair in malignant transformation of human mammary epithelial cells in culture. *Carcinogenesis* 1992; **13**: 1137–41.

9. Shaw JA, Walsh T, Chappell SA et al. Microsatellite instability in early sporadic breast cancer. *Br J Cancer* 1996; **73**: 1393–7.

10. Parsons R, Li G–M, Longley MJ et al. Hypermutability and mismatch repair deficiency in RER + tumour cells. *Cell* 1993; **75**: 1227–36.

11. Modan B, Baidatz D, Mart H et al. Radiation–induced head and neck tumours. *Lancet* 1974; **i**: 277–9.

12. Modan B, Chetrit A, Alfandary E et al. Increased risk of breast cancer after low–dose irradiation. *Lancet* 1989; **ii**: 629–31.

13. Hildreth NG, Shore RE, Dvoretsky PM. The risk of breast cancer after irradiation of the thymus in infancy. *N Engl J Med* 1989; **321**: 1281–4.

14. Lundell M, Mattsson A, Hakulinen T, Holm L–E. Breast cancer after radiotherapy for skin hemangioma in infancy. *Radiation Res* 1996; **145**: 225–30.

15. Shore RE, Hempelmann LH, Kowaluk E et al. Breast neoplasms in women treated with x–rays for acute postpartum mastitis. *J Natl Cancer Inst* 1977; **59**: 913–22.

16. Prince MM, Hildreth NG. The influence of potential biases on the risk of breast tumors among women who received radiotherapy for acute postpartum mastitis. *J Chron Dis* 1986; **39**: 553–60.

17. Mattsson A, Ruden B–I, Hall P et al. Radiation–induced breast cancer: long–term follow–up of radiation therapy for benign breast disease. *J Natl Cancer Inst* 1993; **85**: 1679–85.

18. Travis LP, Curtis RE, Glimelius B et al. Second cancers among long–term survivors of non–Hodgkin's lymphoma. *J Natl Cancer Inst* 1993; **85**: 1932–7.

19. Hancock SL, Tucker MA, Hoppe RT. Breast cancer after treatment of Hodgkin's disease. *J Natl Cancer Inst* 1993; **85**: 25–31.

20. Hrubec Z, Boice JD, Monson RR, Rosenstein M. Breast cancer after multiple chest fluoroscopies: second follow–up of Massachusetts women with tuberculosis. *Cancer Res* 1989; **49**: 229–34.

21. Hoffman DA, Lonstein JE, Morin MM et al. Breast cancer in women with scoliosis exposed to multiple diagnostic x–rays. *J Natl Cancer Inst* 1989; **81**:1307–12.

22. Miller AB, Howe GR, Sherman GJ et al. Mortality from breast cancer after irradiation during fluoroscopic examinations in patients being treated for tuberculosis. *N Engl J Med* 1989; **321**: 1285–9.

23. Goodman MT, Mabuchi K, Morita M et al. Cancer incidence in Hiroshima and Nagasaki, Japan, 1958–87. *Eur J Cancer* 1994; **30A**: 801–7.

24. McGregor DH, Land CE, Choi K et al. Breast cancer incidence among atomic bomb survivors, Hiroshima and Nagasaki, 1950–69. *J Natl Cancer Inst* 1977; **59**: 799–811.

25. Land CE, Hayakawa N, Machado SG et al. A case–control interview study of breast cancer among Japanese A–bomb survivors. I. Main effects. *Cancer Causes Control* 1994; **5**: 157–65.

26. Goodman MT, Cologne JB, Moriwaki H et al. Risk factors for primary breast cancer in Japan: 8-year follow-up of atomic bomb survivors. *Prev Med* 1997; **26**: 144–53.

27. Schapira DV, Clark RA, Wolff PA et al. Visceral obesity and breast cancer risk. *Cancer* 1994; **74**: 632–9.

28. Lea AJ. Dietary factors associated with death rates from certain neoplasms in man. *Lancet* 1966; **ii**: 332–3.

29. Dunn JE. Cancer epidemiology in populations of the United States – with emphasis on Hawaii and California and Japan. *Cancer Res* 1975; **35**: 3240–5.

30. Buell P. Changing incidence of breast cancer in Japanese–American women. *J Natl Cancer Inst* 1973; **51**: 1479–83.

31. Ohgaki H, Takayama S, Sugimura T.

Carcinogenicities of heterocyclic amines in cooked food. *Mutat Res* 1991; **259**: 399–410.

32. Ames BN, McCann J, Yamasaki E. Methods for detecting carcinogens and mutagens with the Salmonella/mammalian–microsome mutagenicity test. *Mutat Res* 1975; **31**: 347–64.

33. Sugimara T, Nagao M, Wakabayashi K. Heterocyclic amines in cooked foods: candidates for causation of common cancers. *J Natl Cancer Inst* 1994; **86**: 2–4.

34. London SJ, Sacks FM, Stampfer MJ et al. Fatty acid composition of the subcutaneous adipose tissue and risk of proliferative benign breast disease and breast cancer. *J Natl Cancer Inst* 1993; **85**: 785–93.

35. Petrek JA, Hudgins LC, Levine B et al. Breast cancer risk and fatty acids in the breast and abdominal adipose tissues. *J Natl Cancer Inst* 1994; **86**: 53–6.

36. Miller AB, Kelly A, Choi NW et al. A study of diet and breast cancer. *Am J Epidemiol* 1978; **107**: 499–509.

37. Graham S, Marshall J, Mettlin C et al. Diet in the epidemiology of breast cancer. *Am J Epidemiol* 1982; **116**: 68–75.

38. Talamini R, La Vecchia CL, Decarli A et al. Social factors, diet and breast cancer in a northern Italian population. *Br J Cancer* 1984; **49**: 723–9.

39. Katsouyanni K, Trichopoulos D, Boyle P et al. Diet and breast cancer: a case–control study. *Int J Cancer* 1986; **38**: 815–20.

40. La Vecchia C, Decarli A, Franceschi S et al. Dietary factors and the risk of breast cancer. *Nutr Cancer* 1987; **10**: 205–14.

41. Hirohata T, Nomura AMY, Hankin JH et al. An epidemiological study on the association between diet and breast cancer. *J Natl Cancer Inst* 1987; **78**: 595–600.

42. Mills PK, Annegers JF, Phillips RL. Animal product consumption and subsequent fatal breast cancer risk among Seventh–day Adventists. *Am J Epidemiol* 1988; **128**: 440–53.

43. Rohan TE, McMichael AJ, Baghurst PA. A population–based case–control study of diet and breast cancer in Australia. *Am J Epidemiol* 1988; **128**: 478–89.

44. Katsouyanni K, Willett W, Trichopoulos D et al. Risk of breast cancer among Greek women in relation to nutrient intake. *Cancer* 1988; **61**: 181–5.

45. Toniolo P, Riboli E, Protta F et al. Calorie–providing nutrients and risk of breast cancer. *J Natl Cancer Inst* 1989; **81**: 278–86.

46. Iscovitch JM, Iscovitch RB, Howe G et al. A case–control study of diet and breast cancer in Argentina. *Int J Cancer* 1989; **44**: 770–6.

47. Shun–Zhiang Y, Rui–Fang L, Da–Dao X, Howe GR. A case–control study of dietary and nondietary risk factors for breast cancer in Shanghai. *Cancer Res* 1991; **50**: 5017–21.

48. Lee HP, Gourley L, Duffy SW et al. Dietary effects on breast cancer risk in Singapore. *Lancet* 1991; **337**: 1197–200.

49. Ingram DM, Nottage E, Roberts T. The role of diet in the development of breast cancer: a case–control study of patients with breast cancer, benign epithelial hyperplasia and fibrocystic disease of the breast. *Br J Cancer* 1991; **64**: 187–91.

50. Holmberg L, Ohlander EM, Byers T et al. A search for recall bias in a case–control study of diet and breast cancer. *Int J Epidemiol* 1996; **25**: 235–43.

51. Hunter DJ, Spiegelman D, Adami H-O et al. Cohort studies of fat intake and the risk of breast cancer – a pooled analysis. *N Engl J Med* 1996; **334**: 356–61.

52. London SJ, Colditz GA, Stampfer MJ et al. Prospective study of relative weight, height, and risk of breast cancer. *JAMA* 1989; **262**: 2853–8.

53. Ziegler RG, Hoover RN, Nomura AMY et al. Relative weight, weight change, height, and breast cancer risk in Asian–American women. *J Natl Cancer Inst* 1996; **88**: 650–60.

54. Sellers TA, Kushi LH, Potter JD et al. Effect of family history, body-fat distribution, and reproductive factors on the risk of postmenopausal breast cancer. *N Engl J Med* 1992; **326**: 1323–9.

55. den Tonkelaar I, Seidell JC, Collete HJA, de Waard F. Obesity and subcutaneous fat patterning in relation to breast cancer in postmenopausal women participating in the Diagnostic Investigation of Mammary Cancer Project. *Cancer* 1992; **69**: 2663–7.

56. Kumar NB, Lyman GH, Allen K et al. Timing of weight gain and breast cancer risk. *Cancer* 1995; **76**: 243–9.

57. Van den Brandt PA, Dirx MJM, Ronckers CM et al. Height, weight, weight change, and postmenopausal breast cancer risk: the Netherlands Cohort Study. *Cancer Causes Control* 1997; **8**: 39–47.

58. Trentham–Dietz A, Newcomb PA, Storer BE et al. Body size and risk of breast cancer. *Am J Epidemiol* 1997; **145:** 1011–19.

59. Grodin JM. Siiteri PK, MacDonald PC. Source of estrogen production in postmenopausal women. *J Clin Endocrinol Metab* 1973; **36:** 207–14.

60. Staszewski J. Breast cancer and body build. *Prev Med* 1977; **6:** 410–15.

61. Adami HO, Rimsten A, Stenkvist B, Vegelius J. Influence of height, weight and obesity on risk of breast cancer in an unselected Swedish population. *Br J Cancer* 1977; **36:** 787–92.

62. Wynder EL, MacCormack FA, Stellman SD. The epidemiology of breast cancer in 785 United States Caucasian women. *Cancer* 1977; **41:** 2341–54.

63. Le Marchand L, Kolonel LN, Earle ME, Mi M–P. Body size at different periods of life and breast cancer risk. *Am J Epidemiol* 1988; **128:** 137–52.

64. Ewertz M. Influence of non–contraceptive exogenous and endogenous sex hormones on breast cancer risk in Denmark. *Int J Cancer* 1988; **42:** 832–8.

65. Folsom AR, Kaye SA, Prineas RJ et al. Increased incidence of carcinoma of the breast associated with abdominal adiposity in postmenopausal women. *Am J Epidemiol* 1990; **131:** 794–803.

66. Kyogoku S, Hirihata T, Takeshita S et al. Anthropometric indicators of breast cancer risk in Japanese women in Fukuoka. *Jpn J Cancer Res* 1990; **81:** 731–7.

67. La Vecchia C, Negri E, Parazzini F et al. Height and cancer risk in a network of case–control studies from Northern Italy. *Int J Cancer* 1990; **45:** 275–9.

68. Lund E, Adami H-O, Bergstrom R, Meirik O. Anthropometric measures and breast cancer in young women. *Cancer Causes Control* 1990; **1:** 169–72.

69. Parazzini F, La Vecchia C, Negri E et al. Anthropometric variables and the risk of breast cancer. *Int J Cancer* 1990; **45:** 397–402.

70. Zhang Y, Rosenberg L, Colton T et al. Adult height and risk of breast cancer among white women in a case–control study. *Am J Epidemiol* 1996; **143:** 1123–8.

71. De Waard F, Baanders–van Halewijn EA. A prospective study in general practice on breast cancer risk in postmenopausal women. *Int J Cancer* 1974; **14:** 153–60.

72. De Waard F, Cornelis JP, Aoki K, Yoshida M. Breast cancer incidence according to weight and height in two cities of the Netherlands and in the Aichi prefecture, Japan. *Cancer* 1977; **40:** 1269–75.

73. Dubin N, Pasternack BS, Strax P. Epidemiology of breast cancer in a screened population. *Cancer Det Prev* 1984; **7:** 87–102.

74. Albanes D, Jones DY, Schatzkin A et al. Adult stature and risk of breast cancer. *Cancer Res* 1988; **48:** 1658–62.

75. Swanson CA, Jones DY, Schatzkin A et al. Breast cancer risk assessed by anthropometry in the NHANES 1 epidemiological follow–up study. *Cancer Res* 1988; **48:** 5363–7.

76. Tornberg SA, Holm LE, Carstensen JM. Breast cancer risk in relation to serum cholesterol, serum beta–lipoprotein, height, weight, and blood pressure. *Acta Oncol* 1988; **27:** 31–7.

77. Swanson CA, Brinton LA, Taylor PR et al. Body size in the breast cancer detection demonstration project. *Am J Epidemiol* 1989; **130:** 1131–41.

78. Tretli S. Height and weight in relation to breast cancer morbidity and mortality. A prospective study of 570,000 women in Norway. *Int J Cancer* 1989; **44:** 23–30.

79. Vatten LJ, Kvinnsland S. Body height and risk of breast cancer. A prospective study of 23,831 Norwegian women. *Br J Cancer* 1990; **61:** 881–5.

80. Hseih C–C, Trichopoulos D, Katsouyuanni K, Yuasa S. Age at menarche, age at menopause, height and obesity as risk factors for breast cancer: associations and interactions in an international case–control study. *Int J Cancer* 1990; **46:** 796–800.

81. Bruning PF, Bonfrer JMG, Hart AAM et al. Body measurements, estrogen availability and the risk of human breast cancer: a case–control study. *Int J Cancer* 1992; **51:** 14–19.

82. Lee HP, Gourley L, Duddy SW et al. Risk factors for breast cancer by age and menopausal status: a case–control study in Singapore. *Cancer Causes Control* 1992; **3:** 313–22.

83. De Stavola BL, Wang DY, Allen DS et al. The association of height, weight, menstrual and other events with breast cancer: results from two prospective studies on the island of Guernsey (United Kingdom). *Cancer Causes Control* 1993; **4:** 331–40.

84. Palmer JR, Rosenberg L, Harlap S et al. Adult height and risk of breast cancer among US black women. *Am J Epidemiol* 1995; **141:** 845–9.

85. Freni SC, Eberhardt MS, Turturro A, Hine RJ. Anthropometric measures and metabolic rate in

association with risk of breast cancer (United States). *Cancer Causes Control* 1996; **7:** 358–65.

86. Mannisto S, Pietinen P, Pyy M et al. Body–size indicators and risk of breast cancer according to menopause and estrogen receptor status. *Int J Cancer* 1996; **68:** 8–13.

87. Wang DY, De Stavola BL, Allen DS et al. Breast cancer risk is positively associated with height. *Breast Cancer Res Treat* 1997; **43:** 123–8.

88. Minton JP, Abou–Issa H, Foecking MK et al. Caffeine and unsaturated fat diet significantly promotes DMBA–induced breast cancer in rats. *Cancer* 1983; **51:** 1249–53.

89. Minton JP, Wisenbaugh T, Matthews RH. Elevated cyclic AMP levels in human breast cancer tissue. *J Natl Cancer Inst* 1974; **53:** 283–7.

90. Fentiman IS, Duhig T, Griffiths A et al. Cyclic AMP inhibits the growth of human breast cancer cells in defined medium. *Mol Biol Med* 1984; **2:** 81–8.

91. Lawson DH, Jick H, Rothman KJ. Coffee and tea consumption and breast disease. *Surgery* 1981; **90:** 801–3.

92. Lubin F, Ron E, Wax Y et al. Coffee and methylxanthines and breast cancer: a case–control study. *J Natl Cancer Inst* 1985; **74:** 569–73.

93. La Vecchia C, Talamini R, Decarli A et al. Coffee consumption and the risk of breast cancer. *Surgery* 1986; **100:** 477–81.

94. Phelps H, Phelps CE. Caffeine ingestion and breast cancer. A negative correlation. *Cancer* 1988; **61:** 1051–4.

95. Smith SJ, Deacon JM, Chilvers CED et al. Alcohol, smoking, passive smoking and caffeine in relation to breast cancer risk in young women. *Br J Cancer* 1994; **70:** 112–19.

96. Williams RR, Horm JW. Association of cancer sites with tobacco and alcohol consumption and socio-economic status of patients: interview study from the Third National Cancer Survey. *J Natl Cancer Inst* 1977; **58:** 525–47.

97. Schatzkin A, Longnecker MP. Alcohol and breast cancer. Where are we now and where do we go from here? *Cancer* 1994; **74:** 1101–10.

98. Longnecker MP, Berlin JA, Orza MJ, Chalmers TC. A meta–analysis of alcohol consumption in relation to risk of breast cancer. *JAMA* 1988; **260:** 652–6.

99. Lowenfeis AB, Zevola SA. Alcohol and breast cancer: an overview. *Alcoholism Clin Exp Res* 1989; **13:** 109–11.

100. Steinberg J, Goodwin PJ. Alcohol and breast cancer risk – putting the current controversy into perspective. *Breast Cancer Res Treat* 1991; **19:** 221–31.

101. Wickramasinghe SN, Gardner B, Barden B. Cytotoxic molecules generated as a consequence of ethanol metabolism in vitro and in vivo. *Lancet* 1986; **ii:** 823–6.

102. Mendelson JH, Mello NK, Teoh SK, Ellingboe J. Alcohol effects on luteinizing hormone releasing hormone–stimulated anterior pituitary and gonadal hormones in women. *J Pharmacol Exp Ther* 1989; **250:** 902–9.

103. Reichman ME, Judd JT, Longcope C et al. Effects of moderate alcohol consumption on plasma and urinary hormone concentrations in premenopausal women. *J Natl Cancer Inst* 1993; **85:** 722–7.

104. Gavaler JS, Love K, Van Thiel D et al. An international study of the relationship between alcohol consumption and postmenopausal estradiol levels. *Alcohol Alcohol* 1991; suppl 1: 327–30.

105. Frimpong NA, Lapp JA. Effects of moderate alcohol intake in fixed or variable amounts on concentration of serum lipids and liver enzymes in healthy young men. *Am J Clin Nutr* 1989; **50:** 987–91.

106. Baron JA. Smoking and estrogen-related disease. *Am J Epidemiol* 1984; **119:** 9–22.

107. MacMahon BE, Trichopoulos D, Cole P et al. Cigarette smoking and urinary estrogens. *N Engl J Med* 1982; **307:** 1062–5.

108. Khaw K-T, Tazuke S, Barrett-Connor E. Cigarette smoking and levels of adrenal androgens in postmenopausal women. *N Engl J Med* 1988; **318:** 1705–9.

109. Kaufman DW, Slone D, Rosenberg L et al. Cigarette smoking and age at natural menopause. *Am J Public Health* 1980; **70:** 420–2.

110. Willet W, Stampfer MJ, Bain C et al. Cigarette smoking, relative weight and menopause. *Am J Epidemiol* 1983; **117:** 651–8.

111. Weiss NS, Farewell VT, Szekely DR et al. Oestrogens and endometrial cancer: effect of other risk factors on the association. *Maturitas* 1980; **2:** 185–90.

112. Daniell HW. Osteoporosis of the slender smoker. *Arch Intern Med* 1976; **136:** 298–304.

113. Valoaras VG, MacMahon BE, Trichopoulos P et al. Lactation and reproductive histories of breast cancer patients in greater Athens. *Int J Cancer* 1969; **4:** 350–63.

114. MacMahon BE, Cole P, Lin TM et al. Age at any birth and breast cancer risk. *Bull WHO* 1970; **43:** 209–21.

115. Lin TM, Chen KP, MacMahon BE. Epidemiologic characteristics of cancer of the breast in Taiwan. *Cancer* 1971; **27:** 1497–504.

116. Mirra AP, Cole P, MacMahon BE. Breast cancer in an area of high parity, Saō Paolo, Brazil. *Cancer Res* 1971; **31:** 77–83.

117. Paffenbarger RS, Kampert JB, Chang H-G. Oral contraceptives and breast cancer risk. *INSERM* 1979; **83:** 93–114.

118. Kelsey JL, Fischer DB, Holford DM et al. Breast cancer and oral contraceptive use: a case–control study. *J Chron Dis* 1983; **36:** 639–46.

119. Vessey M, Baron J, Doll R et al. Oral contraceptives and breast cancer. Final report of an epidemiological study. *Br J Cancer* 1983; **47:** 455–62.

120. Porter JB, Jick H. Breast cancer and cigarette smoking. *N Engl J Med* 1983; **309:** 186.

121. Rosenberg L, Schwingl PJ, Kaufman DW et al. Breast cancer and cigarette smoking. *N Engl J Med* 1984; **310**: 92–4.

122. Janerich DT, Polednak AP, Glebatis DM et al. Breast cancer and oral contraceptive use: a case–control study. *J Chron Dis* 1983; **36:** 639–46.

123. Centers for Disease Control. Long–term oral contraceptive use and the risk of breast cancer. *JAMA* 1983; **249:** 1591–3.

124. Brinton LA, Schairer C, Stanford JL et al. Cigarette smoking and breast cancer. *Am J Epidemiol* 1986; **123:** 614–22.

125. O'Connell DL, Hulka BS, Chambless LE et al. Cigarette smoking, alcohol consumption and risk of breast cancer. *Int J Cancer* 1987; **78:** 229–34.

126. Brownson RC, Blackwell CW, Person DK et al. Risk of breast cancer in relation to cigarette smoking. *Arch Intern Med* 1988; **148:** 140–4.

127. Rohan TE, Baron JA. Cigarette smoking and breast cancer. *Am J Epidemiol* 1989; **129:** 36–47.

128. Schecter MT, Miller AB, Howe GR et al. Cigarette smoking and breast cancer: case–control studies of prevalent and incident cancer in the Canadian National Breast Screening Study. *Am J Epidemiol* 1989; **130:** 213–20.

129. Ewertz M. Smoking and breast cancer risk in Denmark. *Cancer Causes Control* 1990; **1:** 31–7.

130. Schecter MT, Miller AB, Howe GR. Cigarette smoking and breast cancer: a case–control study of screening program participants. *Am J Epidemiol* 1985; **121:** 479–87.

131. Vatten LJ, Kvinnsland S. Cigarette smoking and risk of breast cancer: a prospective study of 24,239 Norwegian women. *Eur J Cancer* 1990; **26:** 830–3.

132. Calle EE, Miracle–McMahill HL, Thun MJ, Heath CW. Cigarette smoking and risk of fatal breast cancer. *Am J Epidemiol* 1994; **139:** 1001–7.

133. Telford HS, Guthrie JE. Transmission of the toxicity of DDT through milk of white rats and goats. *Science* 1945; **102:** 647.

134. Laug EP, Kunze FM, Prickett CS. Occurrence of DDT in human fat and milk. *AMA Arch Indus Hyg Occup Med* 1951; **3:** 245–6.

135. Wolff MS. Occupationally derived chemicals in breast milk. *Am J Ind Med* 1983; **4:** 259–81.

136. Levine R. Recognised and possible effects of pesticides in humans. In: *Handbook of Pesticide Toxicology*, Vol 1. *General principles*. Hayes WJ, Laws ER, eds. San Diego: Academic Press, 1991: 275–360.

137. Robinson AK, Sirbasku DA, Stancel DM. DDT supports growth of an estrogen–responsive tumor. *Toxicol Lett* 1985; **27:** 109–13.

138. Wassermann M, Nogueira DP, Tomatis L et al. Organochlorine compounds in neoplastic and adjacent apparently normal breast tissue. *Bull Environ Contam Toxicol* 1976; **15:** 478–84.

139. Wolff MS, Toniolo PG, Verreault R et al. Blood levels of organochlorine residues and risk of breast cancer. *J Natl Cancer Inst* 1993; **85:** 648–52.

140. Krieger N, Wolff MS, Hiatt RA et al. Breast cancer and serum organochlorines: a prospective study among white, black, and Asian women. *J Natl Cancer Inst* 1994; **86:** 589–99.

141. Van't Veer P, Lobbezoo IE, Martin–Moreno J et al. DDT (dicophane) and postmenopausal breast cancer in Europe: a case–control study. *Br Med J* 1997; **315**: 81–5.

2

Promotion of breast cancer

Felix qui potuit rerum cognoscere causa.
Happy the man who could understand the causes of things.

Virgil

Menstrual cycles • Parity • Twins • Abortion • Lactation • Menopause • Oestrogen • Intratumoral hormone synthesis • Prolactin • Melatonin

Every time that a mammary epithelial cell undergoes mitosis, there is a small probability of faulty DNA replication and, the more cell divisions that occur, the greater the likelihood of either the development of a malignant phenotype or the promotion of the growth of transformed variants. Hence those factors that drive mitosis of breast cells act as potential promoters of breast cancer. Viewed simplistically, this is what the bulk of the epidemiological and endocrine literature on breast cancer is telling us. The longer the duration that breast epithelium is exposed to steroid hormones, particularly in cyclical form, the greater the risk of malignancy. Furthermore, women with higher levels of endogenous or exogenous oestrogens will be more likely to be diagnosed with breast cancer.

MENSTRUAL CYCLES

The number of menstrual cycles that the breast tissue undergoes is a powerful determinant of breast cancer risk so that factors that reduce the number of menses will be protective. This may be achieved by late menarche, early pregnancy, lactation, anovular cycles and early menopause, all of which have been shown to reduce breast cancer risk.

Age at menarche

The main determinant of age at menarche is the attainment of a critical body mass, based on a balance between food intake and exercise.[1] Women who start menstruation before the age of 12 years have a twofold increase in relative risk compared with those whose menarche is after age 13.[2] Apter et al compared the endocrinology of 11 women whose menarche was before the age of 12 years, 14 who menstruated at age 12–12.9, and 19 who started after age 13.[3] When these 44 women were aged 20–31 daily blood samples were taken throughout one menstrual cycle. Those who had menarche before age 12 had increased sex hormone-binding globulin (SHBG) levels during the follicular phase of the cycle and also had elevated follicular oestradiol concentrations. This implies that early menarche may indelibly stamp the individual's ovarian function.

The determinants of age at menarche in 345 Greek students were analysed by Petridou et al, who ascertained energy intake, socioeconomic background, family history and anthropometric variables.[4] The main factors predicting for early menarche were height and body mass index, but additionally there was a correlation between age of mother and daughter at menarche. Moderate

Table 2.1 Lifelong menstrual cycle pattern and risk of breast cancer

Menstrual pattern	Cases	Controls	Relative risk
Regular	2802	2270	1
Irregular	232	293	0.7
Duration ≤ 25 days	402	303	1
Duration 26–30 days	1865	1476	0.9
Duration ≥ 31 days	165	104	1.2
Totally irregular	114	134	0.7

From Parazzini et al.[6]

physical activity and increased total energy intake were both associated with a later start of menstruation.

As a result of the potential negative interaction between age at menarche and early age at first baby, Peeters et al examined the influence of early menarche on breast cancer risk in nulliparous women.[5] A case-control study was conducted with 135 cases and 540 controls derived from the screening projects in Nijmegen and Utrecht. Nulliparous women who had their first period before age 11 had a 2.2 relative risk of breast cancer compared with those who underwent menarche aged more than 12 years.

Parazzini et al collected lifelong menstrual data from 3037 breast cancer cases and 2569 hospital controls.[6] The participants were divided into those who reported lifelong regular cycles and those whose periods had been irregular at some time during their reproductive life. As is shown in Table 2.1, there was a significant reduction in relative risk of breast cancer among women whose menstrual cycle had been totally irregular. In a multivariate analysis this effect remained significant after controlling for age and other breast cancer risk factors.

PARITY

Pregnancy is the major cause of amenorrhoea in women during their reproductive years and so, by sparing the breast from cyclical exposure to oestrogens, could be protective in terms of breast cancer. Against this, there is an increasing concentration of placental oestrogens without the ameliorating effect of progesterone. One of the oldest epidemiological observations about breast cancer was its increased frequency in nuns, which was attributed to their celibate and nulliparous status.

It was MacMahon who first demonstrated that the age at which a woman had her first baby was the main determinant of risk of subsequent breast cancer.[7] For women who had their first baby at age 30 or over, the relative risk of breast cancer was 2.1 compared with those whose first child was born at age 20 or less. The breast cancer risk was greater in parous women who delivered after age 30 than among the nulliparous. It was assumed that the explanation for this effect was the induction of differentiation of terminal end-buds in the breast, thereby causing apoptosis of some cells which had been previously transformed by carcinogens.[8,9]

Rosero-Bixby et al conducted a case-control study in Costa Rica among a multiparous population, comparing 171 breast cancer cases and 826 population-derived controls.[10] Among women aged less than 45, those who were nulliparous had a threefold increase in breast cancer risk. For women aged over 44 years, those with four or more children had a relative risk of 0.3 compared with mothers with one to three children. Those who had their first baby before the age of 20 also had a lower risk of breast cancer.

To determine whether parity and age at first full-term pregnancy were independently

Table 2.2 Odds ratios for breast cancer in relation to age at FFTP and age at LFTP, with progressively refined adjustment

Variable	Adjustment 1	Adjustment 2	Adjustment 3
Age at FFTP (years)			
<20	1.00	1.00	1.00
20–24	1.21	1.08	1.12
25–29	1.63	1.30	1.28
30–34	1.98	1.41	1.25
≥ 35	2.58	1.58	1.82
Age at LFTP (years)			
<25	1.00	1.00	1.00
25–29	1.04	0.98	0.93
30–34	1.05	0.95	0.86
35–39	1.18	1.06	1.00
≥ 40	1.48	1.33	1.18

From Hsieh et al.[14]

protective, Layde et al compared 4599 women with breast cancer participating in the Cancer and Steroid Hormone (CASH) study, with 4536 age-matched women selected by random digit dialling.[11] Taking the odds ratio as unity for those who had their first full-term pregnancy (FFTP) before the age of 18 years, this rose linearly to 1.24 for FFTP at 25, 1.67 at 30 and 1.97 at over 35 years. Within the parous group, after controlling for age at FFTP, there was an additional protective effect seen with increasing pregnancies, with a relative risk of 1 for those with one child. This fell to 0.68 for those with four children and 0.47 in those with more than seven children.

In a Norwegian study it was reported that the effect of age at FFTP disappeared after adjustment for parity and age at last full-term pregnancy (LFTP).[12] To investigate this finding in the context of highly parous women, Kalache et al conducted a case-control study in Brazil of 509 breast cancer patients with two age-matched controls for each.[13] High breast cancer risk was associated with low parity but, after adjustment for parity, both age at FFTP and age at LFTP were significant factors, increasing risk by 1.2 and 1.24 respectively for each 5-year increment. In a multivariate analysis the effect of age at FFTP became insignificant after adjustment for age at LFTP.

This interpretation was criticized by Hsieh et al who considered that women with only one child should be excluded from such analyses because age at FFTP and LFTP is the same.[14] Furthermore, in a high parity group, there may be confounding effects of pregnancies intervening between first and last, with the latter tending to occur late. Using data from a seven-nation collaborative case-control study of high, intermediate and low incidence areas, Hsieh carried out an analysis which was restricted to women with two to nine full-term pregnancies, comprising 3950 cases and 11 510 controls.[14] The results are given in Table 2.2. After the first adjustment, which controlled for age at menarche, menopausal status and body mass index, both age at FFTP and age at LFTP were associated linearly with an increase in risk, although the effect of FFTP carried three times the excess risk of LFTP. In the second adjustment, age at FFTP and LFTP were mutually adjusted together with age at FFTP. At this stage LFTP still retained a significant effect. However, after the third adjustment, which considered only those women with two or more children and controlled for each individual's age at FFTP, the effect of LFTP was lost. For a 5-year delay in age at FFTP, the odds ratio was 1.2 compared with 1.0 for age at LFTP.

In a large Norwegian study of 802 457 parous women, Albrektsen et al studied both the short-term and long-term effects of pregnancy on breast cancer risk.[15] After a follow-up of 16 years, 4787 had developed breast cancer. There was a reduction in incidence during pregnancy but, after delivery, a slight increase in risk for 3–4 years. Thereafter the incidence rate ratio decreased with time, being 0.83 at 10–14 years and 0.63 after more than 20 years. These results suggest that the protective effect of pregnancy on the breast is maximal at a young age. If oral contraceptive formulations could be devised that mimicked the effect of pregnancy this might achieve a significant long-term reduction in incidence of breast cancer.

TWINS

In 1877 Tchouriloff reported that, based on exclusions from military service because of short stature, in countries with taller inhabitants there was a greater proportion of twin births.[16] Subsequent work indicated that mothers of monozygous (MZ) twins did not differ significantly in height from those who had singleton births but those who had dizygous (DZ) twins were significantly taller.[17] From an endocrine viewpoint, mothers of dizygous twins have been found to have higher levels of follicle-stimulating hormone (FSH) and oestradiol.[18] This would suggest that, because of increased height and higher oestrogen concentrations, there could be an increased risk of breast cancer in mothers of DZ twins.

The epidemiological results have not been concordant with this.

Wyshak et al examined the combined records of the Connecticut Twin Registry and the Connecticut Tumor Registry to compare 3982 women who had borne DZ twins and a control group matched pairwise but who had singleton births.[19] There was no excess of breast cancers among the DZ mothers although there was an increased incidence of pancreatic carcinoma (relative risk = 3.2). In the population-based CASH study, Jacobson found that multiple births were reported by 118 out of 3918 cases and 161 of 4047 controls.[20] After adjustment it emerged that, if the last birth was multiple, there was a reduction in risk (odds ratio = 0.6), but no effect of other twin pregnancies (OR = 1.1). However, two subsequent case-control studies did not find any protective effect of DZ twin pregnancies.[21,22]

In contrast, in a reanalysis of an international case-control study, Hsieh reported that there was an increased breast cancer risk in mothers who had multiple births (OR = 1.21) and that this was significantly elevated for up to 15 years after the last multiple birth (OR = 1.76).[23] To examine whether both twin pregnancies and sex of children affected maternal breast cancer risk, Albrektsen et al carried out a prospective study of 802 269 parous Norwegian women, of whom 97 had multiple births.[24] There was a reduction in incidence rate ratio among those who had multiple births (0.89) and this effect was mostly confined to those whose last birth was multiple. There was no effect of the sex of offspring on breast cancer risk.

Thus, contrary to expectation, most of the data suggest a protective rather than a promotional effect for twin pregnancy and breast cancer. Possible explanations are the elevated α-fetoprotein levels in twin pregnancy, which may exert antioestrogenic effect,[20] and the elevated SHBG levels which can reduce the proportion of biologically available oestradiol.[25]

ABORTION

In a case-control study reported in 1981, Pike et al reported that a first trimester spontaneous or

Table 2.3 Case-control studies of abortion and breast cancer risk

Cases	Controls	Odds ratio	Reference
163	326	2.4	Pike et al[26]
3200	4844	1.2	Rosenberg et al[28]
1451	1451	1.9	Howe et al[30]
845	961	1.5	Daling et al[31]
820	1548	2.1	Lipworth et al[32]
918	918	1.9	Rookus and van Leuwen[33]

induced abortion, before first full-term pregnancy, was associated with a 2.4-fold increase in risk of breast cancer in young women.[26] As a result of the widespread use of termination of pregnancy this posed a potentially large public health problem A subsequent cohort study by Hadjimichael et al showed a 3.5-fold increase in risk.[27] In a study of 3200 cases and 4844 controls, Rosenberg reported

that induced abortions in nulliparous women were associated with an increased risk of 1.3.[28] For first trimester terminations the relative risk was 1.4, but 0.9 for an induced termination before FFTP. These data suggested that any risk associated with termination was small. Similarly, data from 49 000 women on the Swedish Abortion Registry showed no increase in risk of breast cancer after induced abortion.[29]

Results of subsequent case-control studies are summarized in Table 2.3.[26,28,30–33] Although the magnitude of the effect varies between studies, all show that the odds ratio is greater than unity and most show a doubling of risk with induced abortion before the first full-term pregnancy. As with the oral contraceptive pill, there is a small but significant increase in risk among a relatively young group of women with a small absolute risk of breast cancer.

LACTATION

When it was originally found that age at FFTP was the major determinant of breast cancer risk associated with pregnancy, controlling for this resulted in any protective effect of lactation disappearing. However, subsequent studies have found that lactation does have an independent effect on breast cancer risk. In a

Table 2.4 Case-control studies of lactation and subsequent breast cancer risk

Cases	Controls	Relative risk		Reference
		Premenopausal	Postmenopausal	
453	1365	0.91	1.8	Byers et al[35]
329	332	0.49	1.0	McTiernan et al[36]
459	1091	0.93	0.85	Siskind et al[37]
521	521	0.64	0.74	Yoo et al[38]
595	616	0.83	–	UK NCCS[39]
1018	1025	0.77	1.25	Yang et al[40]
5878	8216	0.78	1.04	Newcomb et al[41]
452	452	0.66	–	Enger et al[42]

study of Hong Kong boat women, who suckle from only one breast, Ing et al reported that, of 73 who developed subsequent breast cancer, this occurred in the unsuckled breast in 46 (63%).[34] This does suggest that unilateral suppression of lactation may increase the subsequent risk of cancer in that breast.

Case-control studies which have examined the relationship between lactation and breast cancer risk are summarized in Table 2.4.[35–42] Byers reported that, although there was a protective effect of lactation in premenopausal women after controlling for age, parity and age at FFTP, this effect was not seen in the postmenopausal women.[35] Similar results were found by McTiernan et al,[36] but two other studies reported that the protective effect of lactation was also present in postmenopausal women.[37,38]

In the largest case-control study, which consisted of over 5000 cases and 8000 controls, there was a significant protective effect only in premenopausal women.[41] The reason for the apparent lack of effect is uncertain but London has suggested that this may result from a secular trend in that older women were taught to use a more rigid system of timed feeds whereas younger women are more likely to feed on demand.[43] Whatever the explanation, these data can be used to encourage women to breast-feed, not only for their child's sake, but also for their own mammary protection.

MENOPAUSE

After studying age-incidence statistics for breast cancer in Denmark, Clemmesen reported a reduced incidence around the time of the menopause.[44] This became known as the eponymous 'Clemmesen's hook'. The implication of this phenomenon was that the withdrawal of ovarian function led to a regression of some hormonally driven breast cancers. This was investigated by MacMahon and Feinleib who compared the menstrual histories of 340 American women with breast cancer and 340 matched general surgical control cases.[45] An artificial menopause, usually surgically

Table 2.5 Relative risks of breast cancer in relation to age at surgical menopause

Age at surgical menopause (years)	Relative risk
<35	0.36
35–39	0.68
40–44	0.65
45–49	0.73
≥ 50	0.98

From Trichopoulos and MacMahon.[46]

induced, was reported by 16% of the controls but only 8% of the breast cancer cases, indicating a protective effect.

In a larger study of 3887 cases from the Connecticut Cancer Registry and 3581 controls participating in the National Health Examination Survey of 1960–2, Trichopoulos and MacMahon compared the age at menopause and type of menopause of the two groups.[46] Relative risks of breast cancer in relation to age at surgical menopause are shown in Table 2.5. The earlier the age at oophorectomy, the lower the risk of breast cancer, which fell from almost unity at age 50 or more to a relative risk of 0.36 at age less than 35 years.

Other case-control studies also indicated the reduction in risk of breast cancer associated with oophorectomy and hysterectomy performed at a young age.[47,48] Despite this there was imprecision as to whether one or both ovaries had been removed and also the time scale of the protective effect and its relationship to age at surgery. To elucidate these aspects, Schairer et al carried out a record-linkage study on 15 844 women who had undergone gynaecological operations reported to the Uppsala Health Care Region, Sweden.[49] As Table 2.6

Table 2.6 Standardized morbidity ratios of breast cancer by type of operation and years of follow-up in women premenopausal at the time of surgery

Type of operation	Years since operation			
	0–4	5–9	10–14	15–30
Hysterectomy without ovarian surgery	1.2	1.0	1.2	1.9
Unilateral oophorectomy	1.1	0.8	1.4	1.0
Bilateral oophorectomy				
< 50 years	0.5		0.8	
≥ 50 years	1.1		1.8	

From Schairer et al.[49]

Table 2.7 Positive case-control studies of urinary oestrogens and progesterone in premenopausal and postmenopausal women

Hormone assay	Pre-menopausal	Post-menopausal
Urinary oestrogens	3/8	3/7
Urinary progesterone	2/5	–
Plasma oestradiol	3/11	5/11
Plasma progesterone	2/7	0/3
Plasma testosterone	2/3	4/6

From Key and Pike.[53]

shows, in women who underwent unilateral oophorectomy, there was no diminution in breast cancer risk after up to 30 years of follow-up. For those who had a hysterectomy without ovarian surgery, there was an increased risk which became significant after 15 years. For premenopausal women who were aged over 50 at the time of bilateral oophorectomy, no protective effect was seen. Women aged under 50 years had a 50% reduction in breast cancer for up to 9 years after surgery and a 20% reduction between years 10 and 30.

These results confirm the protective effect of bilateral oophorectomy in premenopausal women aged under 50 at the time of surgery and indicate that this effect is particularly apparent within the first 9 years, during which time the risk of breast cancer is halved. This will be achieved at the expense of menopausal symptoms and a possibly increased risk of both coronary heart disease and osteoporosis, but reformulation of hormone replacement therapy might enable these potentially severe side effects to be prevented.

OESTROGEN

Although the epidemiological literature is highly suggestive of an involvement of oestrogen and progesterone in the promotion of breast cancer, direct evidence of endocrine changes predisposing to the disease has been patchy. There have been peaks from which an aetiological link seemed apparent such as pre-existing adrenal androgen deficiency,[50] the inadequate luteal function hypothesis,[51] and the biologically available oestrogen theory.[52] Between times, contradictory data have led many to assume that no consistent endocrine abnormalities have been found that predispose women to breast cancer. This uncertainty prompted Key and Pike to revisit the available endocrine studies.[53] Some of the results are given in Table 2.7, which shows that urinary steroids were very inconsistent, as were plasma levels of progesterone. In contrast there were more studies indicating that postmenopausal breast cancer cases were exposed to higher plasma levels of both oestrogen and testosterone.

Table 2.8 Odds ratios in relation to tertiles of urinary oestrogen excretion

Hormone	Low tertile	Middle tertile	High tertile
Pre-menopausal			
E1	1.0	0.5	0.4
E2	1.0	0.8	0.4
E3	1.0	0.7	0.7
Total	1.0	0.9	0.5
Post-menopausal			
E1	1.0	0.9	1.1
E2	1.0	0.8	1.9*
E3	1.0	1.5	1.8
Total	1.0	0.9	1.9*

E1, oestrone; E2, oestradiol; E3, oestriol;
* $p < 0.05$.
From Key et al.[54]

In a subsequent case-control study nested within the Guernsey prospective project, urinary oestrogens were measured in 38 premenopausal cases and 597 controls and 31 postmenopausal cases with 334 controls.[54] The odds ratios of the tertiles are given in Table 2.8, showing that there was a non-significant trend toward a lowering of risk with increasing urinary oestrogens in premenopausal women. In the postmenopausal woman, there was a significant correlation between oestrogen excretion and risk.

The New York University Women's Health Study is the largest prospective cohort study comprising 14 291 volunteers, aged 35–65, who underwent mammographic screening and gave a blood sample at that time.[55] After 5 years, 130 breast cancers had occurred in postmenopausal participants: for each two age-matched controls were selected randomly and stored serum samples assayed for total E2 (oestradiol), E1 (oestrone), percentage free oestradiol (free E2), SHBG and FSH. The odds ratios for quartiles, after adjustment for Quetelet's index, are shown in Table 2.9, with significant trends for total E1 and E2, together with total free E2, but

Table 2.9 Adjusted odds ratios of breast cancer in relation to quartiles of plasma oestrogens

Oestradiol	Quartile 1	Quartile 2	Quartile 3	Quartile 4
Total E1	1.0	2.2	3.7	2.5*
Total E2	1.0	0.9	1.8	1.8*
% free E2	1.0	1.7	1.9	2.0
Total free E2	1.0	1.4	3.0	2.9†
% albumin-bound E2	1.0	1.3	2.1	3.3†
Total albumin-bound E2	1.0	1.1	2.7	2.2†
% SHBG-bound E2	1.0	0.7	0.4	0.3†
Total SHBG-bound E2	1.0	1.0	1.1	1.3

* p for trend <0.05; † p for trend < 0.001.
From Toniolo et al.[55]

not percentage E2. The percentage of E2 bound to SHBG displayed a significant inverse relationship, indicating a protective effect. These results strongly suggest that endogenous oestradiol is a significant risk factor in postmenopausal women, after adjustment for body mass index.

Confirmatory data were reported from the Guernsey project in a nested case-control study of 61 postmenopausal cases and 179 controls.[56] In the highest tertile of total oestradiol concentration, the odds ratio of breast cancer was 5.3, and this was not significantly altered after adjustment for testosterone or SHBG. Those in the highest tertile of testosterone concentration had an odds ratio of 2.4, unaffected by adjustment for SHBG, but becoming non-significant after adjustment for E2. SHBG levels were inversely related to risk and this remained significant after adjustment for either E2 or testosterone.

For postmenopausal women undergoing mammographic screening, a simultaneous analysis of total E2 could be used to establish a higher-risk group. In these individuals an antioestrogenic intervention would be worthwhile testing in the context of a prospective randomized trial. As an alternative approach, dietary intervention could be useful in order to reduce the peripheral aromatization of adrenal androgens in those with the highest weight. Despite the apparent simplicity of the latter approach, it is more likely that in population terms a pharmacological intervention will be more acceptable than a physiological change in lifestyle.

INTRATUMORAL HORMONE SYNTHESIS

Animal studies have shown that, during pregnancy, there are higher concentrations of oestradiol-17β in the mammary venous blood than the arterial[57] and this synthesis was associated with uptake of androstenedione.[58] Vermeulen measured concentrations of androstenedione in normal and malignant human breast tissue and found that in both the levels were significantly higher than in venous blood.[59] Within the cancers, there were higher concentrations of oestrogen and lower androgen levels than in normal breast tissue.

In a study conducted at Guy's Hospital, lymphatic fluid and peripheral venous blood were collected from 28 women with breast cancer who underwent breast conservation therapy and had a tumorectomy and axillary clearance, with an interstitial boost of 20 Gy to the biopsy site.[60] Histological examination of the biopsy specimen showed that margins were involved in 17 and clear in 11. Among the premenopausal cases who had an incomplete excision so that malignant cells were still present and probably destroyed by interstitial irradiation, there was a significantly elevated level of free testosterone in the lymph during the time of the implant. No differences were found in the blood/lymph ratios of oestradiol, dehydroepiandrosterone sulphate or SHBG.

Osborne et al carried out microdissections of terminal duct lobular units (TDLUs) from normal reduction mammoplasty specimens and from mastectomies for breast cancer.[61] These TDLUs and mammary fat were cultured in vitro and transformation of oestradiol via the C16α-hydroxylation pathway was measured. In the normal tissue, hydroxylation was 1.8 times higher in TDLU than in fat, but in the mastectomy-derived TDLUs the activity was eight times higher. The metabolite 16α-hydroxyoestrone (16αOHE) can induce proliferation and genotoxic damage in vitro and so it is possible that this enhanced production within TDLU cells from patients with breast cancer might be a pre-existing abnormality leading to promotion of malignancy.

PROLACTIN

Although circumstantial evidence links prolactin and breast cancer, it is likely that this hormone is one of many promoters. Prolactin is necessary for the growth and differentiation of the breast, together with the maintenance of lactation and some normal properties, may be maintained in malignant tissue. Women who took reserpine and developed hyperprolacti-

Table 2.10 Adjusted relative risks for breast cancer in prolactin quintiles						
	1	**2**	**3**	**4**	**5**	***p* value**
Premenopausal	1.0	0.7	0.7	1.3	1.1	0.85
Postmenopausal	1.0	1.1	1.8	1.3	1.6	0.97

From Wang et al.[68]

naemia were not at significantly increased breast cancer risk.[62,63] Individuals taking reserpine had blood prolactin levels that were 50% higher than in women taking other drugs for hypertension or untreated age-matched controls.[64] Ross calculated that, in terms of breast cancer, this increase in prolactin would lead to a relative risk of 1.2. Stanford examined duration of reserpine usage and breast cancer risk and found that prolonged use, beyond 10 years, led to a significantly increased relative risk of 4.5.[65]

To examine the relationship between parity and prolactin, Wang performed assays on two cohorts, each comprising 5000 women.[66] There was a significant decrease in prolactin levels with increase in parity among both premenopausal and postmenopausal women, suggesting that this endocrine consequence of parity was a permanent effect. This could explain the benefits of multiparity, and the protection given by late age at final pregnancy. Bulbrook examined the relationship between age and prolactin level and calculated that this fitted a cubic equation.[67] This was consistent with the observed age-incidence curves, and was in favour of prolactin being a promoter rather than an inducer of mammary carcinogenesis.

As a component of the Guernsey project, Wang et al investigated the effect of blood prolactin level on subsequent risk of breast cancer in 2596 premenopausal and 1180 postmenopausal women.[68] Of these 71 premenopausal and 40 postmenopausal women were later diagnosed with breast cancer. Blood levels of prolactin were divided into quintiles and relative risks calculated after adjustment for age, parity, height and prior breast biopsy. The results are given in Table 2.10, and these show that there was no relationship between prolactin level and risk in either premenopausal or postmenopausal women.

These results suggest that, whatever may occur in rodents, variations within the normal range of blood prolactin levels are not a determinant of breast cancer risk in humans. Despite this, before prolactin is written off as a promotional factor in breast cancer, certain complexities have to be considered. Not all the prolactin measured by radioimmunoassay is biologically active as assessed by the NB2 rat lymphoma in vitro system in which mitosis is stimulated by lactogenic hormones.[69] Women with breast cancer have been found to demonstrate a greater surge of bioactive prolactin after thyroid-releasing hormone administration than age-matched controls.[70] Originally, women with a family history of breast cancer were reported to have elevated levels of bioactive prolactin, despite normal radioimmunoassay results,[69] but subsequent studies found no difference.[71,72]

Another problem is that the assays may need to be reanalysed in terms of the different radioimmunoassayable components: 'big-big', 'big' and 'little' prolactin.[73] Also, the glycosylated and non-glycosylated variants of prolactin may exert different physiological effects. The ratio of non-glycosylated/glycosylated prolactin has been reported to rise during pregnancy.[74] Hence, there may be a component of prolactin that does promote breast cancer but, as measured by present radioimmunoassay, elevated levels of the entire hormone do not significantly increase risk.

MELATONIN

Melatonin is synthesized in the pineal gland, predominantly at night, and has pleiotropic activities, some of which might alter the risk of breast cancer. In rats that have been exposed to dimethylbenzanthracene (DMBA), pinealectomy leads to an increased tumour burden which can be prevented by melatonin injection.[75] When melatonin is added to cultures of the human breast cancer cell line MCF-7, it inhibits the growth of the cells in vitro,[76] and also increases oestrogen receptor-binding capacity.[77]

Comparison of mean daytime nadir and night-time peak of plasma melatonin showed no differences between breast cancer patients and controls, although the cases with lower night/day differences were more likely to have oestrogen receptor-positive tumours.[78] Several studies have now shown that there is a seasonal variation in the detection of breast cancer, which is maximally diagnosed in spring and summer.[79–82] To investigate whether melatonin was implicated in seasonal differences, Holdaway et al took blood samples every 2 hours for 24 hours from 20 premenopausal breast cancer cases and nine controls.[83] Samples were drawn within 4 weeks of both the summer and winter solstices and melatonin measured by radioimmunoassay.

The daily secretion of melatonin was similar in patients and controls but among the breast cancer patients there were differences according to the season in which their tumour had been diagnosed. Those women diagnosed in the summer had a mean summer winter difference in amplitude of melatonin of 8 pg/ml, whereas those detected in the winter had an amplitude difference of 22 pg/ml. The significantly greater fall of melatonin level in winter-detected cases could have led to an enhanced tumour growth at that time so that the cancers became clinically detectable.

SYNOPSIS

- Breast cancer risk is increased in relation to number of menstrual cycles with a promotion of malignancy by ovarian hormones.
- Protective factors include age at first pregnancy, lactation and twin pregnancy, but age at last pregnancy is not an independent risk determinant.
- Induced abortion before first-full term pregnancy slightly increases risk whereas early surgical menopause is protective.
- Postmenopausal women with higher blood oestrogen levels are at significantly increased risk of breast cancer.
- There is no relationship between blood prolactin levels and breast cancer risk.
- Melatonin inhibits breast cancer growth in vitro and reduction in summer/winter levels may influence human breast cancer seasonality of diagnosis.

REFERENCES

1. Frisch RE. The right weight: body fat, menarche and fertility. *Proc Nutr Soc* 1994; **53:** 113–29.
2. Hsieh C-C, Trichopoulos D, Katsouyanni K, Yuasa S. Age at menarche, age at menopause, height and obesity as risk factors for breast cancer: associations and interactions in an international case-control study. *Int J Cancer* 1990; **46:** 796–800.
3. Apter D, Reinla M, Vihko R. Some endocrine characteristics of early menarche, a risk factor for breast cancer, are preserved into adulthood. *Int J Cancer* 1989; **44:** 783–7.

4. Petridou E, Syrigou E, Toupadaki N et al. Determinants of age at menarche as early predictors of breast cancer risk. *Int J Cancer* 1996; **68:** 193–8.

5. Peeters PHM, Verbeek ALM, Krol A et al. Age at menarche and breast cancer risk in nulliparous women. *Breast Cancer Res Treat* 1994; **33:** 55–61.

6. Parazzini F, La Vecchia C, Negri E et al. Lifelong menstrual pattern and risk of breast cancer. *Oncology* 1993; **50:** 222–5.

7. Salber EJ, TrichopoulosD, MacMahon B. Lactation and reproductive histories of breast cancer patients in Boston, 1965–66. *J Natl Cancer Inst* 1969; **43:** 1013–24.

8. Russo J, Tay LK, Russo IH. Differentiation of the mammary gland and susceptibility to carinogenesis. *Breast Cancer Res Treat* 1982; **2:** 5–73.

9. Russo J, Gusterson BA, Rogers AE et al. Comparative study of human and rat mammary carcinogenesis. *Lab Invest* 1990; **62:** 244–78.

10. Rosero-Bixby L, Oberle MW, Lee NC. Reproductive history and breast cancer in a population of high fertility, Costa Rica, 1984–5. *Int J Cancer* 1987; **40:** 747–54.

11. Layde PM, Webster LA, Baughman AL et al. The independent associations of parity, age at first full term pregnancy, and duration of breastfeeding with the risk of breast cancer. *J Clin Epidemiol* 1989; **42:** 963–73.

12. Kvåle G, Heuch I. A prospective study of reproductive factors and breast cancer II: age at first and last birth. *Am J Epidemiol* 1987; **126:** 842–50.

13. Kalache A, Maguire A, Thompson SG. Age at last full-term pregnancy and risk of breast cancer. *Lancet* 1993; **341:** 32–5.

14. Hsieh C-C, Chan H-W, Lambe M et al. Does age at the last birth affect breast cancer risk? *Eur J Cancer* 1996; **32A:** 118–21.

15. Albrektsen G, Heuch I, Kvåle G. The short-term and long-term effect of a pregnancy on breast cancer risk: a prospective study of 802,457 parous Norwegian women. *Br J Cancer* 1995; **72:** 480–4.

16. Tchouriloff M. Sur la statistique des naissances gémellaires et leur rapport avec la taille. *Bull Soc Anthrop Paris* 1877; **12:** 440–6.

17. Corney G, Seedburgh D, Thompson B et al. Maternal height and twinning. *Ann Hum Genet Lond* 1979; **43:** 55–9.

18. Martin NG, El Beaini JL, Olsen ME et al. Gonadotropin levels in mothers who have had two sets of DZ twins. *Acta Genet Med Gemellol* 1984; **33:** 131–9.

19. Wyshak G, Honeyman MS, Flannery JT, Beck AS. Cancer in mothers of dizygotic twins. *J Natl Cancer Inst* 1983; **70:** 593–9.

20. Jacobson HL, Thompson WD, Janerich DT. Multiple births and maternal risk of breast cancer. *Am J Epidemiol* 1989; **129:** 865–73.

21. Nasca PC, Weistein A, Baptiste M, Mahoney M. The relation between multiple births and maternal risk of breast cancer. *Am J Epidemiol* 1992; **136:** 1316–20.

22. Hsieh C-C, Goldman M, Pavia M et al. Re 'The relation between multiple births and maternal risk of breast cancer' and 'Multiple births and maternal risk of breast cancer'. *Am J Epidemiol* 1994; **139:** 445–6.

23. Hsieh C-C, Goldman M, Pavia M et al. Breast cancer risk in mothers of multiple births. *Int J Cancer* 1993; **54:** 81–4.

24. Albrektsen G, Heuch I, Kvåle G. Multiple births, sex of children and subsequent breast cancer risk for the mothers: a prospective study in Norway. *Int J Cancer* 1995; **60:** 341–4.

25. Murphy M, Key T, Wang D et al. Multiple births and maternal risk of breast cancer. *Am J Epidemiol* 1990; **132:** 199–200.

26. Pike MC, Henderson BE, Casagrande JT et al. Oral contraceptive use and early abortion risk factors for breast cancer in young women. *Br J Cancer* 1981; **43:** 72–9.

27. Hadjimichael OC, Boyle CA, Meigs JW. Abortion before first livebirth and risk of breast cancer. *Br J Cancer* 1986; **58:** 281–4.

28. Rosenberg L, Palmer JR, Kaufman DW et al. Breast cancer in relation to the occurrence and time of induced and spontaneous abortions. *Am J Epidemiol* 1988; **127:** 981–9.

29. Harris B-ML, Eklund G, Meirik O et al. Risk of cancer of the breast after legal abortion during first trimester: a Swedish register study. *BMJ* 1989; **299:** 1430–2.

30. Howe HL, Senie RT, Bzduch H, Herzfeld P. Early abortion and breast cancer risk among women under age 40. *Int J Epidemiol* 1989; **18:** 300–4.

31. Daling JR, Malone KE, Voigt LF et al. Risk of breast cancer among young women: relationship to induced abortion. *J Natl Cancer Inst* 1994; **86:** 1584–92.

32. Lipworth L, Katsouyanni K, Ekbom A et al. Abortion and the risk of breast cancer. *Int J Cancer* 1995; **61:** 181–4.

33. Rookus MA, van Leeuwen FE. Induced abortion and risk of breast cancer: reporting(recall) bias in a Dutch case-control study. *J Natl Cancer Inst* 1996; **88:** 1759–64.

34. Ing R, Ho JHC, Petrakis NL. Unilateral breast feeding and breast cancer. *Lancet* 1977; **ii:** 124–7.

35. Byers T, Graham S, Rzepka T, Marshall J. Lactation and breast cancer. *Am J Epidemiol* 1985; **121:** 664–74.

36. McTiernan A, Thomas DB. Evidence for a protective effect of lactation on risk of breast cancer in young women. *Am J Epidemiol* 1986; **124:** 353–8.

37. Siskind V, Schofield F, Rice D, Bain C. Breast cancer and breastfeeding: results from an Australian case-control study. *Am J Epidemiol* 1989; **130:** 229–36.

38. Yoo K-Y, Tajima K, Kuroishi T et al. Independent protective effect of lactation against breast cancer: a case-control study in Japan. *Am J Epidemiol* 1992; **135:** 726–33.

39. United Kingdom National Case-Control Study. Breast feeding and risk of breast cancer in young women. *BMJ* 1993; **307:** 17–20.

40. Yang CP, Weiss NS, Band PR et al. History of lactation and breast cancer risk. *Am J Epidemiol* 1993; **138:** 1050–6.

41. Newcomb PA, Storer BE, Longnecker MP et al. Lactation and a reduced risk of premenopausal breast cancer. *N Engl J Med* 1994; **330:** 81–7.

42. Enger SM, Ross RK, Henderson BE, Bernstein L. Breastfeeding history, pregnancy experience and risk of breast cancer. *Br J Cancer* 1997; **76:** 118–23.

43. London SJ. Breastfeeding and breast cancer. *N Engl J Med* 1994; **330:** 1682.

44. Clemmesen J. On the etiology of some human cancers. *J Natl Cancer Inst* 1951; **12:** 1–21.

45. MacMahon B, Feinleib M. Breast cancer in relation to nursing and menopausal history. *J Natl Cancer Inst* 1960; **24:** 733–53.

46. Trichopoulos D, MacMahon B. Menopause and breast cancer risk. *J Natl Cancer Inst* 1972; **48:** 605–13.

47. Brinton LA, Schairer C, Hoover RN, Fraumeni JF. Menstrual factors and risk of breast cancer. *Cancer Invest* 1988; **6:** 245–54.

48. Irwin KL, Lee NC, Peterson HB et al. Hysterectomy, tubal ligation, and the risk of breast cancer. *Am J Epidemiol* 1988; **127:** 1192–1201.

49. Schairer C, Persson I, Falkeborn M et al. Breast cancer risk associated with gynecologic surgery and indications for such surgery. *Int J Cancer* 1997; **70:** 150–4.

50. Bulbrook RD, Hayward JL, Spicer CC, Thomas BS. Abnormal secretion of urinary steroids by women with early breast cancer. *Lancet* 1962; **ii:** 1238-40.

51. Sherman BM, Korenman SG. Inadequate corpus luteum function, A pathophysiological interpretation of human breast cancer epidemiology. *Cancer* 1974; **33:** 1306-12.

52. Siiteri PK, Hammond GL, Nisker JA. Increased availability of serum estrogens in breast cancer: a new hypothesis. In: *Banbury Report 8. Hormones and Breast Cancer*. Pike MC, Siiteri PK, Welsch CW, eds. New York: Cold Spring Harbor, 1981.

53. Key TJA, Pike MC. The role of oestrogens and progestagens in the epidemiology and prevention of breast cancer. *Eur J Cancer Clin Oncol* 1988; **24:** 29–43.

54. Key TJA, Wang DY, Brown JB et al. A prospective study of urinary oestrogen excretion and breast cancer risk. *Br J Cancer* 1996; **73:** 1615–19.

55. Toniolo PG, Levitz M, Zeleniuch-Jacquotte A et al. A prospective study of endogenous estrogens and breast cancer in postmenopausal women. *J Natl Cancer Inst* 1995; **87:** 190–7.

56. Thomas HV, Key TJA, Allen DS et al. A prospective study of endogenous serum hormone concentrations and breast cancer risk in postmenopausal women on the island of Guernsey. *Br J Cancer* 1997; **76:** 401–5.

57. Maule Walker FM, Peaker M. Production of oestradiol-17β by the goat mammary gland in late pregnancy in relation to lactogenesis. *J Physiol* 1978; **284:** 71–3.

58. Prandi A, Gaiani R. Studio *in vitro* ed *in vivo* dell'attivata'steroidogenetica dell mammella della capra nelle ultime della gravidanza. *Atti Soc Ital Sci Vet* 1984; **38:** 194–7.

59. Vermeulen A, Deslyperre JP, Paridaens R et al. Aromatase, 17β-hydroxysteroid dehydrogenase and intratisssular sex hormone concentrations in cancerous and normal glandular breast tissue in postmenopausal women. *Eur J Cancer Clin Oncol* 1986; **22:** 515–25.

60. Hamed H, Caleffi M, Fentiman IS et al. Steroid hormones in lymph and blood from women with early breast cancer. *Eur J Cancer* 1991; **27:** 42–4.

61. Osborne MP, Bradlow HL, Wong GYC, Telang NT. Upregulation of estradiol c16α-hydroxylation in human breast tissue: a potential

biomarker of breast cancer risk. *J Natl Cancer Inst* 1993; **85**: 1917–20.

62. Boston Collaborative Drug Surveillance Program. Reserpine and breast cancer. *Lancet* 1974; **ii**: 669–71.

63. Armstrong B, Skegg D, White G et al. Rauwolfia derivatives and breast cancer in hypertensive women. *Lancet* 1976; **ii**: 8–12.

64. Ross RK, Paganini-Hill A, Krailo M et al. Effects of reserpine on prolactin levels and incidence of breast cancer in postmenopausal women. *Cancer Res* 1984; **44**: 3106–8.

65. Stanford JL, Martin EJ, Brinton LA et al. Rauwolfia use and breast cancer a case-control study. *J Natl Cancer Inst* 1986; **76**: 817–22.

66. Wang DY, De Stavola BL, Bulbrook RD et al. The permanent effect of reproductive events on blood prolactin levels and its relation to breast cancer risk: a population study of postmenopausal women. *Eur J Cancer Clin Oncol* 1988; **24**: 1225–31.

67. Bulbrook RD, Wang DY, Hayward JL et al. Plasma prolactin levels and age in a female population: relation to breast cancer. *Int J Cancer* 1981; **28**: 43–5.

68. Wang DY, De Stavola BL, Bulbrook RD et al. Relationship of blood prolactin levels and the risk of subsequent breast cancer. *Int J Epidemiol* 1992; **21**: 214–21.

69. Love RR, Rose DP. Elevated bioactive prolactin in women at risk for familial breast cancer. *Eur J Cancer Clin Oncol* 1985; **22**: 1553–4.

70. Maddox PR, Jones DL, Mansel RE. Prolactin and total lactogenic hormone measured by micro-bioassay and immunoassay in breast cancer. *Br J Cancer* 1992; **65**: 456–60.

71. Anderson E, Morten H, Wang DY et al. Serum bioactive lactogenic hormone levels on women with familial breast cancer and their relatives. *Eur J Cancer Clin Oncol* 1989; **25**: 1719–25.

72. Love RR, Rose DP, Surawicz TS, Newcombe PA. Prolactin and growth hormone levels in premenopausal women with a strong family history of breast cancer. *Cancer* 1991; **68**: 1401–5.

73. Wang DY. Prolactin and its role in the clinical course and risk of breast cancer. *Rev Endocrine Rel Cancer* 1993; **45**: 25–39.

74. Markoff E, Lee DW, Hollingsworth DR. Glycosylated and nonglycosylated prolactin in serum during pregnancy. *J Clin Endocrinol Metab* 1988; **67**: 519–23.

75. Tamarkin L, Cohen M, Roselle D et al. Melatonin inhibition and pinealectomy enhancement of 7, 12-dimethyl benz-α-anthracene-induced mammary tumors in the rat. *Cancer Res* 1981; **41**: 4432–6.

76. Hill SN, Blask DE. Effects of the pineal hormone melatonin on the proliferation and morphological characteristics of human breast cancer cells (MCF-7) in culture. *Cancer Res* 1988; **48**: 6121–4.

77. Danforth DN, Tamarkin L, Lippman ME. Melatonin increases oestrogen receptor binding activity of human breast cancer cells. *Nature* 1983; **305**: 323–4.

78. Danforth DN, Tamarkin L, Mulvihill JJ et al. Plasma melatonin and the hormone-dependency of human breast cancer. *J Clin Oncol* 1985; **3**: 941-8.

79. Lee JAH. Seasonal alterations and the natural history of breast cancer. *Prog Clin Cancer* 1967; **3**: 96–9.

80. Cohen P, Wax Y, Modan B. Seasonality in the occurrence of breast cancer. *Cancer Res* 1983; **43**: 892–5.

81. Mason BH, Holdaway IM, Mullins PR et al. Seasonal variation in breast cancer detection: correlation with tumour progesterone receptor status. *Breast Cancer Res Treat* 1985; **5**: 171–4.

82. Chelboun JO, Gray BN. The profile of breast cancer in Western Australia. *Med J Aust* 1987; **147**: 331–3.

83. Holdaway IM, Mason BH, Gibbs EE et al. Seasonal changes in serum melatonin in women with previous breast cancer. *Br J Cancer* 1991; **64**: 149–53.

3

Risk factors

Damnosa hereditas – *ruinous inheritance.*

Gaius

Genetics of breast cancer • Benign breast disease

GENETICS OF BREAST CANCER

Breast cancers resulting from a genetic mutation comprise only 5–10% of cases, but individuals considering themselves to be at risk form a disproportionately large part of the workload of breast clinics. Clinicians and geneticists are particularly interested in high-risk cases because of the hope that genetic mutations will reveal mechanisms for the development of sporadic breast cancer. As the molecular biologists have uncovered some of the genetic mutations responsible for familial breast cancer, high-risk women can be identified thereby opening another Pandora's box, given the uncertainty as to the effectiveness of current surveillance or interventions.

Identified genes

The first genetic disorder to be definitely associated with an increased risk of breast cancer was Cowden's disease, the clinical features of which include mandibular and maxillary hypoplasia, facial trichilemmomas and acral keratoses, together with oral mucosal papillomas and fibromas.[1] In a series of 21 women with Cowden's disease, breast cancer developed in 10 while the remainder had multiple fibroadenomas, fibrocystic disease and mammary

hypertrophy.[2] This autosomal dominant condition was also called multiple hamartoma–neoplasia syndrome and was reported by Albrecht et al to be associated with Lhermitte–Duclos disease in which there is abnormal proliferation of cerebellar neuronal elements.[3] At present the location of the susceptibility gene is unknown but study of affected individuals has shown that no germline mutation of *p53* is present.[4]

Ataxia–telangectasia (A-T) is inherited as an autosomal recessive syndrome, with heterozygotes, forming about 1% of the population of the USA.[5] The A-T gene is located on chromosome 11q22–23.[6] Swift et al studied 1599 relatives from 161 families with ataxia–telangectasia and compared their cancer incidence with that of 821 spouses who served as controls.[7] After a follow-up of 6 years, the cancer risk was estimated as 3.5 for heterozygotes compared with that of non-carriers. In terms of breast cancer, the relative risk was 5.1. Based on occupation and history of diagnostic radiographs, those with breast cancer had a six-fold increase in odds ratio for exposure to ionizing radiation. With the population incidence of A-T heterozygotes, such individuals might comprise up to 10% of breast cancer cases.

The combination of soft tissue sarcomas, breast cancers and other early onset carcinomas was first described by Li and Fraumeni in 1969.[8] In a prospective study of 31 members of a family with the eponymous syndrome, five developed breast cancer, four were diagnosed with soft tissue sarcomas and seven with other cancers.[9] The condition was inherited in an autosomal dominant manner and subsequent analysis of skin fibroblasts from members of an affected family indicated that there was a germline mutation of the tumour-suppressor gene *p53* in those with Li–Fraumeni syndrome.[10,11] In a series of 128 breast cancer cases from 109 Swedish families, blood and tumours were screened by constant denaturant gel electrophoresis (CDGE) for mutations of *p53*.[12] No germline mutations were found although 14% of tumours displayed mutant *p53*, indicating that this particular gene does not have a major role in familial breast cancer.

It has been calculated that about half the cases of familial breast cancer and 75% of those with both ovarian and mammary malignancy result from mutations in the *BRCA1* gene, located on chromosome 17q21.[13] This may be an overestimate. Couch et al determined the incidence of *BRCA1* mutations in a group of 263 women with a family history of breast cancer.[14] A pathological mutation was found in 16% although, of those with a family history of breast cancer without ovarian carcinoma, only 7% were carriers of a *BRCA1* mutation.

Multiple mutations of the gene have been described, including deletions, insertions, stop codons and missense substitutions. The gene product is a 190-kDa protein with a zinc finger domain at the amino-terminal region and sequence homology with the granin proteins.[15] BRCA1 protein is membrane associated, passing through the Golgi apparatus before being packaged within secretory vesicles. The protein is post-translationally glycosylated and can be induced by oestradiol. Both in vitro and in vivo, BRCA1 protein inhibits the growth of breast cancer cells whereas the mutant protein has no effect, providing direct evidence that BRCA1 protein is a tumour suppressor.[16]

When the *BRCA1*-coding region was investigated in sporadic breast and ovarian cancers, mutations were rarely found.[17] This suggests that different tumour suppressor genes were involved in most breast cancers. In a series of 80 women who had breast cancer diagnosed when aged less than 35 years, germline mutations of *BRCA1* were found in six (7.5%) and, of the 39 women who had no family history, mutations were found in two (5%).[18] Subsequently, it was found that a specific mutation at position 185 on *BRCA1*, involving a deletion of adenine and guanine (185delAG) was present in 1% of Ashkenazi Jewish women. Fitzgerald et al carried out *BRCA1* mutational analysis in 418 women diagnosed with breast cancer at ages under 40, using automated nucleotide sequencing and a truncated protein assay.[19] *BRCA1* mutations were present in 4 of 30 (13%) women diagnosed at ages under 30, but 185delAG was present in 8 of 39 (21%) Jewish women who had breast cancer at ages under 40.

The other major breast cancer susceptibility gene is *BRCA2*, located on chromosome 13q12–q13, encoding a 3418 amino acid protein of, at present, unknown function.[20] To determine the likelihood of further breast cancer susceptibility genes, Serova et al carried out mutation screening for *BRCA1* and *BRCA2*, together with linkage analysis, in 31 families with 23 site-specific cases.[21] There were four mutations of *BRCA1* and also four *BRCA2* abnormalities. It was predicted that 8–10 breast cancer cases were the result of at least one or more major susceptibility gene.

Breast cancer risk in gene carriers

To estimate the lifetime risk of cancer in women carrying a *BRCA1* pathogenic mutation, Ford et al studied a cohort of 1327 women from 33 families, each of which contained at least four cases of breast or ovarian cancer diagnosed before age 60.[22] Markers examined were D17S250 and D17S579, with prior probability of linkage to *BRCA1* being set at 0.45 for breast cancer families and 0.79 for those with additional ovarian cancer. The estimated cumulative risks are shown in Table 3.1,

Table 3.1 Risk of breast cancer with age in carriers of *BRCA1* mutations

	Cumulative risk (%)			
	Age 40	Age 50	Age 60	Age 70
Unilateral breast cancer	20	50	50	87
Contralateral breast cancer	32	50	55	87

From Ford et al.[22]

showing that the lifetime probability of breast cancer was 0.87. By the age of 50, it was predicted that 50% of *BRCA1* carriers would develop bilateral breast cancer.

The high penetrance of *BRCA1* mutations was also confirmed in a Scottish study of 206 women from 15 families in whom the lifetime risk of breast cancer was 88%.[23] All the cases had developed the disease before the age of 65 years. Nevertheless these results were derived from high-risk families. Struewing et al examined breast cancer risk in 5318 Jewish men and women, among whom 120 were found to be carriers of the 185delAG and 5382insC mutations of *BRCA1* and 6174delT mutation of *BRCA2*.[24] Risk of breast cancer was estimated by comparing the family incidence of the disease among relatives of carriers and non-carriers. The risk by age 70 was calculated as 56% (95% confidence interval = 40–73%), and was of similar magnitude in those with mutations of *BRCA1* and *BRCA2*. This suggests that within this population the lifetime risk was substantially less than that calculated for high-risk families.

Genetic testing

Identification of the *BRCA1* and *BRCA2* tumour-suppressor genes has created a new series of

problems for those who are running family cancer clinics. The most major is to determine who should be offered genetic screening and what information they should be given. There are two available systems for determination of breast cancer risk: the Gail model, originally derived from Breast Cancer Detection Demonstration Project (BCDDP) data,[25] and the Claus model developed from the Cancer and Hormones (CASH) Study.[26] The Gail system uses family history, endogenous oestrogen exposure and clinical risk, whereas the Claus model uses only family history in terms of numbers of relatives with the disease and age at onset. When projected cases from the Gail model were compared with actual numbers, there was an overestimation of risk for premenopausal women.[27] McGuigan et al carried out a direct comparison of the point estimates and 95% confidence intervals of the Gail method and point estimate only from the Claus model to estimate risk for 111 women attending a high-risk breast clinic.[28] There was significant concordance between the two estimates but the major discrepancy was for nulliparous women and those who had had a prior breast biopsy.

Individual perception of breast cancer risk may be inaccurate and is usually an overestimate of likelihood of disease. Smith et al asked 862 women to estimate their lifetime risk and also calculated risk using the Gail model.[29] Most women overestimated their risk by more than 50% and one-third by more than fivefold. Both the youngest and the oldest were the most inaccurate in assessing their own risk. Similar results were reported by Black et al in a survey of women aged under 50 years.[30] In contrast, a study of young women attending a family cancer clinic in Manchester found that 44% estimated their risk within 50% of the Gail prediction, with a quarter underestimating by over 50% and a quarter overestimating by 50%.[31] All these studies indicate the need for education of women attending family clinics and that no assumptions should be made about prior knowledge.

Lerman et al conducted a randomized trial in which specific breast cancer risk counselling was compared with general healthy counselling in 200 women aged over 35 years attending a family cancer clinic.[32] The control group had a structured interview with a nurse educator on health practices, smoking, diet, exercise and cancer screening. The experimental group received a structured interview which covered individual risk factors, personal risk and recommendations for follow-up. Three months later all participants were telephoned and questioned about breast cancer preoccupation, risk comprehension and improvement in understanding. Risk comprehension was significantly better in the experimental group but, in both groups, two-thirds still overestimated their lifetime risk.

At present genetic testing starts not with a woman at risk but with her first-degree relative with breast cancer. As a result of the complexity of mutations of *BRCA1* and *BRCA2*, together with as yet undiscovered susceptibility genes, it is necessary to determine whether a woman with early-onset disease is carrying a pathological mutation. If not, there is no point in testing her sisters and daughters. Almost all the testing that has been conducted so far has been for research rather than as a clinical service. Hence, if a mutation is identified, the individual may or may not wish to know the result. In general terms, those with daughters will be more likely to ask for the result so that their offspring can be either reassured if the result is negative, or possibly tested themselves should a mutation have been identified.

When a young woman with breast cancer is found to be a carrier of a pathological mutation, this may have implications for her own management. If the previous treatment was breast conservation therapy, this means that there will be an increased risk of ipsilateral relapse and the development of a contralateral new primary. Serious consideration should be given to bilateral mastectomy, with or without reconstruction. If a mastectomy has been performed, contralateral prophylactic total mastectomy should be contemplated.

If the affected patient has first-degree relatives who are concerned about their risk, at

what age should testing be performed? No categorical answer can be made to this question. It has been customary to suggest that testing should not be performed before age 30, or 5 years before the age at diagnosis of the mother or sister. By doing this, one possibility for intervention will be missed. If a woman wishes to be tested at age 18, should she be found to be a gene carrier, this would have implications for her subsequent family planning. Use of in vitro fertilization, with polymerase testing of the eight-cell embryo could enable only a mutation-free egg to be implanted. This darwinian approach could lead to the eventual disappearance of *BRCA1* and *BRCA2* mutations from the population.

Surveillance

Before undergoing genetic testing, first-degree relatives must be informed about the available options, should they be found to carry a pathological mutation. At present, options include surveillance, possible prevention trials and prophylactic mastectomy. For many women close surveillance would seem to be the easiest option but individuals need to be made aware that techniques for early detection in premenopausal women are not ideal. There is scant evidence that surveillance saves lives. In a collaborative study of 24 high-risk Dutch families, 78 individuals were diagnosed with breast cancer, of whom 58 presented with symptoms and 18 were detected as a result of screening.[33] The comparative features of the two groups are shown in Table 3.2. The screen-detected cases were less likely to have axillary nodal involvement (52% vs 17%), and none died of metastatic disease compared with 40 of the symptomatic patients.

To assess whether close surveillance conferred any benefit on women considered to be 'at risk', a case-control study was conducted at Guy's Hospital. The subjects were 141 women who attended a follow-up clinic and subsequently developed breast cancer. They were in three categories of risk: first- or second-degree family history, history of recurrent cysts, and

Table 3.2 Comparative features of familial breast cancer cases who were asymptomatic or detected by screening

Feature	Symptomatic	Screened
Number	58	18
Median age	43	43
Nodal involvement (%)	52	17
Deaths	22	0

From Vasen et al.[33]

prior premalignant histological change. Tumour size and stage at diagnosis were compared with that of four age-matched controls, with and without a family history, who presented with symptomatic disease. The patients under surveillance had a better stage at presentation and were less likely to have inoperable tumours (6% compared with 17% of the controls). Tumours were smaller in the surveillance group (median size 2.0 cm vs 2.8 cm). This was associated with a non-significant trend towards improved 5-year survival (85% vs 78%). The results suggest that surveillance may detect some cancers at an earlier stage.

Prevention

Prospects for prevention are discussed in Chapter 23 and include tamoxifen, dietary alteration and retinoids. The pilot study for the tamoxifen prevention trial was conducted at the Royal Marsden Hospital. As part of this, risk perceptions and levels of anxiety in 99 participants were compared with those of 87 women who underwent mammographic screening and had a family history, but were not attending a specialized breast clinic, and 86 women who had been screened but had no family history.[34] All completed a Spielberger trait anxiety inventory and a questionnaire on risk perception. Anxiety

levels were significantly elevated in those women with a family history who were not under surveillance, whereas similar levels were found in those participating in the tamoxifen trial and those without a family history. Participation in prevention studies may reduce rather than increase anxiety in those with a family history, so such individuals should be encouraged to join, when appropriate. Use of agents such as tamoxifen on an *ad hoc* basis is a bad idea because risks and benefits have yet to be determined.

Prophylactic mastectomy

For carriers of susceptibility genes who have experienced the suffering of their relatives who died of metastatic breast cancer, prophylactic mastectomy may be their choice of treatment. If this extreme measure is being considered, every effort should be made to remove all the tissue at risk. Wong et al studied the effectiveness of prophylactic mastectomy in Sprague–Dawley rats with 7,12-dimethylbenzanthracene (DMBA)-induced mammary cancers.[35] Two weeks after administration of DMBA, 50%, 75% and total mastectomies were performed on separate groups. Another group had total mastectomies and the DMBA 2 weeks later. The mean number of breast tumours per rat are shown in Table 3.3, which indicates that the extent of

Table 3.3 Mean number of breast tumours per rat at time of death

Group	Number of tumours per rat
Control	5
50% mastectomy	5
75% mastectomy	5
Total mastectomy	5
Total mastectomy before DMBA	0.2

From Wong et al.[35]

Table 3.4 Studies comparing survival of breast cancer patients with or without a family history

Familial		Sporadic		Reference
Number	Survival rate (%)	Number	Survival rate (%)	
165	70	2833	55	Langlands et al[39]
106	67	ACS	45	Albano et al[40]
556	70	4551	70	Anderson and Badzioch[41]
56	66	235	59	Ruden et al[42]
417	47	3161	50	Slattery et al[43]
35	83	35	61	Porter et al[23]
118	86	615	77	Malone et al[44]

mastectomy after DMBA bore no relationship to subsequent tumour development. Even when a total mastectomy had been attempted, it is likely that some breast tissue remained, and this could be regarded as similar to the situation in humans after a subcutaneous mastectomy.

As it is unlikely that a randomized trial will be conducted to compare total and subcutaneous mastectomy in gene carriers, it is essential that these individuals are registered and followed in order that the relative efficacies can be quantified. In a previous survey of women at varying degrees of risk, who underwent subcutaneous mastectomy, breast cancer occurred subsequently in 0.05%.[36] This percentage could be a considerable underestimate for a high-risk group of women with susceptibility mutations.

Such prophylactic procedures are not without complications. Khouri et al reported a multicentre series of 120 women who underwent simultaneous bilateral mastectomy with transverse rectus abdominis myocutaneous free flaps.[37] The average operating time was 8.6 hours and inpatient stay was 7.6 days. Flap thrombosis occurred in six cases and in one the flap could not be salvaged. Complications including haematoma, partial flap necrosis and wound infection, were reported in 15% of cases,

and abdominal wall weakness or hernia occurred in 12%.

To investigate the probable impact of prophylactic mastectomy on life expectancy in *BRCA1* and *BRCA2* carriers, Schrag et al used a Markov decision analysis model.[38] A series of assumptions was made including stage at diagnosis and prognosis for those with early disease such as probability of different forms of relapse within 10 years. Using a conservative estimate of an 85% reduction in risk of breast cancer after bilateral mastectomy, the estimated increase in life expectancy of 30-year-old women was calculated as being between 2.9 and 5.3 years. With increasing age the gain diminished so that, by the age of 60, the benefit of prophylactic mastectomy was minimal.

Prognosis in familial breast cancer

Some women with a breast cancer susceptibility gene may develop tumours with a better prognosis than those with sporadic disease. Langlands et al examined the survival of 165 breast cancer patients who had an affected first-degree relative and compared this with the outcome for 2833 women with the disease but without any family history.[39] As is shown in Table 3.4, the 5-year survival was better for

Table 3.5 Comparative features of breast cancers in *BRCA1* and *BRCA2* carriers and age-matched sporadic controls

Feature	Sporadic (%)	*BRCA1* (%)	Odds ratio	*BRCA2* (%)	Odds ratio
Ductal I	24	9	1.0	11	1.0
Ductal II	40	35	1.7	48	2.7
Ductal III	36	66	4.4	41	2.6
Lobular	10	3	0.4	10	1.0
Tubular	5	2	0.5	0	–
Medullary	2	13	5.2	3	1.6

familial cases and this may have been attributable to a significantly increased proportion of stage I cases in the familial group.

A similar study from the USA compared the outcome of 106 breast cancer cases from 18 affected families and audited results from the American College of Surgeons (ACS).[40] Once more the survival of the familial group was better despite there being no difference between the stage at diagnosis of both groups. Anderson and Badzioch compared the survival of a larger group of familial cases and found no difference when compared with 4551 sporadic cases.[41] In a cohort of 291 breast cancer patents, of whom 56 gave a family history, Ruder et al reported a slightly better survival for that group.[42] Among those without a family history (after adjustment for stage, ethnic origin, body mass index, occupation, menopausal status and age at menarche), there was a relative risk of 1.4 of dying of breast cancer. This difference did not achieve statistical significance.

Using the Utah Population Database, Slattery et al examined the influence of family history of breast cancer on survival after diagnosis of the disease in 3578 women, of whom 417 had a first-degree family history.[43] Those whose mother had breast cancer had an increased risk of dying of the disease (hazard ratio 1.4), and individuals who had a family history and were

diagnosed before age 50 had a relative risk of 1.5 of death from breast cancer. One possible explanation for these discrepant findings was that a heterogeneous population had been studied, some of whom were gene carriers with a variety of susceptibility genes.

Porter et al compared the 5-year survival of 35 women with *BRCA1*-linked breast cancer and age-matched sporadic breast cancer cases.[23] For the *BRCA1* carriers the 5-year survival rate was 83% compared with 61% for age-matched cases. In addition, the survival of 17 women with familial cancer unlinked to *BRCA1* was 59%, indicating that not all mutations predispose to a less aggressive disease.

Malone et al analysed survival in 733 breast cancer cases reported to the Cancer Surveillance System of Washington State and found that there was a 50% reduction in relative risk of dying among those with a first-degree family history.[44] Those with a second-degree family history had a similar prognosis to those without a family history. After adjustment for tumour stage, age at diagnosis and tumour size, the protective effect of a first-degree family history was still present.

The Breast Cancer Linkage Consortium compared the histopathology of tumours from women having *BRCA1* and *BRCA2* mutations with cancers from women without a family history.[45] There were 118 women with *BRCA1*

Table 3.6 Risk of breast cancer in relation to benign histology and family history

Histology	Number	Cancers	Relative risk
Epithelial hyperplasia without atypia (EHWA)	1693	73	1.9
Atypical hyperplasia (AH)	232	30	5.3
EHWA without family history	1498	61	1.9
EHWA with family history	195	12	2.0
AH without family history	193	20	4.3
AH with family history	39	10	8.4

From Dupont and Page.[49]

mutations, 78 carriers of *BRCA2* and 440 age-matched controls. As shown in Table 3.5, the *BRCA1* carriers were more likely to have grade III ductal cancers, less likely to have lobular lesions and had a greater proportion of medullary or atypical medullary tumours. *BRCA2* carriers had tumours of higher grade and were less likely to have tubular cancers.

Mutations of *BRCA1* causing truncation of protein before exon 13 were found to be associated with an increased likelihood of ovarian cancer.[46] Following this, Sobol et al examined the locus of *BRCA1* mutation and the mitotic index of the tumour in 28 breast cancer cases.[47] Rapidly proliferating cancers occurred mainly in women with mutations towards the two terminal domains of the BRCA1 protein, suggesting that these highly conserved regions play an important role in mammary cell growth control. Individuals with these mutations are more likely to develop cancers that may have a short preclinical phase as a result of rapid growth, and thus screening mammography may need to be arranged more frequently.

BENIGN BREAST DISEASE

More than 150 years ago, Astley Cooper described the coexistence of breast cysts and malignancy.[48] Since that time a large body of clinicopathological research has tried to examine the relationship between benign breast disease and breast cancer. Unfortunately the phrase 'benign breast disease' has often been used without either clinical or pathological definition, compounded by the tendency of some radiologists to report mammographic densities as 'dysplasia'. Hence it had been impossible to determine whether biopsied benign lesions or aspirated cysts constituted risk factors for subsequent development of malignancy.

The seminal studies conducted by David Page at Vanderbilt University, Nashville have illuminated our understanding of premalignant breast histology, so that women at risk can be identified and most biopsied cases can be reassured and spared unnecessary follow-up. Dupont and Page reported a follow-up study of 3303 women who had had a breast biopsy and were followed up for a minimum of 17 years.[49] Of these individuals, 1925 (58%) had biopsies that on review had shown epithelial hyperplasia (epitheliosis). Of the entire group, 134 subsequently developed breast cancer. Relative risks of breast cancer in relation to histology of the original benign biopsy are shown in Table 3.6. The presence of epithelial hyperplasia led to almost a doubling of risk compared with those without hyperplasia. Atypical hyperplasia was

Table 3.7 Postmortem findings in relation to racial group and breast cancer risk			
Feature	Caucasian	Hispanic	Native American
Breast cancer rate (per year)	89/100 000	46/100 000	25/100 000
EH+++ aged 45–54 (%)	10	12	0
EH+++ aged >54 (%)	5	0	0
From Bartow et al.[52]			

associated with a fivefold risk which rose to 8.4 when those with atypical hyperplasia and a first-degree family history were compared with women with epithelial hyperplasia without atypia (EHWA) and a family history. What this study did was to delineate a small group of women with atypical hyperplasia and a family history, 39 out of 3303 (1%), with a very high risk.

In subsequent work the relationship between other breast cancer risk factors such as parity and age at first baby was examined in those with and without epithelial hyperplasia and atypical hyperplasia.[50] Of those who were nulliparous, 9% had atypical hyperplasia compared with 6% of the parous cases ($\chi^2 = 6.4$, $p < 0.01$). For those women with atypical hyperplasia who had their first baby aged 20 years or less, the relative risk of breast cancer was 1.6, which rose to 4.5 for those who gave birth aged over 20, and 4.9 for the nulliparous. In addition, the influence of breast size and epithelial hyperplasia was studied. Women were asked to describe their breast size as small, medium or large and, if hesitant, were assigned to the middle category. For women without epithelial hyperplasia, the relative risk in relation to breast size did not differ significantly from unity but, when epithelial hyperplasia was present, the relative risk for those with small breasts was 1.8, that for medium 2.1, rising to 3.0 for those with large breasts. This last finding was consistent with results from a postmortem study of Japanese women living in Hawaii in whom the

volume of breast tissue was greater in those with epithelial hyperplasia.[51]

In a forensic postmortem series of 519 women from New Mexico and eastern Arizona, histological changes in the breast were examined in relation to racial origin: Caucasian, Hispanic and Native American.[52] As is shown in Table 3.7, there was a similar percentage of severe epithelial hyperplasia in both the Caucasian and Hispanic women but none in the Native Americans. After age 54, when most would have been postmenopausal, only the Caucasian women were found to have severe epithelial hyperplasia.

Dupont and Page carried out a reanalysis of their data to determine whether there was a time-dependent aspect of breast cancer risk in women with EHWA and atypical hyperplasia.[53] For both atypical hyperplsia and EHWA half of the subsequent breast cancers had occurred within 10 years of the biopsy. With a constant cancer incidence rate in those with atypical hyperplasia, and a rising incidence with age in the rest of the population, this means that there is a reduction in relative risk with time. In practical terms, if a woman with atypical hyperplasia has lived more than 10 years after diagnosis, without developing breast cancer, she can be reassured that her risk is not materially greater than that of other women and therefore she does not have to remain under close surveillance.

Several other follow-up studies have examined histological features and breast cancer risk. Tavassoli and Norris reported a long-term follow-up of 117 women with epithelial hyperplasia and 82 with atypical hyperplasia.[54] After 8 years, invasive breast cancer occurred in three (3%) of those with epithelial hyperplasia, and eight (10%) of those with atypical hyperplasia, equating to a relative risk of 3.8. In a case-control study nested within the Nurses Health Study, London et al reviewed benign biopsy specimens from 121 women who were subsequently diagnosed with breast cancer and 488 controls.[55] Slides were reviewed blindly and adjustment was made for menopausal status, age at menarche, age at first baby, parity and first-degree family history. Compared with women who did not have hyperplasia on the original biopsy specimen those with epithelial hyperplasia had an adjusted relative risk of 1.6 and those with atypical hyperplasia an adjusted relative risk of 3.7.

One of the larger personal series of benign cases was that of Haagensen, which included both public and private patients who consulted him between 1930 and 1982.[56] Bodian et al reviewed the histopathology of 1799 cases, of whom 1521 (85%) had evidence of epithelial hyperplasia. Those with epithelial hyperplasia had a twofold increase in risk of breast cancer. There was no significant association between degree of atypia and breast cancer risk, but moderate or severe atypical hyperplasia was associated with a relative risk of 3, and severe ductal atypia with a relative risk of 3.9.

Within the Breast Cancer Detection and Prevention Project (BCDDP), which comprised over 280 000 women, a nested case-control study was conducted on 1467 who underwent a benign biopsy.[58] Results of this were remarkably similar to the original study from Vanderbilt University. Epithelial hyperplasia had a relative risk of 1.3, and atypical hyperplasia was associated with a relative risk of 4.3. A first-degree family history increased breast cancer risk by 2.4 and there was a synergy between familial hyperplasia and atypical hyperplasia.

All these studies suggest that atypical epithelial hyperplasia is a rare but real risk factor for breast cancer. Women who have had a benign biopsy with evidence of atypical hyperplasia should remain under surveillance for up to 10 years. They are potential candidates for prevention studies but should not be given agents such as tamoxifen on an *ad hoc* basis. Until such time as there is proof from prospective trials of an effective intervention, close clinical follow-up with regular breast imaging will have to remain the most appropriate management of women with atypical hyperplasia.

Breast cysts

In Haagensen's series of 1693 women with aspirated breast cysts, 72 (4%) subsequently developed breast cancer compared with an expected 17 in the New York population, giving a relative risk of 4.[56] Nevertheless, in Dupont and Page's original paper, histological evidence of cysts was not associated with a significant increase in relative risk.[49] This suggests that there is a subgroup of women with cysts that also have atypia.

In a follow-up study of 3809 Italian women with aspirated breast cysts, Ciatto et al reported that the observed/expected ratio of breast cancers was 1.8, a significant but modest increase in risk.[59] In a similar study from Cardiff, Bundred et al reported 15 breast cancers in a series of 644 women with aspirated cysts.[60] Using age-specific incidence data from the same period, the women with cysts had a 4.4 relative risk of breast cancer. Those that had bilateral or multiple cysts were significantly more likely to have associated atypical hyperplasia and to develop breast cancer.

In another Italian study, Bruzzi et al reported on a 6-year follow-up of a cohort of 802 women with aspirated breast cysts.[61] The potassium/sodium (K^+/Na^+) ratio, as measured in the cyst fluid since previous work, had indicated that type I cysts with a K^+/Na^+ ratio of over 1.5 had a higher risk of developing breast cancer compared with those with type II cysts ($K^+/Na^+ < 1.5$).[62] After adjustment for breast cancer risk factors the relative risk of malignancy in those with type I cysts was 4.2 times that of women with type II cysts.

These results suggest that women with a single breast cyst do not need routinely to be kept under surveillance but should be asked to return if a new lump develops. For those with recurrent cysts, measurement of K^+/Na^+ ratio may be worthwhile because those with type II cysts can be reassured and those with type I cysts kept under more structured follow-up.

SYNOPSIS

• Genetic mutations are responsible for 5–10% of breast cancers and known susceptibility genes include those for Cowden's disease, ataxia–telangectasia, Li–Fraumeni syndrome and *BRCA1* and *BRCA2*.
• Gene carriers have a lifetime probability of 0.87 for developing breast cancer and half the cases will be diagnosed before age 50.
• Individuals' perception of risk can be very inaccurate with both under- and overestimation compared with using predictions from the Gail or Claus models.
• Genetic testing should be confined to those women with first-degree relatives in whom pathogenic mutations have been detected.
• The role of surveillance in gene carriers is unproven although there is some evidence of benefit.
• It is likely that total mastectomy will substantially reduce breast cancer incidence and that subcutaneous procedures will be less effective, but no data are currently available.
• Individuals seeking prevention should be encouraged to participate in on-going trials rather than being treated in an *ad hoc* manner.
• Some women with breast cancer susceptibility genes may develop cancer with a better prognosis than among those with sporadic disease.
• Histological markers of increased risk are atypical ductal and lobular hyperplasia and individuals with these lesions and a family history are at high risk of breast cancer.
• Women who develop multiple breast cysts are at a two- to threefold increased risk of breast cancer and should be encouraged to report all new lumps.

REFERENCES

1. Lloyd KM, Dennis M. Cowden's diseases. A new symptom complex with multiple system involvement. *Ann Intern Med* 1963; **58:** 136–42.
2. Brownstein MH, Wolf M, Bikowski JB. Cowden's disease. A cutaneous marker of breast cancer. *Cancer* 1978; **41:** 2393–8.
3. Albrecht S, Haber RM, Goodman JC, Duvic M. Cowden syndrome and Lhermitte–Duclos disease. *Cancer* 1992; **70:** 869–76.
4. Eng C, Murday V, Seal S et al. Cowden syndrome and Lhermitte–Duclos disease in a family: a single genetic syndrome with pleiotropy. *J Med Genet* 1994; **31:** 458–61.
5. Swift M, Morrell D, Croamartie E et al. The incidence and frequency of ataxia-telangectasia in the United States. *Am J Hum Genet* 1986; **39:** 573–83.
6. Gatti RA, Berkel I, Boder E et al. Localisation of an ataxia telangectasia gene to chromosome 11q22–23. *Nature* 1988; **336:** 577–80.
7. Swift M, Morrell D, Massey RB, Chase CL. Incidence of cancer in 161 families affected by ataxia-telangectasia. *N Engl J Med* 1991; **325:** 1831–6.
8. Li FP, Fraumeni JF. Soft-tissue sarcomas, breast cancer, and other neoplasms. A familial syndrome? *Ann Intern Med* 1969; **71:** 747–52.
9. Li FP, Fraumeni JF. Prospective study of a family cancer syndrome. *JAMA* 1982; **247:** 2692–4.
10. Malkin D, Li FP, Strong LC et al. Germ line p53 mutations in a familial syndrome of breast cancer, sarcomas, and other neoplasms. *Science* 1990; **250:** 1233–8.
11. Srivastava S, Zou Z, Pirollo K et al. Germ-line transmission of a mutated p53 gene in a cancer-prone family with Li–Fraumeni syndrome. *Nature* 1990; **348:** 747–9.
12. Zelada-Hedman M, Børresen-Dale A-L, Claro A et al. Screening for TP53 mutations in patients and tumours from 109 Swedish breast cancer families. *Br J Cancer* 1997; **75:** 1201-4.

13. Miki Y, Swensen J, Shattuck-Eidens D et al. A strong candidate for the breast and ovarian cancer susceptibility gene BRCA1. *Science* 1994; **266:** 66-71.

14. Couch FJ, DeShano ML, Blackwood MA et al. BRCA1 mutations in women attending clinics that evaluate the risk of breast cancer. *N Engl J Med* 1997; **336:** 1409-15.

15. Jensen RA, Thompson ME, Jetton TL et al. BRCA1 is secreted and exhibits properties of a granin. *Nature Genet* 1996; **12:** 303–8.

16. Holt JT, Thompson ME, Szabo C et al. Growth inhibition and tumour inhibition by BRCA1. *Nature Genet* 1996; **12:** 298–302.

17. Futreal PA, Liu Q, Shattuck-Eidens D et al. BRCA1 mutations in primary breast and ovarian carcinomas. *Science* 1994; **266:** 120–2.

18. Langston AX, Malone KE, Thompson JD et al. BRCA1 mutations in a population-based sample of young women with breast cancer. *N Engl J Med* 1996; **334:** 137–42.

19. Fitzgerald MG, MacDonald DJ, Krainer M et al. Germ-line BRCA1 mutations in Jewish and non-Jewish women with early onset breast cancer. *N Engl J Med* 1996; **334:** 143–9.

20. Wooster R, Bignell G, Lancaster G et al. Identification of the breast cancer gene BRCA2. *Nature* 1995; **378:** 789–91.

21. Serova OM, Mazoyer S, Puget N et al. Mutations in BRCA1 and BRCA2 in breast cancer families: are there more breast-cancer susceptibility genes? *Am J Hum Genet* 1997; **60:** 486–95.

22. Ford D, Easton DF, Bishop DT et al. Risks of cancer in BRCA1 mutation carriers. *Lancet* 1994; **343:** 692–5.

23. Porter DE, Cohen BB, Wallace MR et al. Breast cancer incidence, penetrance and survival in probable carriers of BRCA1 gene mutation in families linked to BRCA1 on chromosome 17q12–21. *Br J Surg* 1994; **81:** 1512–15.

24. Struewing JP, Hartge P, Wacholder S et al. The risk of cancer associated with specific mutations of BRCA1 and BRCA2 among Ashkenazi Jews. *N Engl J Med* 1997; **336:** 1401–8.

25. Gail MH, Brinton LA, Byar DP et al. Projecting individualized probabilities of developing breast cancer for white females who are being examined annually. *J Natl Cancer Inst* 1989; **81:** 1879–86.

26. Claus EB, Risch N, Thompson WD. Autosomal dominant inheritance of early-onset breast cancer. Implications for risk projection. *Cancer* 1994; **73:** 643–51.

27. Bondy ML, Lustbader ED, Halabi S et al. Validation of a breast cancer risk assessment model in women with a positive family history. *J Natl Cancer Inst* 1994; **86:** 620–5.

28. McGuigan KA, Ganz PA, Breant C. Agreement between breast cancer risk estimation methods. *J Natl Cancer Inst* 1996; **88:** 1315–7.

29. Smith BL, Gadd MA, Lawler C et al. Perception of breast cancer risk among women in breast center and primary care settings: correlation with age and family history of breast cancer. *Surgery* 1996; **120:** 297–303.

30. Black WC, Nease RF, Tosteson ANA. Perceptions of breast cancer risk and screening effectiveness in women younger than 50 years of age. *J Natl Cancer Inst* 1995; **87:** 720–1.

31. Evans DGR, Burnell LD, Hopwood P, Howell A. Perception of risk in women with a family history of breast cancer. *Br J Cancer* 1993; **67:** 612–14.

32. Lerman C, Lustbader E, Rimer B et al. Effects of individualized breast cancer risk counselling: a randomized trial. *J Natl Cancer Inst* 1995; **87:** 286–92.

33. Vasen HFA, Beex LVAM, Cleton FJ et al. Clinical heterogeneity of hereditary breast cancer and its impact on screening protocols: the Dutch experience on 24 families under surveillance. *Eur J Cancer* 1993; **29A:** 1111–14.

34. Thirlaway K, Fallowfield L, Nunnerley, Powles T. Anxiety in women 'at risk' of developing breast cancer. *Br J Cancer* 1996; **73:** 1422–4.

35. Wong JH, Jackson CF, Swanson JS et al. Analysis of the risk reduction of prophylactic mastectomy in Sprague–Dawley rats with 7, 12-dimethylbenzanthracene-induced breast cancer. *Surgery* 1986; **99:** 67–71.

36. Pennisi VR, Capozzi A. The incidence of obscure carcinoma in subcutaneous mastectomy. Results of a national survey. *Plast Reconstr Surg* 1975; **56:** 9.

37. Khouri RK, Ahn CY, Salzhauer MA et al. Simultaneous bilateral breast reconstruction with the Transverse Rectus Abdominis Musculocutaneous free flap. *Ann Surg* 1997; **226:** 25–34.

38. Schrag D, Kuntz KM, Garber JE, Weeks JC. Decision analysis – effects of prophylactic mastectomy and oophorectomy on life expectancy among women with BRCA1 and BRCA2 mutations. *N Engl J Med* 1997; **336:** 1465–71.

39. Langlands AO, Kerr GR, Bloomer SM. Familial breast cancer. *Clin Oncol* 1976; **2:** 41–5.

40. Albano WA, Recarbaren JA, Lynch HT et al. Natural history of hereditary cancer of the breast and colon. *Cancer* 1982; **50:** 360–3.

41. Anderson DE, Badzioch MD. Survival in familial breast cancer patients. *Cancer* 1986; **58:** 360–5.

42. Ruder AM, Moodie PE, Nelson NA, Choi NW. Does family history of breast cancer improve survival among patients with breast cancer? *Am J Obstet Gynecol* 1988; **158:** 963–8.

43. Slattery MI, Berry TD, Kerber RA. Is survival among women diagnosed with breast cancer influenced by family history of breast cancer? *Epidemiology* 1993; **4:** 543–8.

44. Malone KE, Daling JR, Weiss NS et al. Family history and survival of young women with invasive breast cancer.*Cancer* 1996; **78:** 1417–25.

45. Breast Cancer Linkage Consortium. Pathology of familial breast cancer: differences between breast cancers in carriers of BRCA1 and BRCA2 mutations and sporadic cases. *Lancet* 1997; **349:** 1505–10.

46. Gayther SA, Warren W, Mazoyer S et al. Germline mutations of the BRCA1 gene in breast and ovarian cancer families provide evidence for a genotype–phenotype correlation. *Nat Genet* 1995; **11:** 429–33.

47. Sobol H, Stoppa-Lyonett D, Bressac-de-Paillerets B et al. Truncation at conserved terminal regions of BRCA1 protein is associated with highly proliferating hereditary breast cancers. *Cancer Res* 1996; **56:** 3216–19.

48. Cooper AP. *The Anatomy and Diseases of the Breast*. 1845.

49. Dupont WD, Page DL. Risk factors for breast cancer in women with proliferative breast disease. *N Engl J Med* 1985; **312:** 146–51.

50. Dupont WD, Page DL. Breast cancer risk associated with proliferative disease, age at first birth, and a family history of breast cancer. *Am J Epidemiol* 1987; **125:** 769–79.

51. Sasano N, Tateno H, Stemmermann GN. Volume and hyperplastic lesions of breasts of Japanese women living in Hawaii and Japan. *Prev Med* 1978; **7:** 196–204.

52. Bartow SA, Pathak DR, Black WC et al. Prevalence of benign, atypical and malignant breast lesions in populations at different risk for breast cancer. *Cancer* 1987; **60:** 2751–60.

53. Dupont WD, Page DL. Relative risk of breast cancer varies with time since diagnosis of atypical hyperplasia. *Hum Pathol* 1989; **20:** 723–5.

54. Tavassoli FA, Norris HJ. A comparison of the results of long-term follow-up for atypical intraductal hyperplasia and intraductal hyperplasia of the breast. *Cancer* 1990; **65:** 518–29.

55. London SJ, Connolly JL, Schnitt SJ, Colditz GA. A prospective study of benign breast disease and the risk of breast cancer. *JAMA* 1992; **267:** 941–4.

56. Haagensen CD. *Diseases of the Breast*, 3rd edn. Philadelphia: WB Saunders, 1986.

57. Bodian CA, Perzin KH, Lattes R et al. Prognostic significance of benign proliferative breast disease. *Cancer* 1993; **71:** 3896–907.

58. Dupont WD, Parl FF, Hartmann WH et al. Breast cancer risk associated with proliferative breast disease and atypical hyperplasia. *Cancer* 1993; **71:** 1258–65.

59. Ciatto S, Biggeri A, Del Turco MR et al. Risk of breast cancer subsequent to proven gross cystic disease. *Eur J Cancer* 1990; **26:** 555–7.

60. Bundred NJ, West RR, Dowd JO et al. Is there an increased risk of breast cancer in women who have had a breast cyst aspirated? *Br J Cancer* 1991; **64:** 953–5.

61. Bruzzi P, Dogliotti L, Naldoni C et al. Cohort study of risk of breast cancer with cyst type in women with gross cystic disease of the breast. *BMJ* 1997; **314:** 925–8.

62. Miller WR, Scott WN, Phil M et al. Using biological measurements, can patients with benign breast disease who are at high risk of breast cancer be identified? *Cancer Detect Prev* 1992; **16:** 13–20.

4

Presenting features

*What a book a devil's chaplain might write on the clumsy, wasteful,
blundering, low, and horribly cruel works of nature.*

Charles Darwin

Clinical history • Clinical examination • Nipple discharge • Pitfalls

As the diagnosis of breast cancer is, for many women, a living nightmare, despite improvements in treatment and prolongation of survival, new breast symptoms or signs can provoke a psychological emergency. The panic and uncertainty resulting from a delay of just a few days before being seen by a specialist does not impact on prognosis, but may change a normally composed person into a sleep-deprived petrified wretch. One of the tasks of those who work in breast clinics is to educate both general practitioners and their patients in terms of what does constitute a valid reason for consultation and referral. Each time publicity is generated on delays in diagnosis, particularly in young women, breast clinics are deluged with worried 30-year-old women, thus causing delay in assessing those older women who are more likely to have an underlying malignant cause for their symptoms.

There are protean clinical manifestations of breast cancer but the most common by far is a painless lump. The Yorkshire Breast Group reported signs and symptoms of 1205 women presenting with operable breast cancer.[1] These are summarized in Table 4.1. Over 75% of the patients had a lump and, although only 5% had pain as a presenting feature, closer questioning revealed one-third to have some pain associated with the lump either spontaneously or after palpation.

Table 4.1 Presenting symptoms in 1205 patients with operable breast cancer

Symptom	Percentage
Lump	76
Swelling	8
Pain	5
Nipple retraction	4
Paget's disease	3
Nipple bleeding/discharge/crusting	2
Skin puckering	1
Lump in axilla	1

From Yorkshire Breast Group.[1]

Reintgen et al compared the mammographic and clinical findings in 553 women diagnosed with breast cancer to examine the anatomy of missed lesions.[2] Patients were a combination of both symptomatic and screened cases, with overall, 58% of the lesions being palpable. The

Table 4.2 Relationship between patho-logical size and palpability of breast cancers

Pathological tumour size (mm)	Percentage palpable
1–5	0
6–10	19
11–15	48
16–20	82
21–25	91
26–30	83
31–35	89
36–40	90
41–45	100
46–50	100
>50	96
All	58

From Reintgen et al.[2]

relationship between the pathologically measured tumour size and palpability is shown in Table 4.2. None of the cancers with a diameter of 1–5 mm were palpable and only one in five of those measuring 6–10 mm could be felt preoperatively. It was only when the cancers measured more than 40 mm that all were palpable. Experienced clinicians were unable to detect most breast cancers until they measured over 16 mm in size.

CLINICAL HISTORY

For a clinical consultation to reach a satisfactory conclusion three criteria have to be met: taking an appropriate and sympathetic history, performing a thorough examination, and giving a comprehensible explanation to the patient. Failure to achieve any of these objectives will lead, at the very least, to an increase in anxiety and frustration on the patient's part and possi-bly to the beginning of a chain of communica-tion lapses, perhaps culminating in threats of litigation. At the very onset of the consultation, when a patient is most anxious, the manner of taking the clinical history can make or break the doctor–patient relationship. Most women attending symptomatic breast clinics will not have breast cancer but, if symptoms such as breast pain or nodularity are dismissed as inconsequential by the doctor, great patient frustration may be induced.

Breast pain, with or without nodularity, is the most common cause of general practice consul-tations on matters mammary.[3] Most of these patients are not referred to hospital because their symptoms are self-limiting but, even so, they comprise most of those attending breast clinics. In premenopausal women, cyclical endocrine changes are usually responsible for mastalgia whereas among postmenopausal cases, most breast pains are rib-cage derived. When taking a history, the location and lateral-ity of breast pain should be sought together with duration of symptoms. Severity can be difficult to assess but interference with social and sexual function may indicate a chronic problem for which treatment could be benefi-cial. It is worthwhile asking the patient if she has attended for reassurance that there was no sinister underlying cause, or because the pain was of such severity and chronicity that specific treatment was being sought.

For women who complain of a breast lump, the duration of the symptoms and method of detection should be determined together with the presence or absence of associated pain. In addition, the patient should be asked about alterations in the shape of the breasts, particu-larly the nipples, together with nipple discharge and skin changes.

Many centres ask a battery of questions such as age at menarche, or age at first full-term delivery, collected for epidemiological projects that often never materialize and have no bearing on the individual patient's breast cancer risk. If this information is going to be collected it is probably best to get patients to complete a brief questionnaire before being seen so that the clinician can concentrate on the more important aspects of the history and examination.

Core information, which may aid diagnosis, should include menopausal status, date of last menstrual period, lactation and family history. In addition, the prior history of breast operations and other serious illnesses should be sought. Although it is customary to determine the length of time for which oral contraceptives were taken, it is more important to ascertain any use of hormone replacement therapy, which can maintain a premenopausal breast structure and susceptibility in women who would be biologically postmenopausal.

CLINICAL EXAMINATION

There is no single correct method of breast examination: of utmost importance is the examiner having a systematic approach involving observation, elevation of the arms, thorough palpation of the breast tissue, and assessment of the axillae and cervical lymph nodes. Elevation of the head-end of the couch to 45° is more comfortable for older cases and avoids towering over patients. The examination room should be warm and well lit because subtle changes of skin tethering or peau d'orange may be missed in a Stygian milieu and the patient will be uncomfortable if she is cold.

The patient should be asked to identify the site of symptoms and, if complaining of a lump, the position in which it can most easily be felt. That having been done, the contralateral breast should be examined first in order that attention is not diverted by clinical signs on the affected side from clinical exclusion of bilateral breast cancer (which affects 5% of cases with malignancy). Should a lump be found its dimensions should be measured using calipers with the vertical and horizontal extent being recorded. Mobility must be determined and, if there appears to be some tethering, this should be noted in relation to both skin and underlying muscle.

The upper outer quadrant and axillary tail can best be palpated with the patient lying half

on her side towards and away from the examiner. If, in addition, the arm is placed by her side, the axilla can be examined because the suspensory ligament will have been relaxed by this procedure. If malignancy is suspected, the patient can be laid flat so that abdominal palpation can be performed, followed by an examination of the chest for localized tenderness or pleural effusion. For cases with mastalgia, other potential painful loci can be checked including ribs, costochondral junctions and vertebrae. At this time the patient can be placed into one of four diagnostic categories:

- Benign, lump-free
- Benign lump/localized nodularity
- Malignant lump
- Possibly malignant lump.

Benign, lump-free

This will comprise the largest group seen at breast clinics, many of whom had discomfort or nodularity that settled before they were seen. It was customary to carry out routine mammography on those who were aged 35 years or over and to review the patient 6 weeks later. That was before it was known which age group benefited from mammographic screening and before the expression 'one stop clinic' was coined. Now the pressure is on to get all the investigations carried out on the first visit to the clinic and discharge those deemed to be normal.

Substantial numbers of women seen at breast clinics are in their 30s and, provided that no lumps are palpable, do not require any investigations. Such patents can be reassured and told that that they do not have to be seen again unless a new problem occurs. There is no value to using breast ultrasonography as a so-called screening test for breast cancer in young women: this investigation is sometimes being used as a palliative procedure under circumstances where a reasonable explanation and reassurance would have been more effective.

It is women aged under 35 with equivocal changes of localized nodularity who pose a greater problem. Neither mammography nor ultrasonography is useful and this is a situation in which fine needle aspiration cytology (FNAC) will be of value. When the cytologist is prepared to provide an instant report, the patient can be reassured and discharged if this is C2. More problematic is the acellular report (C1) but this may also be regarded as normal if the lesion is suspected to be fatty, and fat cells rather than epithelial cells are seen. Should there be an unexpected report of atypical (C3), severely atypical (C4) or malignant (C5) cells, the clinician is faced with a dilemma. How much should the patient be told at her first visit? It has to be remembered that cytologists will sometimes revise their diagnosis upon reflection and so it may be better to tell the patient that the result is uncertain and arrange to see her again with the final cytology report.

Which patients with no abnormal physical signs should have mammograms? There is no simple answer to this. Most centres order mammograms in women over 35 or 40 but it can be argued that the lower age limit could be 50. Women over 50 should be encouraged to participate in screening programmes and not subjected to extra mammography. Women over 65 are not invited for screening and because they comprise the age group from which 50% of cancers are derived, they should have mammography when attending breast clinics with symptoms such as breast pain arising from the rib cage.

Benign lump

Fibroadenoma is the most common cause for a mobile lump in women aged under 30 years. This is a diagnosis usually suspected on clinical grounds but which must be confirmed either cytologically or histologically. Although there has been a trend towards conservative management of such lesions, it is essential these patients should be properly investigated: disaster may follow delayed diagnosis of a cancer thought to be a fibroadenoma. Every time this happens the will is weakened to adopt a non-

operative stance towards these lesions. As paradoxically, it is the smaller (<5 mm) lumps that are the more likely to be misdiagnosed and inadequately sampled, it could be argued that these should all be removed (in the luteal phase of the cycle).

If the patient wishes to have the lump removed, there is no point in carrying out FNAC or ultrasonography. These should be reserved for women who wish to avoid surgery for a putative fibroadenoma. If both FNAC and ultrasonography are indicative of fibroadenoma, a watch and wait policy can be adopted but, as a few of these lesions will still prove to be malignant, patients should be followed for at least a year. Even with a conservative approach, about 50% of younger patients with breast lumps will have these excised.[4]

Breast cysts are unusual in women aged under 30, unless they are lactating, in which case a suddenly appearing lump may be a galactocele. The diagnosis and treatment are by aspiration and, provided that this yields milk, with resolution of the lump, no further treatment is necessary. Cystic disease of the breasts is more common in women aged 35–50, an age at more risk of breast cancer, so it is important that certain precautions are taken when dealing with suspected cysts. After the dimensions of the cyst(s) have been measured, aspiration is performed. If non-blood-stained fluid is obtained, and the lump disappears, the diagnosis has been made. When there is either blood in the aspirate or a residual lump, fluid should be sent for cytology.

It is for these reasons that cyst fluid aspiration should not be undertaken by general practitioners, because there may be haematoma formation after failed aspiration which will change the dimensions of the lump and alter other clinical signs. Aspiration should be carried out by the person who will be responsible for further treatment, should the lump prove to be non-cystic. Any benefit from avoidance of a hospital appointment will be offset by the potential for upstaging and therefore possibly over-treating a breast cancer that was originally thought to be a cyst.

Table 4.3 Confirmation of the diagnosis of cancer in relation to menstrual status and tumour stage

Tumour stage	Premenopausal	Postmenopausal
Operable ≤ 4 cm	Luteal wide excision	FNAC + core biopsy
Operable > 4 cm	Luteal core biopsy	FNAC + core biopsy
Inoperable	Core biopsy	FNAC + core biopsy

Malignant lump

Clinical suspicion that a lump is malignant will be suggested by a hard irregular contour, evidence of tethering to superficial or deep structures, or skin infiltration and peau d'orange. Unilateral nipple inversion with an associated lump is suspicious although inflammatory lesions can produce similar physical signs. At this time the patient should be told that the findings are suspicious and may be caused by cancer, but that investigations will be necessary to confirm the diagnosis. It is probably best that bilateral mammograms are taken immediately, before any other invasive tests, and thus before the breast architecture has been disturbed by iatrogenic intervention.

Once breast radiographs have been taken, further investigations will depend upon the patient's menopausal status and tumour stage. Final treatment decisions will depend upon confirmation that the lump is an invasive carcinoma and the simplest way in which this can be achieved is a core biopsy using Tru-Cut or Biopty-Cut needle.[5,6] Using a combination of core biopsy and FNAC, a diagnosis of malignancy can be made in up to 90% of breast cancers, so that in most cases a single stage operation can be performed.

If the patient is premenopausal, a luteal phase wide excision biopsy may be the safest method of making the diagnosis, as discussed in Chapter 7. The situation is complicated in premenopausal women with larger primaries in

whom first-line chemotherapy might be required in order to perform breast-conserving surgery. For these cases a luteal phase core biopsy provides an opportunity to make the diagnosis, while leaving assessable tumour in order that response to chemotherapy can be monitored. It could be argued that the systemic therapy might be able to destroy tumour microemboli shed by the trauma of core biopsy, but this remains contentious.

For premenopausal patients with inoperable disease, timing of biopsy is unlikely to alter the already dire prognosis and so either FNAC or core biopsy should be performed, with measurement of oestrogen receptor/progesterone receptor (ER/PR), which enables selection of either endocrine or cytotoxic palliative therapy. Table 4.3 gives suggestions for diagnosis of malignancy in both premenopausal and postmenopausal cases and, in the latter group, whenever possible a combination of FNAC and core biopsy should be used. If neither modality confirms the diagnosis of malignancy, an open biopsy is mandatory, which may of course place a constraint on subsequent treatment options.

Possibly malignant lump

Even the most experienced surgeons may sometimes have difficulty determining whether an area of localized nodularity is benign or malignant. Both FNAC and mammography may be of help. The latter may show trabecular

Table 4.4 Histopathology in 284 microdochectomy operations

Histology	No. (%)	Hb-positive	Hb-negative
Intraduct papilloma	126 (44)	107 (85)	19 (15)
Duct ectasia	92 (32)	67 (73)	25 (27)
Cystic disease	28 (10)	13 (46)	15 (54)
No abnormality	22 (8)	12 (55)	10 (45)
Carcinoma	16 (6)	16 (100)	0

From Chaudary et al.[7]

distortion or localized irregular microcalcification. In the absence of these changes and with an unequivocally normal C2 cytology report, it is unlikely that malignancy is being missed. A few patients with invasive lobular cancers will have so few malignant cells in Indian file pattern that these are difficult to sample cytologically and undetectable radiologically, while giving rise to minimal clinical signs.

If there is doubt on clinical grounds and there is little help from standard investigations, the patient may be best served by a surgical biopsy which will end the period of uncertainty so that she can either be reassured or the appropriate treatment for breast cancer can be started. Although every surgeon is trying to reduce the number of unnecessary (benign) biopsies, each one results in a reassured patient and those that confirm malignancy have led to an earlier diagnosis.

NIPPLE DISCHARGE

For the patient, a blood-stained nipple discharge is a serious problem, which she may fear is a manifestation of cancer. Luckily most nipple discharges are not caused by underlying malignancy. When a patient has a palpable lump and a discharge, almost invariably determining the nature of the lump explains the discharge and the diagnosis can be made by FNAC or excision biopsy.

In the absence of a lump, the most important first-line investigation is testing the discharge for haemoglobin, using standard urine-testing sticks. If no haemoglobin is present, surgical intervention is almost never necessary. Milky discharge usually results from incomplete involution after lactation and extensive investigation is not needed in women with a regular cycle because hyperprolactinaemia from a prolactinoma usually leads to galactorrhoea with irregular periods. Only under the latter circumstances is it necessary to measure serum prolactin and image the pituitary fossa.

After lactation, the most common cause of nipple discharge is duct ectasia, in which normal breast secretions lie stagnant within dilated ducts and discharge either spontaneously or during washing. Typically, several ducts are involved and the disease is often bilateral, with discharge varying in colour from pale straw through to blue/brown. Although all the discharge in duct ectasia may contain no haemoglobin, sometimes there is one duct containing Hb-positive material. Irrespective of the colour, if Hb-positive discharge emanates from one duct, patients at Guy's Hospital are advised to undergo microdochectomy. The histological findings in relation to discharge haemoglobin content in a series of 284 microdochectomies are summarized in Table 4.4.[7] Carcinoma was responsible for only 6% of the nipple discharges with 50% being ductal carcinoma in situ (DCIS) and 50% invasive. All the cancers had Hb-positive discharge compared with 85% of those caused by intraduct papilloma and 73% of those with duct ectasia. Microdochectomy specifically removes the affected duct, stops the discharge and reveals the underlying pathology, which in most cases is benign.

PITFALLS

Missed breast cancers represent a tragedy for the patient and a rebuke to the surgeon, possibly followed by expensive litigation. Although in some cases the cancer was undiagnosable at the time of presentation, for a few there is evidence that vital clinical clues were missed, or the diagnosis of benignity was based on inadequate investigation. As the major risk factor for cancer is age, clinical suspicion may be diminished when assessing younger women, a few of whom will have malignancy, probably presenting as either an apparently benign lump or a seemingly benign area of nodularity. Hence it is essential to obtain at least a cytological diagnosis of a discrete lesion in a young woman.

Surgeons such as Sir Hedley Atkins believed that no woman should be allowed to retain a breast lump and so every probable fibroadenoma was excised. Things have changed in the brave new world of breast surgery. The advent of FNAC, and budgetary pressure to avoid removal of benign tissue, have led to more lumps being retained, some of which will be malignant. If the patient is adamant that she does not wish to have a lump removed, and these are relatively few (having been appraised of the facts), there must be unequivocal proof that the lump is benign. This should comprise, at very least, a C2 cytology, and better still a core biopsy showing typical fibroadenoma histology. Failure to obtain cytology or to repeat an acellular smear could be construed as negligence should the lump subsequently prove to be a cancer.

Younger women are more likely to have poorly differentiated cancers and these, together with invasive lobular carcinomas, may give rise to localized nodularity rather than a discrete lump. For this reason, FNAC should be carried out even when mammography or ultrasonography show no apparent abnormality. Clinical distinction between diffuse malignancy and nodularity may be impossible, whereas cyclical changes such as swelling and discomfort do not automatically rule out malignancy.

One of the most satisfying conclusions for a clinical consultation is the successful drainage of a breast cyst. Routine cytological examination of cyst fluid is redundant, provided that it is not blood-stained and the lump has completely resolved. Such patients are usually seen a few weeks later to ensure that recurrence of the cyst has not occurred. In a series of 400 patients with cysts treated at Guy's Hospital and seen again 6 weeks later, there was a lump at the site of cyst aspiration in 64 (16%).[8] In addition, there was a new cyst at another site in 22 (5%). Of the residual lumps complete aspiration was possible in 44 (69%) and, of the 20 (31%) with a residual mass after second aspiration, all had a biopsy with two being found to have invasive cancers.

Patients who develop recurrent breast cysts do carry an increased risk of breast cancer which means that they should be told to return if new lumps develop and not to assume that a new lump is cystic. It is incumbent upon the surgeon to aspirate these lumps, including the smaller ones and, if no fluid is obtained, to send cells for cytology. Dismissing a discrete lump as being a cyst without aspirational or ultrasonic confirmation is an unacceptably high-risk activity.

SYNOPSIS

- Most breast cancers present as a lump but this may be associated with pain in up to one-third of cases.
- To convince women that they do not have

a serious breast condition, it is necessary to take a sympathetic history, perform a thorough examination and give a comprehensible explanation of the situation.

• If possible women without lumps, or with minimal nodularity, should be assessed and have appropriate investigations without a need to return for follow-up.

• Discrete lumps or localized nodularity should not be regarded as benign unless there is unequivocal cytological or histological evidence.

• Patients with a haemoglobin-containing breast discharge need a microdochectomy to determine the underlying diagnosis which will usually be benign.

REFERENCES

1. The Yorkshire Breast Group. Symptoms and signs of operable breast cancer 1976–1981. *Br J Surg* 1983; **70:** 350–1.
2. Reintgen D, Berman C, Cox C et al. The anatomy of missed breast cancers. *Surg Oncol* 1993; **2:** 65–75.
3. Nichols S, Waters WE, Wheeler MJ. Management of female breast disease by Southampton General Practitioners. *BMJ* 1980; **281:** 1450–3.
4. Cant PJ, Madden MV, Close PM et al. Case for conservative management of selected fibroadenomas of the breast. *Br J Surg* 1987; **74:** 857–9.
5. Fentiman IS, Millis RR, Hayward JL. Value of needle biopsy in outpatient management of breast cancer. *Arch Surg* 1980; **115:** 652–4.
6. Barretto V, Hamed H, Griffiths AB et al. Automatic needle biopsy in the diagnosis of early breast cancer. *Eur J Surg Oncol* 1991; **17:** 237–9.
7. Chaudary MA, Millis RR, Davies GC et al. Nipple discharge. The diagnostic value of testing for occult blood. *Ann Surg* 1982; **196:** 651–5.
8. Hamed H, Cody A, Chaudary MA et al. Follow-up of patients with aspirated breast cysts. Is it necessary? *Arch Surg* 1989; **124:** 253–5.

5

Making the diagnosis

To observations which ourselves we make,
We grow more partial for th' Observer's sake.

Alexander Pope

Mammography • Ultrasonography • Fine needle aspiration cytology • Needle biopsy • Comparative studies • Automated core biopsy

Most patients with breast problems who are sent for specialist opinion will not have breast cancer, although many will be in great fear that their symptoms are the result of malignancy. Often, after a careful clinical evaluation has not revealed any abnormality, the only requirement is to explain and reassure the patient, without recourse to any investigation. At the other extreme are women with classic signs of cancer such as a hard tethered lump, in whom the diagnosis is obvious to even the least experienced. Although there is a necessity to obtain histological or cytological confirmation before proceeding to definitive treatment, there is little uncertainty and the patient can be told immediately that she has a suspicious breast lump.

More problematic are those women with less definite signs such as coarse nodularity or localized nodularity at the borderline between lump and lumpiness. It is under these circumstances that triple assessment (clinical evaluation, cytology/core biopsy and breast imaging) is essential to avoid missing breast cancers that can lead to potentially severe consequences for both patient and doctor. Triple assessment is also mandatory in women with clinically benign lumps, if these are to be managed conservatively.

MAMMOGRAPHY

X-rays were first used to image the breasts by Warren who reported the results of sagittal views of 100 breast cancer cases in 1930.[1] The particular radiological signs which he described were scarring and irregularity of the tissue around the tumours, some of which were so advanced that direct pleural infiltration could be seen. With palpable tumours and a relatively high radiation dosage the sensitivity of the technique was 75% and the specificity 100%.

The typical appearance of a spiculated density was first described by Leborgne in a monograph entitled *The Breast in Roentgen Diagnosis*.[2] In addition, he indicated the diagnostic value of microcalcifications on films: 'calcifications in carcinoma are generally tiny, dot-like or somewhat elongated, innumerable and irregularly grouped very close together in an area of the breast, resembling a powdering of fine grains of salt.' This pattern of microcalcification was present in 30% of the breast cancers that he imaged.

Mammography moved from being an experimental technique into mainstream radiology largely as a result of the work of Egan.[3] In a series of 1000 cases, a sensitivity of 97% was

Table 5.1 Sensitivity of mammography in women with palpable breast lumps in relation to age

Age ≤ 50		Age > 50		Reference
Number	**Sensitivity (%)**	**Number**	**Sensitivity (%)**	
154	70	366	83	Elegy and Urban[4]
157	78	185	92	Young and Sadowsky[5]
139	56	360	87	Eideken[6]

achieved, indicating the potential value of mammography both in the assessment of breast lesions and for screening asymptomatic women. The major radiological features suggestive of malignancy are an irregular opacity associated with trabecular distortion and associated irregular microcalcification. Such signs are typical of ductal carcinomas as a result of stromal invasion inducing a fibrous reaction and because of the intraductal necrosis and calcification of malignant cells. For some patients with infiltrating lobular carcinomas, the mammographic changes may be more subtle or even non-existent are a result of the single file pattern of infiltration which may be undetectable mammographically or manifest as minor asymmetry.

Hence some palpable breast lumps may not be detected mammographically. Three series that reported sensitivity of mammography in relation to age (≤ 50 and > 50) in women with palpable breast lumps are summarized in Table 5.1.[4-6] For women aged over 50 years the mean sensitivity was 87% and this fell to 68% in those aged 50 or younger. Even after optimal mammography up to one-third of cancers will be missed in those aged 50 or younger and 10% of malignancies in those over 50 years. This underlines the fact that a woman with a palpable lump and a normal mammogram needs experienced evaluation and not false reassurance.

To maximize the value of mammography and enhance the radiologist's interpretation it is essential that high quality films are taken. Eklund et al stressed the need for taking a good clinical history and a team approach to management of breast problems and also summarized the important radiological factors for quality assurance.[7] These comprised: visualizing the area of interest, optimal breast tissue inclusion, adequate exposure, high contrast, high resolution, proper compression and freedom from artefacts. In addition, correct labelling and optimal viewing conditions are needed to achieve consistently good results.

Optimal inclusion

If there is doubt as to whether the clinical abnormality has been included in the films, a small radio-opaque skin marker should be placed over the palpable abnormality so that, if necessary, extended views can be taken. Should it not be possible to include the site of the abnormality, ultrasound may need to be considered. To ensure that almost all the breast tissue has been included on the mediolateral oblique (MLO) view, there should be pectoralis major fibres visible at the nipple level, and the inframammary fold should be included in the image. The axillary tail should be seen over the pectoral muscle and retromammary fat should be visible, with the anterior margin of the pectoral muscle showing a convex margin. For a complete craniocaudal (CC) view, both the lateral and medial breast tissue should be included and retromammary fat should be seen. If the inframammary fold has been elevated, there will be pectoral muscle at the margin of the film.

Adequate exposure

The aim of mammography, particularly in women with dense glandular tissue, is to achieve sufficient penetration so that fibrous strands and vasculature can be distinguished from the breast parenchyma. Underexposure will increase the risk of missing relatively non-contrasting lesions. This is better achieved by a slightly higher radiation exposure because prolongation of exposure time may increase the risk of blurring as a result of involuntary movement.

High contrast

To improve the contrast between glandular tissue, fibrous bands fat and microcalcifications, extended processing can be used to achieve optimal image development. Additionally, scatter of X-rays can be minimized by reducing as far as possible the kilovolt peak setting, so that the image is as sharp as possible. Use of a grid can sharpen the image but with an increased radiation exposure. Despite this, Eklund et al have argued that the risk to the patient of an increased radiation dose is more than offset by the benefit of not missing a cancer.[7]

Breast compression

The aim of breast compression is to reduce the amount of overlap of glandular and fibrous tissue and minimize the crowding of structures on the film. Although greater compression will improve the clarity of the films and reduce the chance of cancers being missed in dense breasts, there must be a balance so that the procedure is not too painful. An unpleasant experience during screening mammography might lead to

rejection of subsequent invitations. To investigate this problem, Bennett et al conducted a questionnaire survey of 1000 women attending a screening centre at the Royal Women's Hospital in Brisbane, Australia.[8] Mammography was reported as being comfortable or non-painful by 64% and uncomfortable in 35%. Only 1% found the procedure very uncomfortable with 0.2% saying that the pain was intolerable. This suggests that, when mammography is carried out by experienced radiographers, the compression is acceptable to 99% of screened women.

Reducing false-positive cases

When the radiologist reports trabecular distortion or localized microcalcification, this is usually accompanied by the suggestion that a biopsy should be performed. As a result some will undergo an operation after which a benign diagnosis is made (false-positive). The ratio of benign/malignant biopsies has been reported as being as high as 4:1 in the USA,[9,10] although in the UK screening programme this has now fallen to 0.3:1.[11]

As mammography had not been shown to reduce mortality in screened women aged under 50 years, Kerlikowske et al examined the positive predictive value (PPV) of biopsied radiographic lesions in women aged 40–49 and 50 or over.[12] They found an apparent sudden jump in PPV at age 50 and this prompted Kopans et al to examine PPV and age in 4778 women who had a biopsy for a mammographic abnormality at Massachusetts General Hospital.[13] In this large series there was a gradual increase in PPV from 12% at age 40 rising to 46% at age 79.

To try and improve the positive predictive value of mammography, Lo et al used an artificial neural network (ANN) based on mammographic findings and patient age.[14] Nine input features were used in a three-layer, back-propagation, feed-forward ANN. These included distribution, number and type of calcifications, mass size, margin, shape, density and associated findings, and special features.

Table 5.2 Sensitivity and specificity of ultrasonography in patients with palpable breast lumps

No. of patients	No. of cancers	Sensitivity (%)	Specificity (%)	Reference
235	120	83	93	Jellins et al[15]
268	97	90	94	Schmidt et al[16]
77	31	68	93	Egan and Egan[17]
148	45	87	90	Hayashi et al[18]
223	166	93	74	Warwick et al[19]
400	174	97	94	Perre et al[20]
		86	**90**	**Total**

Mammograms from 254 patients who underwent biopsy were reviewed by radiologists who had been blinded to the pathological findings. Of the biopsies, 96 confirmed malignancy and the network was able to distinguish between ductal carcinoma in situ (DCIS) and invasive cancers. All 28 DCIS cases were correctly identified (specificity 100%) and 48 of 61 invasive cancers were diagnosed appropriately (sensitivity 70%). This might provide a useful non-invasive technique for planning surgery in women with mammographic lesions and might avoid the need for stereotactic needle biopsy. In addition, use of ANN might help to improve the PPV in younger women with radiographic abnormalities.

ULTRASONOGRAPHY

Most clinicians who manage breast problems acquire some skills in the interpretation of breast radiographs but relatively few achieve the same competence with ultrasonography, unless they are regularly carrying out sonographic examinations themselves. Ultrasonography is above all an investigation that is dependent on operator skill and on being present when the imaging is performed. There is no problem identifying a cyst on a hard copy of an ultrasonography but the subtleties of echo pattern within a small lesion may be lost on the casual observer.

One of the major roles for ultrasonography is distinction between solid or cystic lesions, particularly those that are impalpable. A cyst may be diagnosed with confidence when there is sonographic evidence of smooth contour, a well-defined posterior wall, and absent internal echoes other than anterior sound reverberations. Such lesions can be left without further cytological or surgical investigation. Another useful role is the assessment of putative fibroadenomas when the patient would prefer not to have an excision biopsy. When ultrasonography shows a mass lesion with displacement of breast architecture and well-defined internal echoes and borders, it is likely that the lump is a fibroadenoma. Notwithstanding this, cytological confirmation is mandatory because some breast cancers may mimic fibroadenomas both clinically and sonographically.

Several ultrasonic features have been described as being diagnostic of malignancy.

- Irregularity of margins
- Heterogeneous internal echoes
- Disruption of normal tissue planes
- Ultrasonic shadowing
- Depth/width ratio > 1
- Increased echoes in superficial layer.

Table 5.3 Results of FNAC when specimen was taken by a clinician

Number	Cancers (%)	Sensitivity (%)	Specificity (%)	Reference
3545	10	89	83	Kline et al[22]
861	32	77	85	Strawbridge et al[23]
1183	43	65	96	Azzarelli et al[24]
683	46	83	96	Dixon et al[25]
1731	91	83	83	Eisenberg et al[26]
1283	54	83	93	Barrows et al[27]
9286	**46**	**80**	**89**	**Total**

All or none of these features may be present in association with a palpable lump so that ultrasonography should be regarded as a complementary investigation and not used in the exclusion of malignancy. Results of ultrasonic investigation of palpable breast lumps in five series are given in Table 5.2.[15–20] Overall, the sensitivity was 86% and the specificity 90%. In other words, almost one in five breast cancers will not have ultrasonic features of malignancy and one in ten of lesions that appear malignant on ultrasonography will prove to be benign on histological examination.

In experienced hands ultrasonography can be a very useful adjunct to mammography, even with small tumours. Hirst reviewed 137 hard copies of ultrasonic examinations from women with breast cancers which pathologically measured 10 mm or less.[21] Of the cases two-thirds were symptomatic. At least one feature of malignancy was noted in 129 (94%). The most common abnormalities were irregular margins and heterogeneous internal echoes. Hence, under these circumstances, ultrasonography can be a useful tool in terms of indicating the need for further cytological or histological characterization of a small or impalpable breast lesion. If the intention is to demonstrate that a palpable lump is benign, a normal sonographic report cannot be taken as absolute confirmation.

FINE NEEDLE ASPIRATION CYTOLOGY

Fine needle aspiration cytology (FNAC) is the most widely used technique for making a preoperative diagnosis of breast cancer and as such it is important that the limitations of the methodology are clearly understood. Failure to take other factors into account may lead to the late diagnosis of breast cancer, occasional misdiagnosis of benign lesions as malignant and overtreatment of women with non-invasive disease. Optimal results will be achieved by those who are experienced in aspiration, providing fully trained cytologists with adequate specimens.

The results of the larger series (>500 cases), in which the FNAC samples were taken by clinicians, are summarized in Table 5.3.[22-27] This shows that the average sensitivity of FNAC was 80%, when taking as a positive report either a malignant (C5) or probable malignant (C4) result. The mean specificity was 89%, but a false-positive diagnosis of malignancy was made in 8 of 5904 (0.1%). Overall, there were insufficient cells for diagnosis (C1) in 18% of samples taken by clinicians.

Table 5.4 summarizes some of the larger series of FNAC results in which the specimens were taken by cytopathologists, rather than clinicians.[28-32] The sensitivity rose from 80% to

Table 5.4 Results of FNAC when specimen was taken by a cytopathologist

Number	Cancers (%)	Sensitivity (%)	Specificity (%)	Reference
2077	51	92	93	Linsk et al[28]
2670	64	92	94	Zajdela et al[29]
1145	22	83	84	Bell et al[30]
594	26	87	87	Smith et al[31]
670	73	96	95	Palombini et al[32]
7156	**47**	**90**	**91**	**Total**

90%, but there was little increase in specificity (91% vs 89%). There were 4 of 3626 (0.1%) false-positive results. When FNAC was performed by cytologists, only 12% of the specimens were inadequate as compared with 18% of those taken by clinicians ($\chi^2 = 66.1$, $p < 0.00001$). This underlines the need for experience in taking FNAC specimens, in order to minimize the percentage of inadequate samples. An additional advantage of a cytopathologist taking FNAC specimens is the opportunity to check the aspirate immediately to determine whether cells are present in sufficient numbers and, if not, to repeat the procedure.

Not only can FNAC be used to make a diagnosis of malignancy but also cytological grading can be performed which correlates well with histological grade.[33] Robinson et al devised a cytological grading system based on cell dissociation, size, uniformity, nucleolar morphology, nuclear margin and chromatin pattern.[34] Using these criteria three grades were established, and applied to cytology from 377 invasive cancers. The cytological grade was compared with the grade of the excised tumour as determined by the Elston modification of Bloom and Richardson's classification.[35]

The results are given in Table 5.5, which shows that, although there was a statistically significant correlation between the two grading systems, nevertheless precision was lost on

Table 5.5 Comparison of cytological and histological grade of invasive cancers

Cytological grade	Histological grade*		
	I	II	III
1	59 (64)	34 (28)	3 (4)
2	28 (30)	65 (54)	30 (43)
3	5 (6)	21 (18)	36 (53)

* Numbers in parentheses are percentages.
From Robinson et al.[34]

cytological grading. Thus, of those tumours graded cytologically as 1, only 64% proved to be histologically grade I. Likewise only 53% of cytologically grade 3 specimens were derived from histologically grade III cancers. If treatment is going to be based on a preoperative grading, it may be better if this is derived from a core biopsy rather than a cytological specimen.

It can sometimes be useful to measure the oestrogen and progesterone receptor status (ER/PR) of the tumour if first-line systemic treatment is being considered. In studies in which the cytological ER has been measured immunocytochemically and compared with that of the excised tumour, the mean sensitivity was 95% and the specificity 87%.[36–39] Thus cases suitable for endocrine therapy can be fairly accurately identified by ER/PR status of a cytological aspirate. To try and improve the predictive power of cytological ER assessment, Horsfall et al applied automated image analysis to nuclei in cytological specimens from 35 patients with breast cancer.[40] Cells were stained with an ERICA kit and then scanned with an image analysis system to determine the staining pattern of at least 250 nuclei. When these results were compared with the final ER results on histological specimens, the sensitivity was 91% and the specificity 100%. More widespread use of imaging technology might improve the predictive power of ER estimations on cytological specimens.

A further problem with FNAC is the potential distortion on subsequent mammograms. To assess the magnitude of this effect, Horobin et al compared mammograms taken before FNAC and also within 5 days of the procedure.[41] There were 52 patients in the study and all mammograms were reviewed blindly by one radiologist. A difference between the two sets of radiographs was found in 10 (19%). In six cases there was a reduction in size or disappearance of a density as a result of aspiration of a cyst. In four patients there was an increase in density in the post-aspiration films as a result of haemorrhage from the procedure. This could result in an overestimate of the size of a tumour, or obscure a small carcinoma. Whenever possible, mammography should be performed before any invasive procedures are conducted.

NEEDLE BIOPSY

Even after a C5 cytology has been reported, in many cases this will not have sufficiently characterized the cancer so that a treatment plan can be discussed with the patient when she is told that her breast lump is malignant. In the absence of clinical signs of infiltration, such as skin tethering or nipple retraction the possibility exists that the lesion is DCIS. An additional complication is that some non-invasive cancers will induce a fibrotic reaction with skin tethering to the lump. As there are different options for invasive cancer and DCIS, it is better to obtain a histological diagnosis when the patient is first seen in the clinic.

This is the rationale for core needle biopsy, originally performed using the Tru-Cut needle under local anaesthesia. Series reporting sensitivity and specificity are summarized in Table 5.6.[42–49] The mean sensitivity was 83% and the

Table 5.6 Results of core needle biopsy in women with breast lumps				
No. of cases	No. cancers (%)	Sensitivity (%)	Specificity (%)	Reference
102	87 (85)	74	100	Roberts et al[42]
368	278 (76)	73	100	Elston et al[43]
151	135 (89)	79	100	Fentiman et al[44]
162	103 (64)	75	100	Gonzalez et al[45]
194	170 (88)	89	96	Bradbeer[46]
151	112 (74)	88	100	Minkowitz et al[47]
140	130 (93)	95	100	Baildam et al[48]
145	126 (87)	90	100	Vega et al[49]
		83	**100**	**Mean**

Table 5.7 Comparison of fine needle aspiration and Tru-Cut core biopsy in the diagnosis of palpable breast lumps

Number	Cancers (%)	FNAC Sensitivity (%)	Specificity (%)	Tru-Cut Sensitivity	Specificity	Reference
131	73	52	96	74	100	Davies et al[51]
81	62	92	100	68	100	Shabot et al[52]
56	100	52	100	70	100	Sadler et al[53]
103	69	80	97	84	100	Scoupa et al[54]
	Average	**69**	**98**	**74**	**100**	

specificity 100%. The only series in which false-positive diagnoses of malignancy were reported used a combination of Tru-Cut and frozen section.[46] Causes of false-negative Tru-Cut results include highly fibrotic tumours, crush artefact rendering pathological interpretation impossible and operator inexperience. Once competence with the technique has been achieved, it is acceptable to both the surgeon and patient.[44] Not only can a histological diagnosis be obtained preoperatively but also ER/PR status and flow cytometry can be performed on Tru-Cut specimens.[50]

COMPARATIVE STUDIES

Various studies have directly compared FNAC and Tru-Cut in patients with palpable breast lumps and these are outlined in Table 5.7.[51–54] Davies et al reported that both the sensitivity and specificity were significantly better when Tru-Cut was used.[51] Of the benign cases, five were originally regarded as malignant on cytological examination. Shabot et al came to a contrary conclusion.[52] In a relatively small study of 50 malignant and 31 benign lesions, the sensitivity of FNAC was 92% whereas that of Tru-Cut was only 68%. Three separate FNAC specimens were taken from each patient and

passed through a millipore filter to entrap epithelial cells, and these additional steps may have led to the very high sensitivity of FNAC in this study.

Sadler et al compared the results of Tru-Cut and FNAC in 56 patients with infiltrating lobular carcinomas and showed that core biopsy was a better method of making the correct diagnosis preoperatively (sensitivity 70% versus 52%).[53] In the study of Scoupa et al the sensitivity of FNAC was only marginally lower than that of Tru-Cut but three suspicious FNAC reports were issued concerning lumps which subsequently proved to be benign.[54] Overall, these comparative studies demonstrated a slightly better sensitivity and specificity for Tru-Cut biopsy. In an attempt to obtain the best quality core biopsies, with minimal crush artefact, automated systems have been developed in order that the instrument may be operated with one hand, leaving the other free to either fix the tumour or alternatively to hold an ultrasonic probe for localization of impalpable lesions.

AUTOMATED CORE BIOPSY

In a pilot study at Guy's Hospital, 107 patients with palpable breast lumps had a core biopsy

Table 5.8 Results of randomized trials comparing Bioptycut needle gauges and Tru-Cut biopsy

Number	Tru-Cut		Bioptycut 14 G		Bioptycut 18 G		Reference
	Sensitivity (%)	Specificity (%)	Sensitivity (%)	Specificity (%)	Sensitivity (%)	Specificity (%)	
151	68	100	88	100	96	100	McMahon et al[57]
122	–	–	98	100	93	100	Hamed et al[58]

performed using the Bioptycut system.[55] Of these lumps 90% proved to be malignant where the sensitivity of Bioptycut was 65% and the specificity 100%. This study demonstrated the learning curve associated with the technique. Dividing the cases into four equal groups sequentially, for the first quarter the sensitivity was 50%, for the next 63%, for the third quarter 63% and for the final quarter 83%. In another study from Gras, Austria, 109 patients with breast lumps had a core taken using the BIP High Speed Multi 22 system.[56] Of the lumps, 74% were malignant: the sensitivity of the technique was 99% and the specificity 100%.

Different gauges of Bioptycut needles are available and two trials have compared the results using 14 and 18 gauge needles.[57,58] In the first study, conducted at Galloway Royal Infirmary, Scotland, 151 patients with palpable breast lumps were randomized to one of three core biopsy methods: Tru-Cut (14 gauge), Bioptycut (14 G) or Bioptycut (18 G).[57] Results are shown in Table 5.8. Bioptycut samples were substantially better than those produced by Tru-Cut with an inadequate sample in 22% of the Tru-Cut biopsies compared with 4% of the Bioptycut 18 G and none of the Bioptycut 14 G samples. Pain scores were measured immediately after the biopsy and Tru-Cut was more painful than Bioptycut 18 G and marginally more so than Bioptycut 14 G.

In the Guy's Hospital trial there was a comparison of 14 G and 18 G Bioptycut.[58] The 14 G needle proved to have a sensitivity of 98% against 93% for 18 G. Taking the results of these two trials, Bioptycut 14 G should be used for preoperative diagnosis because, in experienced hands, this can achieve histological confirmation in almost all patients with palpable breast cancers. However, it should be stressed that experience with the system is necessary before these very good results can be attained routinely.

SYNOPSIS

• Even with optimal mammography up to 40% of cancers will be missed in women aged less than 50 and up to 15% in those over 50 years.

• In patients with palpable lumps, ultra-sonography has a sensitivity of 86% and a specificity of 90%.

• If taken by experienced clinicians, fine needle aspiration cytology has a sensitivity and specificity of 90%.

• Core needle biopsy has a sensitivity of 83% which rises to over 90% when an automated system is used.

REFERENCES

1. Warren SL. A roentgenologic study of the breast. *Am J Roentgenol Rad Ther* 1930; **24:** 113–24.

2. Leborgne RA. *The Breast in Roentgen Diagnosis.* Montevideo: Impresora Uraguaya, 1953.

3. Egan RL. Experience with mammography in a tumour institute. Evaluation of 1000 studies. *Radiology* 1960; **75:** 894–900.

4. Elegy RA, Urban DU. Mammography in symptomatic women 50 years of age or under, and those over 50. *Cancer* 1979; **43:** 878–82.

5. Young JO, Sadowsky NL, Young JW, Herman L. Mammography of women with suspicious breast lumps. *Arch Surg* 1986; **121:** 807–9.

6. Eideken S. Mammography and palpable cancer of the breast. *Cancer* 1988; **61:** 263–5.

7. Eklund GW, Cardenoss G, Parsons W. Assessing adequacy of mammographic image quality. *Radiology* 1994; **190:** 297–307.

8. Bennett IC, Robert DA, Osborne JM, Baker CA. Discomfort during mammography: a survey of women attending a breast screening center. *Breast Dis* 1994; **7:** 35–41.

9. Kopans D. The positive predictive value of mammography. *AJR* 1992; **158:** 521–6.

10. Knutzen AM, Gisvold JJ. Likelihood of malignant disease for various categories of mammographically detected, nonpalpable breast lesions. *Mayo Clin Proc* 1993; **68:** 454–60.

11. NHS Breast Screening Programme. *NHS Breast Screening Review 1995.*

12. Kerlikowske K, Grady D, Barclay J et al. Positive predictive value of screening mammography by age and family history of breast cancer. *JAMA* 1993; **270:** 2444–50.

13. Kopans DB, Moore RH, McCarthy KA et al. Positive predictive value of breast biopsy as a result of mammography: there is no abrupt change at age 50 years. *Radiology* 1996; **200:** 357–60.

14. Lo JY, Baker JA, Kornguth PJ et al. Predicting breast cancer invasion with artificial neural networks on the basis of mammographic findings. *Radiology* 1997; **203:** 159–63.

15. Jellins J, Reeve TS, Croll J et al. Results of breast echographic examinations in Sydney, Australia 1972–1979. *Semin Ultrasound* 1982; **3:** 58–62.

16. Schmidt W, van Kaick G, Muller A et al. Ultrasonic diagnosis of malignant and benign human breast lesions. *Ultrasound Med Biol* 1983; **Suppl 2:** 407–14.

17. Egan RL, Egan KL. Detection of breast carcinoma: comparison of automated waterpath whole-breast sonography, mammography and physical examination. *Am J Radiol* 1984; **143:** 493–7.

18. Hayashi N, Tamaki N, Yonekura Y et al. Real-time sonography of palpable breast masses. *Br J Radiol* 1985; **58:** 611–15.

19. Warwick DJ, Smallwood JA, Guyer PB et al. Ultrasound mammography in the management of breast cancer. *Br J Surg* 1988; **75:** 243–5.

20. Perre CI, Koot VCM, de Hooge P, Leguit P. The value of ultrasound in the evaluation of palpable breast tumours: a prospective study of 400 cases. *Eur J Surg Oncol* 1994; **20:** 637–40.

21. Hirst C. Sonographic appearance of breast cancers 10 mm or less in diameter. In *Breast Ultrasound Update.* Madjar H, Teubner J, Hackelöer B-J, eds. Basel: Karger, 1994: 127–39.

22. Kline TS, Joshi LP, Neal HS. Fine-needle aspiration of the breast: diagnoses and pitfalls. A review of 3545 cases. *Cancer* 1979; **44:** 1458-64.

23. Strawbridge HTG, Basset AA, Foldes I. Role of cytology in management of lesions of the breast. *Surg Gynecol Obstet* 1981; **152:** 1–7.

24. Azzarelli A, Guzzon A, Pilotti S et al. Accuracy of breast cancer diagnosis by physical, radiologic and cytologic combined examinations. *Tumori* 1983; **69:** 137–41.

25. Dixon JM, Anderson TJ, Lamb J et al. Fine needle aspiration cytology in relationship to clinical examination and mammography in the diagnosis of a solid breast mass. *Br J Surg* 1984; **71:** 593–6.

26. Eisenberg AI, Haidu SI, Wilhelmus J et al. Preoperative aspiration cytology of breast tumors. *Acta Cytol* 1986; **30:** 135–46.

27. Barrows GH, Anderson TJ, Lamb JL et al. Fine needle aspiration of breast cancer: relationship of clinical factors to cytology results in 689 primary malignancies. *Cancer* 1986; **58:** 1493–8.

28. Linsk I, Kreuzer G, Zajicek J. Cytologic diagnosis of mammary tumors from aspiration biopsy smears: II. Studies on 210 fibroadenomas and 210 cases of benign dysplasia. *Acta Cytol* 1972; **16:** 130–8.

29. Zajdela A, Ghossein NA, Pilleron JP, Ennuyer A. The value of aspiration cytology in the diagnosis of breast cancer: experience at the Fondation Curie. *Cancer* 1975; **35:** 499–506.

30. Bell DA, Hajdu SI, Urban JA, Gaston JP. Role of aspiration cytology in the diagnosis and management of mammary lesions in office practice. *Cancer* 1983; **51**: 1182–9.
31. Smith C, Butler J, Cobb C, State D. Fine-needle aspiration cytology in the diagnosis of primary breast cancer. *Surgery* 1988; **103**: 178–83.
32. Palombini L, Fulciniti F, Vetrani A et al. Fine-needle aspiration biopsies of breast masses: a critical analysis of 1956 cases in 8 years. *Cancer* 1988; **61**: 2273–7.
33. Hunt CM, Ellis IO, Elston CW et al. Cytological grading of breast carcinoma – a feasible proposition? *Cytopathology* 1990; **1**: 287–95.
34. Robinson IA, McKee G, Nicholson A et al. Prognostic value of cytological grading of fine-needle aspirates from breast carcinomas. *Lancet* 1994; **343**: 947–9.
35. Elston CW. Grading of invasive carcinoma of the breast. In: *Diagnostic Histopathology of the Breast.* Page D, Anderson T, eds. Edinburgh: Churchill Livingstone, 1987.
36. Crawford DJ, Lope-Pihie A, Cowan S et al. Re-operative determination of oestrogen receptor status in breast cancer by immunocytochemical staining of fine needle aspirates. *Br J Surg* 1985; **72**: 991–3.
37. Flowers JL, Cox EB, Geisinger KR et al. Use of monoclonal antioestrogen receptor antibody to evaluate estrogen receptor content in fine needle aspiration breast biopsies. *Ann Surg* 1986; **203**: 250–4.
38. Azavedo E, Baral E, Skoog L. Immunohistochemical analysis of estrogen receptors in cells obtained from human carcinomas. *Anticancer Res* 1986; **6**: 263–5.
39. Marrazzo A, La Bara G, Taormina P, Bazan P. Determination of oestrogen receptors with monoclonal antibodies in fine needle aspirates of breast carcinoma. *Br J Cancer* 1989; **59**: 426–8.
40. Horsfall DJ, Jarvis LR, Grimbaldeston MA et al. Immunocytochemical assay for oestrogen receptor in fine needle aspirates of breast cancer by video image analysis. *Br J Cancer* 1989; **59**: 129–34.
41. Horobin JM, Matthew BM, Preece PE, Thompson AJ. Effects of fine needle aspiration on subsequent mammograms. *Br J Surg* 1992; **79**: 52–4.
42. Roberts JG, Preece PE, Bolton PM et al. The 'Tru-Cut' biopsy in breast cancer. *Clin Oncol* 1975; **1**: 297–303.
43. Elston CW, Cotton RE, Davies CJ et al. A comparison of the use of trucut needle and fine needle aspiration cytology in the pre-operative diagnosis of carcinoma of the breast. *Histopathology* 1978; **2**: 239–54.
44. Fentiman IS, Millis RR, Hayward JL. Value of needle biopsy in outpatient diagnosis of carcinoma of the breast. *Arch Surg* 1980; **115**: 652–3.
45. Gonzalez E, Grafton WD, Morris DR et al. Diagnosing breast cancer using frozen sections from trucut needle biopsies. *Ann Surg* 1985; **202**: 696–701.
46. Bradbeer JW. Outpatient diagnosis of breast cancer. *Breast J Surg* 1985; **72**: 927–8.
47. Minkowitz S, Moskowitz R, Khafif RA et al. Trucut needle biopsy of the breast. An analysis of its specificity and sensitivity. *Cancer* 1986; **57**: 320–3.
48. Baildam AD, Turnbull L, Howell A et al. Extended role for needle biopsy in the management of carcinoma of the breast. *Breast J Surg* 1989; **76**: 553–8.
49. Vega A, Garijo F, Ortega E. Core needle aspiration biopsy of palpable breast masses. *Acta Oncologica* 1995; **34**: 31–4.
50. Baildam AD, Turnbull L, Howell A et al. Extended role for needle biopsy in the management of carcinoma of the breast. *Br J Surg* 1989; **76**: 553–8.
51. Davies CJ, Elston CW, Cotton RE et al. Preoperative diagnosis in carcinoma of the breast. *Br J Surg* 1977; **64**: 326–8.
52. Shabot MM, Goldberg IM, Schick P et al. Aspiration cytology is superior to Tru-Cut needle biopsy in establishing the diagnosis of clinically suspicious breast masses. *Ann Surg* 1981; **196**: 122–6.
53. Sadler GP, McGee S, Dallimore NS et al. Role of fine needle aspiration cytology and needle-core biopsy in the diagnosis of lobular carcinoma of the breast. *Br J Surg* 1994; **81**: 1315–17.
54. Scoupa CD, Koukoras D, Spiliotis J et al. Comparison of fine needle aspiration and Tru-cut biopsy of palpable mammary lesions. *Cancer Detect Prev* 1996; **20**: 620–4.
55. Barreto V, Hamed H, Griffiths AB et al. Automatic needle biopsy in the diagnosis of early breast cancer. *Eur J Surg Oncol* 1991; **17**: 237–9.
56. Cerwenka H, Hoff M, Rosanelli G et al. Experience with a high speed biopsy gun in breast cancer diagnosis. *Eur J Surg Oncol* 1997; **23**: 206–7.

57. McMahon AJ, Lutfy AM, Matthew A et al. Needle core biopsy of the breast with a spring-loaded device. *Br J Surg* 1992; **79:** 1042–5.

58. Hamed H, de Freitas R, Rasbridge S et al. A prospective randomised study of two gauges of Biopty-cut needle in diagnosis of early breast cancer. *The Breast* 1995; **4:** 135–6.

6

Biopsy

We are more sensible of one little touch of the surgeon's lancet than of twenty wounds with a sword in the heat of fight.

Michel de Montaigne

Excision biopsy • Frozen section • Needle localization biopsy • Stereotactic needle biopsy • Staging investigations • Steroid receptors • Flow cytometry • Tumour characterization

EXCISION BIOPSY

Despite the increasing use of preoperative fine needle aspiration cytology (FNAC) and core biopsy, about 80% of lumps excised are benign.[1] Although this could be construed as a substantial waste of surgical time and potential morbidity for patients, there are often good reasons for excising a breast lesion. Some are objective such as an inadequate FNAC specimen or the cytological presence of atypical cells. More subjective are patient concern because of her family history or the recent diagnosis of malignancy in a friend or neighbour. The surgeon may have just treated a young woman with a lump that had been presumed to be a fibroadenoma and yet proved to be malignant, which will have lowered the threshold for recommending a biopsy. True fibroadenomas may enlarge and cause pain and this usually prompts the patient to ask for surgical removal.

The indications for biopsy are doubt on the part of the surgeon as to the nature of a breast lesion, or because of the wish of the patient to be rid of a lump. More litigation occurs as a result of failure to excise a lump than from overzealous excision of benign lesions. The object of assessment of a breast lump is to estab-lish its nature and, if this cannot be achieved by triple assessment, a biopsy is mandatory.

There is still considerable debate on whether breast biopsies should be performed under local or general anaesthesia. Most surgeons will excise small superficial lesions under local anaesthesia but balk at deeper larger lesions. This is a result of the difficulty in achieving good local anaesthesia within the breast, and the safety and accessibility of day-case general anaesthesia. Bellantone et al reviewed their experience of using local anaesthesia for excision of 460 clinically benign lumps, and general anaesthesia for 360 suspicious cases.[1] Of the clinically benign group, only 4% proved to be malignant and, of the suspicious cases, 98% were malignant. This represented very accurate preoperative diagnosis, enabling a more extensive procedure to be performed for those with malignancy. What is not recorded is the patient view of excision under local anaesthesia.

It is traditional to site breast incisions along Langer's lines in the belief that this will cause least gaping of subsequent scars. However, as has been pointed out by Benson, these do not correlate well with skin tension in the living which are better described by resting skin tension lines (RSTLs).[2] Rather than running

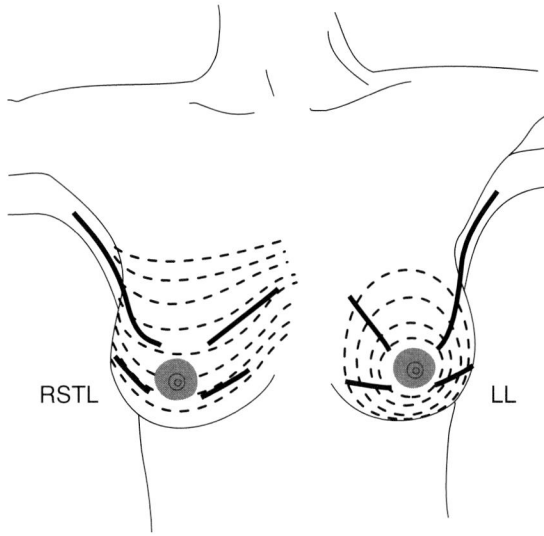

Fig. 6.1 Comparison of resting skin tension lines and Langer's lines. (Reproduced with permission from Benson.[2])

circumferentially, RSTLs are transverse and oblique laterally, as shown in Fig. 6.1. Hence, radial incisions should run parallel with RSTL with a better cosmetic result achieved if breast conservation therapy is the aim or mastectomy may be easier if this is to be the definitive surgery.

Avoidance of haematoma formation is best achieved by meticulous haemostasis, but this is a counsel of perfection and may be impossible in some patients. It has been questioned whether the use of deep sutures to approximate the breast tissue can reduce haematoma formation. Paterson et al examined 162 mastectomy specimens for haematoma at the biopsy site and compared those in which deep sutures had been used with others in which the cavity had not been closed.[3] There were significantly more haematomas in the unsutured group (31% vs 54%).

In a randomized trial conducted at the Westminster Hospital, London, 98 women undergoing breast biopsy had either no drain or a Penrose drain inserted.[4] There was a similar incidence of postoperative wound complications (haematoma and infection) in both groups. Subsequently, 202 patients were randomized to have a vacuum drain or no drain and to have the cavity either closed with absorbable sutures or left unsutured. The lowest incidence of wound complications (8%) occurred in those who had both a drain and suturing of the biopsy cavity. This was followed by drain without suture (11%), no drain with suturing (14%), with the highest incidence of 27% complications in those who had neither a drain nor sutures. There was a relationship between length of wound and complications which were noted in 16% of those with incisions 6 cm or less, and 32% of those with wounds over 6 cm. Of the obese patients 42% developed complications but only 19% of those who were thin or normal. Not surprisingly, the experience of the surgeon also determined the complication rate which was 8% for operations performed by consultant or senior registrar and 17% in those conducted by registrars.

Warren et al conducted a randomized trial in which 107 patients undergoing breast biopsy were randomized to no drainage (55) or insertion of a suction drain (52).[5] There was no difference in the incidence of wound infections (one in each group), but there were more haematomas in the undrained group (87% vs 65%). The median pain score and duration of pain were similar in both groups. Thus, although the measured incidence of haematoma formation is greater if no drain is inserted, this does not have an significant influence on either postoperative pain or wound infection.

In another study which examined the relationship between haematoma formation and subsequent wound infection, Lipshy et al reviewed 289 breast cancer cases treated by mastectomy half of whom had been diagnosed by FNAC and half by open biopsy.[6] Wound infection after mastectomy occurred in 7% of those diagnosed by excision biopsy but in only 2% of those who had FNAC diagnosis. This illustrates further the advantage of a preoperative diagnosis of malignancy.

FROZEN SECTION

It is paradoxical that, after years of trying to dissuade surgeons from pressurizing their pathologists to give hurried answers on suboptimally processed frozen section material, the procedure is undergoing a renaissance. This arises from the use of FNAC to make a preoperative diagnosis and the desire to perform one-stage procedures. Even with a C5 cytological diagnosis definitive treatment cannot be undertaken unless there is unequivocal clinical or radiological evidence of invasion. Under these circumstances the pathologist may be asked for a frozen section diagnosis of invasion to avoid unnecessary axillary surgery in patients with ductal carcinoma in situ (DCIS). This may place an intolerable burden on the pathologist who, quite reasonably, may refuse to give a definitive answer under these conditions.

Mistakes are made with frozen section diagnosis. In a long-term follow-up study of 230 cases, all of whom were diagnosed by frozen section and went on to immediate mastectomy, review of paraffin sections showed benign changes only in three (1%).[7] In a series of 672 cases with impalpable breast lesions, frozen section was used in all but no diagnosis could be made in 22 (3%).[8] In 27 cases the diagnosis was modified after paraffin section examination, with three false-positive diagnoses and 24 false negatives.

There can be few surgeons who now believe that a diagnosis of breast cancer is a surgical emergency with any delay having an impact on prognosis. However, the timing of surgery may have an impact as discussed in Chapter 7. In addition, incomplete excision may worsen survival. In a series of 3264 patients with breast cancer treated by the Danish Breast Cancer Cooperative Group with excision biopsy, frozen section and immediate modified radical mastectomy, 48% were found subsequently to have residual carcinoma at the biopsy site.[9] There was a significantly better survival among those who had no residual cancer in the mastectomy. A situation that exists for only 10–30 minutes (residual cancer while awaiting mastectomy) may exert a profound impact on prognosis, possibly because the trauma of cutting through the cancer may enable tumour cells to metastasize.

Frozen section should be used only as a last ditch measure when other methods of making a preoperative diagnosis have failed. Its routine use is potentially dangerous. From the patient's point of view it is better to be aware of the histological diagnosis before definitive treatment is undertaken, in order that options can be discussed. Thankfully, frozen section is another disappearing example of the depersonalization of medicine and the disenfranchisement of patients from the decision-making process concerning their future.

NEEDLE LOCALIZATION BIOPSY

With increasing frequency breast surgeons are being sent women with impalpable lesions, picked up as a result of mammographic screening, either of an unknown nature or with a cytological or histological diagnosis. For those with histologically confirmed invasive cancer the aim of surgery will be to remove the lesion completely and perform axillary surgery. Those with a C5 cytology will require a complete local excision. In the undiagnosed cases, the surgeon has to remove the lesion without taking an excessive amount of normal tissue which could lead to a poor cosmetic outcome in a patient with benign histology.

To achieve the best results, the close cooperation of the surgeon, radiologist and pathologist is essential. The method of localization is a matter of personal preference and experience. Originally some centres used methylene blue dye or charcoal to mark the lesion but most localizations are now performed with hook wires. Although the operation can be carried out under local anaesthesia, most surgeons prefer a general anaesthetic. In a study from the University of Colorado, 81 needle localization biopsies were performed under local anaesthetic and 36 under general anaesthetic.[10]

Among those biopsied under local anaesthesia only 78% of the target lesions were successfully removed compared with 92% of those who had a general anaesthetic. It was concluded that general anaesthesia should be used in terms of efficiency and patient comfort.

There are no guidelines for the best localization of an impalpable lesion. Kopans et al suggested that the tip of the marker wire should lie within 5 mm of the abnormality,[11] whereas others have suggested that a distance of 1–2 cm is acceptable.[12,13] From a surgical viewpoint, any marker that is more than 2 cm from the lesion may be of little use other than serving to indicate the laterality of the abnormality.

To reduce the radiation exposure of the breast, it is potentially enticing to use ultrasonography rather than X-ray mammography to localize an impalpable lesion. The results have, however, been patchy. Weber et al reported that ultrasonography was able to localize only 25% of mammographic masses and 14% of microcalcifications – a total success rate of 18%.[14] In contrast, Perre et al successfully localized 93% of lesions.[15] In a different approach, Di Giorgio et al used an intraoperative ultrasonic probe which identified the lesion in all cases.[16] Similarly Memon and Berstock found that about 50% of mammographic abnormalities were detectable ultrasonographically and, in 20 intraoperative ultrasonic localizations, the lesion was successfully identified and removed.[17]

As magnetic resonance imaging (MRI) is being used with greater frequency for breast examination, so more women are being diagnosed with enhancing lesions but without clinical or radiological signs. The nature of the MRI system makes localization difficult, with a need for non-ferrous markers. Desouza et al devised a frameless stereotactic localization technique, outside the MRI scanner, using an ultrasonic probe and were able to place the needle successfully within 2 mm of the lesion in eight of nine (89%) cases and at a second attempt in one patient.[18]

Alexander et al reviewed the outcome in 932 needle localization biopsies, performed at the Memorial Sloan-Kettering Cancer Centre, New York, between 1981 and 1984, and a second

series carried out in 1987.[19] For the localization, a combination of a radiopaque dye and methylene blue was used. The earlier series comprised 311 cases of whom 29% had malignancy and the second series consisted of 220 patients of whom 29% also had cancer. In the entire series there were seven (1.3%) missed lesions. Perdue et al reported a series of 536 needle localization biopsies where the abnormality was not present in the specimen radiograph in 5%.[20]

In a large consecutive series of 1182 needle localizations performed in Florence, 427 (36%) were found to have invasive cancer, 121 (10%) had in situ cancer, 22 (2%) had atypia and 612 (52%) were diagnosed with benign lesions.[21] Of those aged less than 50, 33% had cancer, compared with 46% of those aged 50–69 and 63% of women aged over 59 years. The most common radiological sign of malignancy was a stellate opacity (73%), followed by irregular opacities (62%), localized microcalcifications (42%), parenchymal distortion (20%) and regular opacities (8%).

Needle localization biopsy is not without complications: Rappaport et al reported 144 consecutive procedures with wound infections developing in 11 (8%), compared with an institutional clean surgical operation infection rate of 1%.[22] When a drain was inserted as part of the biopsy procedure, the infection rate rose from 5% o 25%. Diathermy burns were recorded in seven cases (5%). The lesion of interest was not removed in four women (3%), and incompletely removed in another four. Additional use of methylene blue dye, in 54 cases, resulted in a 100% success rate in removal of the abnormality.

STEREOTACTIC NEEDLE BIOPSY

If the nature of a mammographic abnormality could be determined without recourse to surgery, some patients with benign lesions, such as radial scars, could be spared an unnecessary operation. Furthermore, if proof of invasive cancer could be achieved preoperatively, definitive surgery could be planned as a

Table 6.1 Comparison of results from stereotactic core biopsy and surgical excision in patients with impalpable breast lesions

Number	Cancer (%)	Stereotactic		Surgical		Reference
		Sensitivity (%)	Specificity (%)	Sensitivity (%)	Specificity (%)	
122	19	96	100	96	100	Parker et al[25]
100	36	97	100	97	100	Elvecrog et al[26]
231	55	94	100	100	100	Brenner et al[27]
Mean		**96**	**100**	**98**	**100**	

one-stage procedure. The technique of stereotactic cytological diagnosis was originally developed by Bolmgren et al at the Karolinska Institute.[23] Subsequently, Gent et al reported a series of 543 patients with impalpable lesions who underwent stereotactic cytological diagnosis.[24] The needle tip was placed within 1 mm of the lesion in 90% of cases and a subsequent surgical biopsy was performed in 187. The sensitivity of cytology was 98% and the specificity 95%.

The disadvantage of a stereotactic diagnosis of malignancy in an occult lesion is the same as with a palpable lump: non-invasive tumours cannot be distinguished from invasive cancers. Increasing demands for more specific preoperative information prompted the use of stereotactic core biopsies. Three series which compared the results of stereotactic biopsy with needle localization biopsy are shown in Table 6.1.[25-27] Parker et al used an automated 14 gauge cutting needle and showed that the sensitivity of stereotactic and surgical biopsy was the same, with one cancer being missed by each technique.[25] Similar results were obtained by Elvecrog et al, who showed that stereotactic needle biopsy could be as accurate as needle localization biopsy for making both benign and

malignant diagnoses.[26] Commenting on these results, Kopans stressed the need for vertical accuracy in needle placement because a small error in the horizontal aiming points could lead to a substantial error in calculation of depth.[28] With a variance of 5 mm in calculation this could lead to a depth error of 1 cm, resulting in failure to sample the lesion of interest.

Brenner et al examined the influence of the number of stereotactic samples and operator experience in terms of diagnostic accuracy.[27] The first core biopsy correctly identified 84% of cancers, rising to 90% by the third core biopsy and 94% by the fifth. When the technique was first used, the sensitivity of a first core was 78% and this rose to 92% by the fifth biopsy. The success of core biopsy in making the diagnosis of malignancy was dependent on the mammographic appearances. These were divided into mass lesions, clustered microcalcifications, masses with microcalcifications, focal asymmetry and trabecular distortion. Results are shown in Table 6.2 which indicates that malignant mass lesions with microcalcification could be correctly diagnosed after only two core biopsies. In contrast, trabecular distortion as a result of cancer was identified in only 86% of cases after five cores had been taken. As

Table 6.2 Percentage detection of impalpable cancers by stereotactic biopsy in relation to number of cores taken and type of mammographic abnormality

Mammographic abnormality	Core 1 (%)	Core 2 (%)	Core 3 (%)	Core 4 (%)	Core 5 (%)
Mass	96	96	97	97	98
Microcalcifications	69	77	80	91	92
Mass and microcalcifications	87	100	100	100	100
Focal asymmetry	60	80	80	100	100
Trabecular distortion	64	86	86	86	86
Overall	**84**	**89**	**90**	**94**	**94**

From Brenner et al.[27]

trabecular distortion may be caused by either malignancy or a radial scar, a benign result cannot be taken as confirmation that the lesion is non-malignant, even after five negative core biopsies.

STAGING INVESTIGATIONS

Fashions change with time and this has been true of staging investigations for patients with apparently early breast cancer. As a result of the known risk of subsequent systemic relapse, particularly in bone, extensive work was carried out using skeletal scintigraphy before surgery in order to detect occult metastatic disease.[29] After the first enthusiasm had worn off, many clinicians started looking critically at the value of bone scanning in patients with operable disease. In a review of 1074 bone scans performed on breast cancer patients at Guy's Hospital, London, the rate of positive bone scans in 271 with stage I disease was 0%.[30] Among 593 with stage II disease the positivity rate was 3%, and this rose to 7% in 179 with stage III breast cancer. Following this review it was decided that patients with single tumours up to 4 cm in diameter would not undergo

routine preoperative skeletal scintigraphy, unless they had specific bone symptoms.

Most centres now have a small core of staging tests: chest radiograph, full blood count and biochemical screen. With normal liver function tests hepatic ultrasonography is unnecessary. The value of preoperative staging tests has been studied prospectively by the Italian Task Force for Breast Cancer (FONCaM).[31] The study group comprised 3627 patients with early breast cancer, and sensitivity and specificity of the various tests is shown in Table 6.3. All the tests had both a sensitivity and positive predictive value (PPV) of less than 50%. Restricting the analysis to those with stage I/II disease the detection rate was 0.2% for chest radiographs, 0.2% for bone scans and almost zero for liver ultrasonography and scintigraphy.

For an otherwise fit patient with operable breast cancer, the only mandatory preoperative test is bilateral mammography and, if mastectomy is going to be performed, only contralateral radiographs need to be taken. Almost all patients will have had mammography as part of their routine diagnostic work-up, but a few younger women may have escaped this investigation. It is necessary in order to confirm that

Table 6.3 Value of preoperative staging tests in patients with early breast cancer

Investigation	Sensitivity (%)	Specificity (%)	PPV (%)
Chest radiograph	31	99	44
Skeletal survey	35	99	32
Bone scintigraphy	48	95	15
Liver ultrasonography	29	99	33
Liver scintigraphy	20	97	8

From Ciatto et al.[31]

the disease is unifocal within the affected breast and that there is no contralateral evidence of breast cancer.

STEROID RECEPTORS

In 1989, a paper was published in *The Lancet* entitled 'Who needs oestrogen receptor assays?', in which it was argued that appropriate decisions about management of early and advanced breast cancer could be made without knowledge of the oestrogen receptor/progesterone receptor (ER/PR) status.[32] As results of further clinical trials have emerged and with new methods of treatment coming into vogue, this hawkish position needs modification.

In terms of selection of patients for adjuvant treatment, there is now clear evidence of the benefit of ovarian suppression in premenopausal women.[33] Furthermore the Scottish adjuvant trial, which compared ovarian suppression with chemotherapy for premenopausal node-positive patients, showed that patients with ER-positive tumours had a better survival if treated by ovarian ablation rather than chemotherapy.[34] Thus knowledge of the ER status might influence the decision as to

whether hormonal or cytotoxic adjuvant treatment was more appropriate.

Nevertheless, if the type and grade of the primary tumour had been reported by the pathologist, this would be a good guide as to the likelihood of endocrine positivity.[35] Tumours that are well or moderately differentiated (tubular, mucoid, lobular, ductal grade I/II) are usually ER-positive whereas poorly differentiated cancers (ductal grade III or medullary) are ER-negative. It is likely that a similar effect would be seen in postmenopausal patients and that selection of patients with ER-negative or grade III tumours would be more likely to benefit from cytotoxic chemotherapy than tamoxifen.

An ER/PR assay could also be useful in the selection of appropriate primary systemic therapy for patients with large operable or locally advanced cancers. Under these circumstances it is possible to make an attempt at grading either a cytological or a core biopsy specimen, but this may prove difficult because of the sparseness of malignant cells. Hence it may be necessary to use an immunocytochemical assay to measure ER/PR status of the cancer cells.

Table 6.4 Relationship of S-phase fraction, ploidy and prognosis in breast cancer

Number	Follow-up (years)	Univariate	Multivariate	Reference
565	10	SPF/ploidy	Ploidy	Cornelisse et al[37]
490	6	Ploidy	–	Hedley et al[38]
308	8	Ploidy	–	Kallioniemi et al[39]
345	7	Ploidy	Ploidy	Clark et al[40]
472	6	SPF	–	Stål et al[41]
351	25	Ploidy	–	Toikkanen et al[42]
398	10	SPF	SPF	Fisher et al[43]
293	8	–	–	Stanton et al[44]

In terms of ER/PR status and outcome in early breast cancer, it is now generally accepted that these are at best weak prognostic factors. In a recent study of 2257 patients with operable disease, followed for a median of 8.5 years, it was found that both ER and PR were significant prognostic indicators in a univariate analysis.[36] In a multivariate model, the major significant variables were grade, nodal status and tumour size with ER status being just significant. A time-dependent analysis was undertaken which showed that ER status declined in prognostic significance by 20% per year and after 8 years it had lost prognostic power.

FLOW CYTOMETRY

The major prognostic variables in patients with breast cancer are tumour size, grade and axillary nodal status. Among patients with histologically negative axillary nodes, a substantial amount of work has been done in an attempt to delineate a high-risk group who might benefit from systemic adjuvant therapy. One of the major candidates as an independent prognostic factor has been cell proliferation, as measured by S-phase fraction (SPF) and DNA ploidy. The larger studies which have examined SPF and prognosis are summarized in Table 6.4.[37–44] These indicate that ploidy is a signifi-

cant univariate factor, with patients having diploid tumours surviving better than those with aneuploid lesions. However in only two studies was ploidy a significant variable on multivariate analysis.[37,40] Similarly, S-phase fraction was significant in three studies,[37,41,43] as a univariate factor but in only one multivariate analysis.[43]

It is likely that S-phase fraction and ploidy lose significance in multivariate analyses when tumour grade is entered as a prognostic variable. In the analysis of Clark et al[40] tumour grade was not known and this may explain why ploidy remained significant in the multivariate model. The predictive power of both S-phase and DNA ploidy is weak and can be replaced by tumour grade, which should be quantified by all pathologists reporting malignant breast biopsies.

TUMOUR CHARACTERIZATION

As well as steroid hormone receptors and indicators of proliferation, multiple other tumour characteristics, which might have prognostic power, have been measured and evaluated. One such was epidermal growth factor receptor (EGFR). Original work suggested that EGFR-positive tumours were more aggressive, irrespective of histological subtype.[45] However, subsequent work with more cases and longer follow-up indicated that EGFR did not have prognostic significance. In a study of 229 women with early breast cancer, followed for a median of 34 months, the only significant prognostic variables were tumour size, type and pathological node status.[46] Murray et al also confirmed that EGFR was not of prognostic significance, and neither was transforming factor α (TGF-α), although tumours that had high levels of transforming factor β (TGF-β) were associated with a longer disease-free survival, in a univariate analysis.[47]

The *c-erb-2* gene (neu), which shows extensive homology with EGFR, has been found to be amplified and over-expressed in up to 20% of breast cancers.[48] Amplification of the oncogene and over-expression of gene product were reported to be associated with a worsening of prognosis.[48,49] Yet again, subsequent work indicated that *c-erbB-2* amplification and protein over-expression were not independent prognostic factors.[50,51]

Cathepsin D is a lysosomal acid protease, the secretion of which is stimulated by oestrogens.[52] Originally described in the MCF-7 cell line it has been found to be present in both breast epithelial and stromal cells. As synthesis of a protease might enable malignant cells to invade and metastasise, it was studied as a prognostic marker and found to be associated with a worse survival relapse-free and overall survival.[53,54] Subsequent studies which included multivari-

ate analyses have shown that higher concentrations of cathepsin D, in either tumour or stromal cells, is not a significant prognostic marker.[55,56]

All these negative studies on sophisticated aspects of tumour behaviour indicate that the present best prognostic variables are those provided by the histopathologist. Tumour grade represents an integration of the aggressive features of a cancer and any putative prognostic factor has to stand the test of multivariate analysis which includes this measure of malignant differentiation. Likewise the axillary nodal status is a measure of both the aggressiveness of the tumour together with length of time that it has existed and the capacity to metastasize. These are the gold standards against which all new prognostic variables have to be judged.

SYNOPSIS

- With experience, stereotactic core biopsy is as accurate as needle localization biopsy for most mammographic abnormalities.
- Mammography is the only mandatory staging investigation in otherwise well women with operable breast cancer.
- The most important prognostic variables in patients with early breast cancer are tumour type, grade size and pathological axillary nodal status.

REFERENCES

1. Bellantone R, Rossi S, Lombardi CP et al. Excisional breast biopsy: when, why and how? *Int Surg* 1995; **80**: 75–8.
2. Benson EA. Breast incisions for conservation surgery. *Ann R Coll Surg Engl* 1997; **79**: 233.
3. Paterson ML, Nathanson SD, Havstad S. Hematomas following excisional breast biopsies for invasive breast carcinoma: the influence of deep suture approximation of breast parenchyma. *Am Surg* 1994; **60**: 845–8.
4. Law NW, Lamont PM, Johnson CD, Ellis H. Drainage or suture of the cavity after breast biopsy. *Ann R Coll Surg Engl* 1990; **72**: 11–13.
5. Warren HW, Kaye B, Griffith CDM et al. Should breast biopsy cavities be drained? *Ann R Coll Surg Engl* 1994; **76**: 39–41.
6. Lipshy KA, Neifeld JP, Boyle RM et al. Complications of mastectomy and their relationship to biopsy technique. *Ann Surg Oncol* 1996; **3**: 290–4.

7. Fentiman IS, Millis RR, Chaudary MA et al. Which patients are cured of breast cancer? *Br Med J* 1984; **289**: 1198–211.

8. Bianchi S, Palli D, Ciatto S et al. Accuracy and reliability of frozen section diagnosis in a series of 672 nonpalpable breast lesions. *Anat Pathol* 1995; **103**: 199–205.

9. Andersen JA, Blichert-Toft M, Jjaergaard J et al. Prognostic significance of residual cancer tissue after diagnostic biopsy in breast carcinoma. Three-year short-term results. *Eur J Cancer* 1984; **20**: 765–70.

10. Norton LW, Zeligman BE, Pearlman NW. Accuracy and cost of needle localization breast biopsy. *Arch Surg* 1988; **123**: 947–50.

11. Kopans DB, Waitzkin ED, Linetsky L et al. Localization of breast lesions identified on only one mammogram view. *AJR* 1987; **149**: 39–41.

12. Yanskakas BC, Knelson MH, Albernethy ML et al. Needle localization biopsy of occult lesions of the breast. Experiences in 199 cases. *Invest Radiol* 1988; **23**: 729–33.

13. Adler OB, Engel A. Mammographic wire-guided biopsies in non-palpable breast lesions. *Eur J Radiol* 1989; **11**: 108–11.

14. Weber WN, Sickles EA, Callen PW, Filly RA. Nonpalpable breast lesion localization: limited efficacy of sonography. *Radiology* 1985; **155**: 783–4.

15. Perre CI, de Hooge P, Hoynck van Papendrecht AAGM, Muller JWT. Locating and marking non-palpable, mammographically suspicious breast lesions with the aid of ultrasound. *Eur J Surg Oncol* 1991; **17**: 477–9.

16. Di Giorgio A, Alessi GP, Arnone P, Canavese A. Ultrasonically guided excisional biopsy of non-palpable breast lesions. *Br J Surg* 1996; **83**: 103.

17. Memon MA, Berstock DA. Ultrasound-guided excision of impalpable breast lesion. *Ann R Coll Surg Engl* 1996; **78**: 61–2.

18. Desouza NM, Coutts GA, Puni RK, Young IR. Magnetic resonance imaging guided biopsy using a frameless stereotactic technique. *Clin Radiol* 1996; **51**: 425–8.

19. Alexander HR, Candela FC, Dershaw DD, Kinne DW. Needle-localized mammographic lesions. Results and evolving treatment strategy. *Arch Surg* 1990; **125**: 1441–4.

20. Perdue P, Page D, Nellestein M et al. Early detection of breast carcinoma: a comparison of palpable and nonpalpable lesions. *Surgery* 1992; **111**: 656–9.

21. Ciatto S, Del Turco MR, Bonardi R et al. Non-palpable lesions of the breast detected by mammography – review of 1182 consecutive histologically confirmed cases. *Eur J Cancer* 1994; **30A**: 40–4.

22. Rappaport W, Thompson S, Wong R et al. Complications associated with needle localization biopsy of the breast. *Surg Gynecol Obstet* 1991; **172**: 303–6.

23. Bolmgren J, Jacobson B, Nordenstrom R. Stereotaxic instrument for needle biopsy of the mammogram. *Am J Roentgenol* 1977; **129**: 121–5.

24. Gent HJ, Sprenger E, Dowlatshi K. Stereotaxic needle localization and cytological diagnosis of occult breast lesions. *Ann Surg* 1986; **204**: 580–4.

25. Parker SH, Lovin JD, Jobe WE et al. Nonpalpable breast lesions: stereotactic automated large-core biopsies. *Radiology* 1991; **180**: 403–7.

26. Elvecrog EL, Lechner MC, Nelson MT. Nonpalpable breast lesions: correlation of stereo-taxic large-core needle biopsy and surgical biopsy results. *Radiology* 1993; **188**: 453–5.

27. Brenner RJ, Fajardo L, Fisher PR et al. Percutaneous core biopsy of the breast: effect of operator experience and number of samples on diagnostic accuracy. *AJR* 1996; **166**: 341–6.

28. Kopans DB. Review of stereotaxic large-core needle biopsy and surgical biopsy results in nonpalpable breast lesions. *Radiology* 1993; **189**: 665–6.

29. Galasko CSB. The significance of occult skeletal metastases detected by skeletal scintigraphy in patients with otherwise apparently 'early' breast cancer. *Br J Surg* 1975; **62**: 694–6.

30. Coleman RE, Rubens RD, Fogelman I. Reappraisal of the baseline bone scan in breast cancer. *J Nucl Med* 1988; **29**: 1045–9.

31. Ciatto S, Spacini P, Azzini V et al. Preoperative staging of primary breast cancer. A multicentre study. *Cancer* 1988; **61**: 1038–40.

32. Barnes DM, Fentiman IS, Millis RR, Rubens RD. Who needs oestrogen receptor assays? *Lancet* 1989; **i**: 1126–7.

33. Early Breast Cancer Trialists' Collaborative Group. Systemic treatment of early breast cancer by hormonal, cytotoxic, or immune therapy. *Lancet* 1992; **339**: 1–15; 71–84.

34. Scottish Cancer Trials Breast Group and ICRF Breast Unit, Guy's Hospital, London. Adjuvant ovarian ablation versus CMF chemotherapy in premenopausal women with pathological stage

II breast carcinoma: the Scottish Trial. *Lancet* 1993; **341**: 1293–8.

35. Millis RR. The relationship between the pathology of breast cancer and hormone sensitivity. *Rev Endocrinol Rel Cancer* 1987; **20**(suppl): 13–18.

36. Pichon MF, Broet P, Magdelenat H et al. Prognostic value of steroid receptors after long-term follow-up of 2257 operable breast cancers. *Br J Cancer* 1996; **73**: 1545–51.

37. Cornelisse C, van der Velde C, Caspers R et al. DNA ploidy and survival in breast cancer patients. *Cytometry* 1987; **8**: 225–34.

38. Hedley DW, Rugg C, Gelber R. Association of DNA index and S-phase fraction with prognosis of node positive early breast cancer. *Cancer Res* 1987; **47**: 4729–35.

39. Kallioniemi O-P, Blanco G, Alavaikko M et al. Improving the prognostic value of DNA flow cytometry in breast cancer by combining DNA index and S-phase fraction. A proposed classification of DNA histograms in breast cancer. *Cancer* 1988; **62**: 2183–90.

40. Clark GM, Dressler LG, Owens MA et al. Prediction of relapse or survival in patients with node-negative breast cancer by DNA flow cytometry. *N Engl J Med* 1989; **320**: 627–33.

41. Stål O, Wingren S, Carstensen J et al. Prognostic value of DNA ploidy and S-phase fraction in relation to estrogen receptor content and clinicopathological variables in primary breast cancer. *Eur J Cancer* 1989; **25**: 301–9.

42. Toikkanen S, Joensuu H, Klemi P. The prognostic significance of nuclear DNA content in invasive breast cancer – a study with long-term follow-up. *Br J Cancer* 1989; **60**: 693–700.

43. Fisher B, Gunduz N, Constantino PH et al. DNA flow cytometric analysis of primary operable breast cancer. Relation of ploidy and S-phase fraction to outcome of patients in NSABP B-04. *Cancer* 1991; **68**: 1465–75.

44. Stanton PD, Cooke TG, Oakes SJ et al. Lack of prognostic significance of DNA ploidy and S phase fraction in breast cancer. *Br J Cancer* 1992; **66**: 925–9.

45. Sainsbury JRC, Nicholson S, Angus B et al. Epidermal growth factor receptor status of histo-logical sub-types of breast cancer. *Br J Cancer* 1988; **58**: 458–60.

46. Bolla M, Chedin M, Colonna M et al. Lack of prognostic value of epidermal growth factor receptor in a series of 229 T1/T2. N0/N1 breast cancers, with well defined prognostic parameters. *Breast Cancer Res Treat* 1994; **29**: 265–70.

47. Murray PA, Barrett-Lee P, Travers M et al. The prognostic significance of transforming growth factors in human breast cancer. *Br J Cancer* 1993; **67**: 1408–12.

48. Slamon DJ, Clark GM, Wong SG et al. Human breast cancer: correlation of relapse and survival with amplification of the HER-2/neu oncogene. *Science* 1987; **235**: 177–82.

49. Paik S, Hazan R, Fisher ER et al. Pathologic findings from the National Surgical Adjuvant Breast and Bowel Project: prognostic significance of c-erbB-2 protein overexpression in primary breast cancer. *J Clin Oncol* 1990; **8**: 103–12.

50. Van der Vijver MJ, Peterse JL, Mooi WJ et al. Neu-protein overexpression in breast cancer. Association with comedo-type ductal carcinoma in situ and limited prognostic value in stage II breast cancer. *N Engl J Med* 1988; **319**: 1239–45.

51. Ottestad L, Andersen TI, Nesland JM et al. Amplification of *c-erbB-2*, *int-2*, and *c-myc* genes in node negative breast carcinomas. *Acta Oncol* 1993; **32**: 289–94.

52. Westley B, Rochefort H. Estradiol induced proteins in the MCF-7 human breast cancer cell line. *Biochem Biophys Res Commun* 1979; **90**: 410–16.

53. Spyratos F, Maudelonde T, Brouillet JP et al. Cathepsin D: an independent prognostic factor for metastasis of breast cancer. *Lancet* 1989; **ii**: 1115–18.

54. Tandon A, Clark G, Chirgwin J, McGuire WL. Cathepsin D and prognosis in breast cancer. *N Engl J Med* 1990; **322**: 297–302.

55. Ravdin PM, Tandon AK, Allred DC et al. Cathepsin D by western blotting and immunohistochemistry: failure to confirm correlations with prognosis in node-negative breast cancer. *J Clin Oncol* 1994; **12**: 467–74.

56. Joensuu H, Toikkanen S, Isola J. Stromal cell cathepsin D expression and long-term survival in breast cancer. *Br J Cancer* 1995; **71**: 155–9.

7

Timing of surgery

Carpe diem.

Background • Unopposed oestrogen hypothesis • Endocrine studies • Pathological studies • Meta-analysis • Present situation

The attitude of surgeons towards breast cancer has largely been influenced by the prevailing philosophy of the time. In an age when it was believed that the major site of metastatic disease was in the locoregional nodes, it was hoped that the most radical surgery would lead to the greatest likelihood of cure. Subsequently, it was mooted that axillary nodal metastases were merely an indicator of metastatic potential and that most patients had metastatic disease at the time of diagnosis: their only hope of cure lay in the use of adjuvant systemic treatment and, by implication, local treatment had no influence on outcome.

Present evidence suggests that this latter hypothesis is fallacious because not only tumour features, such as size, type and grade, but also patient characteristics may influence outcome. After controlling for tumour size and axillary nodal status, postmenopausal women who are obese have a worse prognosis than thinner patients.[1] In addition, tumour manipulation during surgery may lead to shedding of malignant cells which are detectable in bone marrow[2,3] Although it could be argued that such cells are non-viable and do not have prognostic significance, it has been found that perioperative chemotherapy can lead to an improvement in prognosis.[4]

Taken together these findings suggest that metastatic disease after primary surgery might not have arisen from pre-existing micrometastases but could be a direct consequence of attempted tumour extirpation, and that the modification of hormonal influences acting on the breast might well lead to a reduction, or abolition, of tumour cell shedding perioperatively.

BACKGROUND

Both patients and doctors are aware that hormonal fluctuations during the normal menstrual cycle lead to functional and structural alterations within the breast, particularly premenstrual fullness and discomfort, sometimes amounting to pain. If this is prolonged, it may require treatment that can be achieved with antioestrogens such as tamoxifen.[5] Within the normal breast, there is an increase in growth rate at a cellular level, as measured by the thymidine labelling index (TLI), during the luteal phase of the cycle.[6]

In view of these cyclical changes, Ratajzak et al postulated that the behaviour of breast cancers might be influenced by manipulation at different phases of the menstrual cycle and used the mouse C3HeB/Fe model to test this hypothesis.[7] This mouse allows the growth of a spontaneous murine mammary cancer that is rich in oestrogen receptors. A suspension of malignant cells was implanted in the hind leg

Table 7.1 Recurrence in relation to time of tumour excision in mice

	Near oestrus (%)	Post oestrus (%)
1 month:		
Relapsed	60	84
Non-relapsed	40	16
3 months:		
Relapsed	73	88
Non-relapsed	27	12

From Ratajzak et al.[7]

and the tumour size was measured after 14–17 days, with the leg subsequently being amputated. The stage of the oestrous cycle was determined by daily vaginal smear cytology for the next 28 days, after which the animals were sacrificed. The size and extent of lung metastases were measured in all animals with evident disease. In those without evident metastases the lungs were minced and a cell suspension injected subcutaneously into syngeneic mice which were observed for the next 4 months for the presence and size of tumour at the inoculation site. Results are given in Table 7.1.

The phase of the menstrual cycle during which the tumour was implanted had no impact on the incidence of pulmonary metastases but there were significantly more mice with no evidence of disease when the tumour was excised during the 'near oestrous' phase. As a result of this interaction between the hormonal environment and likelihood of metastatic disease in mice, Ratajzak et al postulated that it might be possible to determine the time of the menstrual cycle in women at which tumour excision carried the greatest probability of surgical cure.

Following this, Hrushevsky et al reviewed the outcome of 41 premenopausal patients who had breast cancers resected at known times in the menstrual cycle.[8] Of the 19 who had surgery in the perimenstrual period (days 0–6 and 21–36), recurrence occurred in eight (42%) compared with only three of 22 (14%) of those who had mid-cycle surgery (days 7–20). In a multivariate analysis of prognostic factors (time of surgery, tumour size, lymph node status and steroid receptor status), timing of surgery emerged as an independent predictor of relapse-free and overall survival. When other groups examined outcome in relation to timing of surgery they were unable to replicate the original finding.[9–11] As an example, an analysis of 279 premenopausal patients treated at the Centre Rene Huguenin showed that, of 136 women undergoing perimenstrual surgery, the 5-year mortality rate was 20% compared with 31% for the 143 who had mid-cycle surgery.[11] It would appear that, yet again, results obtained in a rodent model system were not directly applicable to human malignancy.

UNOPPOSED OESTROGEN HYPOTHESIS

There is a substantial body of evidence that oestrogens can influence the behaviour of breast cancer. The original demonstration by Beatson that bilateral oophorectomy could lead to regression of advanced disease was the inspiration for much of the clinical and laboratory research on breast cancer this century.[12] The action of oestrogens on both malignant and normal breast tissue was shown to be modulated by oestrogen receptors.[13] In vitro studies have shown that oestrogens could not only stimulate cell proliferation, but also induce the synthesis of proteases, possibly leading to a greater probability of invasion and establishment of viable micrometastases.[14]

For these reasons, it was postulated that unopposed oestrogen could adversely affect some breast cancers, leading to an increased risk of viable cells being shed at the time of attempted tumour excision. Within the menstrual cycle, there are very low levels of oestrogen during the early cycle, while, after ovulation, oestrogens are opposed by proges-

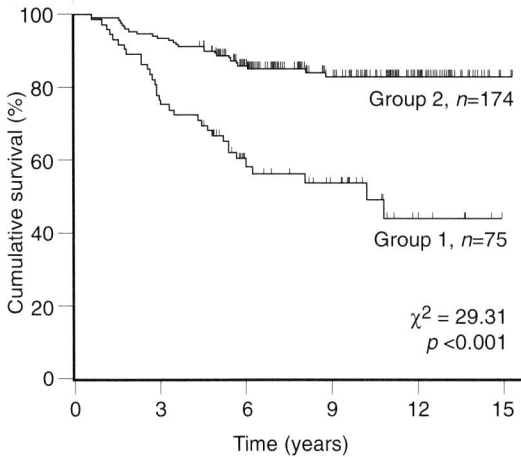

Fig. 7.1 Overall survival of premenopausal women undergoing tumour excision in the follicular phase (days 3–12) and at other times in the menstrual cycle (days 1–2, 13–28).

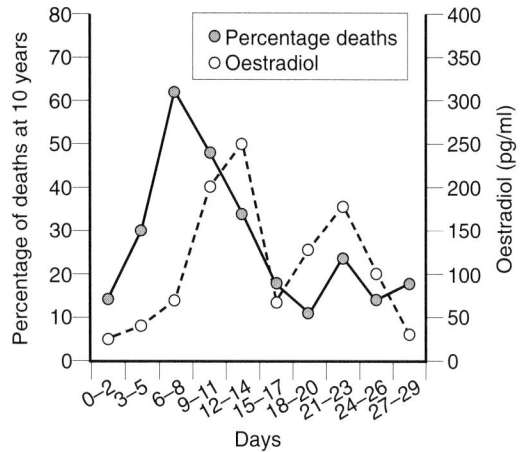

Fig. 7.2 Ten-year mortality rates by timing of surgery in the menstrual cycle. Group 1, surgery days 3–12; group 2, surgery on other days of menstrual cycle.

terone secreted by the corpus luteum. This was the basis of the analysis which was conducted at Guy's Hospital, London.[15] The study group comprised 560 premenopausal women with operable breast cancer treated at the Guy's Hospital Breast Unit, between 1975 and 1985. The original hospital notes of all the patients were examined to determine the date of last menstrual period (LMP) before the day of tumour excision. This information was available for 249 cases. Of the other 311, the reasons for exclusion were: LMP data unavailable (151), irregular periods (96), hysterectomy (24), using oral contraceptives (22), and miscellaneous (18) for reasons such as pregnancy lactation and hormone replacement therapy. The overall survival of those with known LMP and those with unknown LMP was found to be similar, indicating that there was no bias in the availability of LMP data.

Those with known LMP were divided into two groups based on phase of the cycle at the time of surgery. The first group of 75 women had tumours resected at a time of unopposed oestrogen (days 3–12), and the second of 174 underwent surgery at a time of low oestrogen (days 1–2) or in the luteal phase (days 13–28). A comparison of known prognostic factors, such as tumour size, tumour type, axillary nodal status, steroid receptor status and primary and adjuvant treatment, showed a similar distribution in both groups.

As is shown in Fig. 7.1, there was a significant difference in the survival of the groups after 10 years with 58% of those treated between days 3 and 12 being alive compared with 84% of those undergoing surgery at other times. Although there was a slight difference in node-negative cases operated on at the two different times, the main effect was seen in node-positive women. Only 33% were alive when tumour excision was performed between days 3 and 13 compared with 78% treated at other times of the cycle. The magnitude of this effect was greater than that of any known form of adjuvant therapy.

When the various prognostic subgroups were examined, it emerged that there was a significant effect of timing of surgery in patients with grade I/II tumours as well as those with grade III lesions, although less so in the latter group. The magnitude of the effect was similar in patients with ER/PR-positive and -negative tumours. In terms of tumour size, no effect was found in patients with cancers greater than 4 cm in diameter. A multivariate analysis of prognostic factors for survival showed that the significant independent variables were: number of involved axillary nodes ($\chi^2 = 33.3$); LMP day ($\chi^2 = 33.1$); tumour type/grade ($\chi^2 = 23.5$); and patient age ($\chi^2 = 4.6$). Figure 7.2 gives the 10-year mortality rates for patients grouped in 3-day intervals of operation during the cycle and shows clearly the pattern of mortality which is very similar to the expected oestradiol levels at these times. This supports the hypothesis of a relationship between unopposed oestrogen and prognosis.

To follow up these remarkable findings, a second study examined outcome in 150 premenopausal patients treated between 1985 and 1990.[16] Again there was a highly significant difference in relapse-free survival of those treated between days 3 and 13, and those operated on at other times of the cycle. The magnitude of the effect was less than that seen in the previous study. One aspect of management had changed during that time. An increasing use was made of core needle biopsy to make a preoperative diagnosis of malignancy with the result that some who had excision performed at a 'favourable' time of the cycle had previously had a core needle performed at an 'unfavourable' time. Figure 7.3 shows the relapse-free survival of those patients undergoing excision at a 'favourable time'. It shows that, among the albeit small group who had previously undergone core biopsy between days 3 and 13, all had relapsed within 3 years compared with none who underwent needle biopsy at other times. This suggests that the trauma of core biopsy might have been responsible for releasing viable metastatic cells from the primary tumour. A multivariate analysis of factors predicting recurrence in the group undergoing surgery at a favourable time

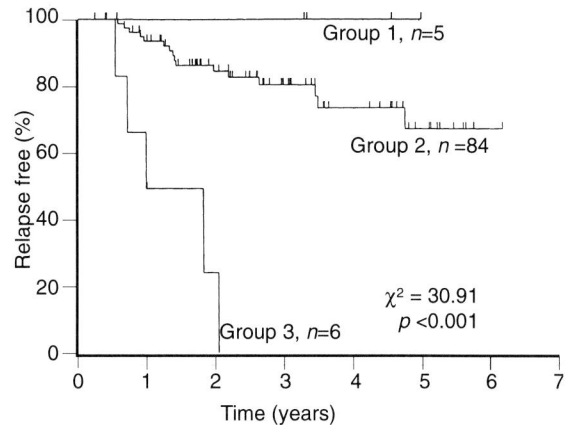

Fig. 7.3 Relapse-free survival of women undergoing tumour excision at a favourable time. Group 1, core biopsy also at a favourable time; group 2, no core biopsy; and group 3, core biopsy at an unfavourable time.

showed that the significant variables were: tumour type/grade ($\chi^2 = 6.9$); needle biopsy ($\chi^2 = 4.9$); tumour size ($\chi^2 = 4.6$); and lymph node status ($\chi^2 = 4.5$).

By this time, Senie et al had published confirmatory findings from the Sloan-Kettering Cancer Center.[17] In a study of 283 women treated by mastectomy and axillary clearance, of those who had surgery in the follicular phase (days 1–13) relapse occurred in 43% compared with 29% in those having luteal phase surgery (days 14–28). A significant effect was observed only in those patients with positive axillary nodes. In an accompanying editorial, McGuire expressed scepticism about this finding because it was based on a retrospective rather than a prospective study and concluded that, if sufficient subgroups or time intervals within the cycle were analysed, a statistically significant association might arise by chance.[18]

Gregory et al countered this by arguing that the results found followed an a priori hypothesis and were not the result of a 'data-dredging exercise'.[19] Furthermore, the level of signifi-

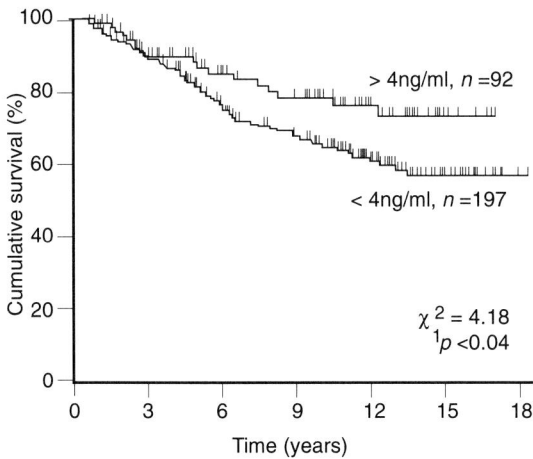

Fig. 7.4 Overall survival of breast cancer patients based on progesterone 4 ng/ml or less and more than 4 ng/ml.

cance found in the Guy's study[15] was 6×10^{-8}, so that the probability of a chance finding was less than one in a million. Using a random assignment of results with a p value of 0.05 there were 28% positive cases, whereas with the p value of 6×10^{-8}, there were no positive results in 10 000 further repetitions. Finally, a meta-analysis of the 10 papers reporting studies at that time showed that, overall, there was a significant overall effect of timing of surgery (p = 0.003). Testing for heterogeneity however gave a p value of 0.009, suggesting that the differences between the results from various centres could not be explained by chance and were not the result of a normal distribution.

ENDOCRINE STUDIES

All the published results on timing of surgery had been based on calculations derived from the LMP before surgery. However, it could be argued that it is the next menstrual period after surgery that is important, because the stress of surgery and a diagnosis of malignancy could

lead to delay in ovulation or possibly an anovular cycle. The hormonal status at the time of tumour excision could be the most important determinant of outcome. Luckily, at Guy's Hospital, as part of a study of prognostic factors in early breast cancer, blood had been taken and frozen serum stored from 471 premenopausal patients.[20] In 289 (61%), this had been taken within 4 days of surgery. The date of the LMP was known in 234 (81%).

Both oestradiol (E2) and progesterone (P) were measured by radioimmunoassay. For those patients with known LMP there was no relationship between phase of the cycle and serum E2, because of wide interindividual variations. However, P levels did show a correlation, with P levels 4 ng/ml or less in 92% of those in the follicular phase and over 4 ng/ml in 56% of those in the putative luteal phase. When the patients were subdivided on a basis of progesterone – 4 ng/ml or less and over 4 ng/ml, it was found that there was a significant difference in overall survival, as shown in Fig. 7.4. This was true both for the entire group and when subdivided into node-negative and node-positive cases. The relationship between outcome of surgery in relation to phase of the menstrual cycle was demonstrated independently.

PATHOLOGICAL STUDIES

The impact of menstrual phase on prognosis suggests that cohesiveness of malignant cells might be modified, either as a direct effect on the tumour or possibly because of endocrine stimulation of hormone-sensitive peritumoral normal tissue. Whatever the explanation, this might be manifest in histopathological changes in or around the tumour. For this reason histopathological review was conducted to determine whether there were detectable changes in specimens removed from patients at different times in the menstrual cycle.[21] The study comprised specimens from 363 premenopausal patients which were reviewed to determine the incidence of vascular invasion around the tumours together with axillary

Table 7.2 Pathological features and timing of surgery		
	Group 1 (days 3–12)	Group 2 (other days)
Node-positive (%)	62	47
Vascular invasion positive (%)	47	33

Table 7.3 Multivariate analysis of prognostic factors for survival		
Factor	χ^2	p value
Node number	40.7	<0.0001
Tumour type/grade	36.8	<0.0001
LMP day	27.5	<0.0001
Tumour size	3.9	0.05
Age	2.0	0.16
Vascular invasion	2.0	0.15

lymph node status in those undergoing surgery on days 3–12, and those at other times in the cycle. The results are summarized in Table 7.2.

There was a significant increase in axillary nodal positivity in those undergoing surgery between days 3 and 12 ($p = 0.01$), despite there being no difference in distribution of tumour size or histological grade in the two groups. The mean number of involved nodes was 4.2 in group 1 and 2.6 in group 2. It is possible that some axillary micrometastases might have arisen perioperatively from disseminated tumour emboli. That there was a difference in cancer cell cohesiveness is manifested by the difference in incidence of vascular invasion: 33% in group 1 and 47% in group 2. The presence of tumour emboli within lymphatics and veins may indicate that, in some cases, this may be a 'snapshot' of tumour dissemination caused by the trauma of surgery.

Although it could be argued that the observed effects of timing of surgery result from a chance skewed distribution of prognostic variables so that the observed endocrine effects were spurious, Table 7.3 shows a multivariate analysis of prognostic factors demonstrating that LMP is an independently significant variable.

This study showed that the likelihood of both local vascular invasion and the presence of axillary nodal micrometastases might be influenced by the phase of the menstrual cycle, with those undergoing surgery at a time of

unopposed oestrogen being more likely to suffer tumour spread. It was of interest therefore to determine whether any similar effect could be observed in postmenopausal cases.

Survival in postmenopausal breast cancer patients has been shown to be inversely related to body weight in most studies,[22–27] but such a relationship is less obvious in premenopausal women.[28] Although there is a relationship between body weight and other prognostic factors such as tumour size and axillary lymph node involvement, the effect of obesity remains an independent factor on multivariate analysis.[22,26] The mechanism through which menopausal status and body weight influence survival is uncertain, although it is known that most circulating oestrogens in postmenopausal women are derived from peripheral aromatization of adrenal androgens in subcutaneous fat. Thus more obese women have higher plasma levels of oestrogens.[29]

A review was conducted of 393 postmenopausal women with operable breast cancer treated in Guy's Hospital Breast Unit between 1987 and 1991.[30] Weight was measured at the time of diagnosis and vascular invasion was recorded as being present or absent. Vascular invasion (VI) was seen in slightly more of the 50 perimenopausal patients than in the 343 postmenopausal cases (44% vs 36%). In the tumour specimens from postmenopausal patients weighing 50 kg or less, VI was observed in 11% as compared with 45% of those

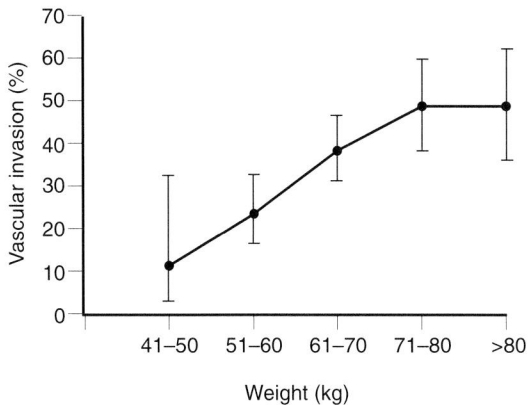

Fig. 7.5 Body weight and vascular invasion in postmenopausal women with breast cancer.

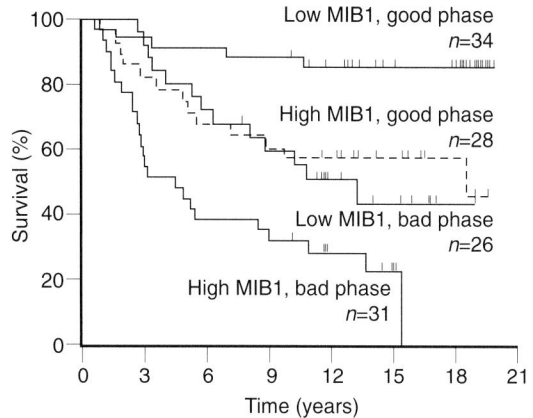

Fig. 7.6 Overall survival of premenopausal breast cancer patients in relation to MIB1 score and timing of surgery.

weighing more than 80 kg ($p = 0.02$). There was a close relationship between body weight and incidence of vascular invasion as shown in Fig. 7.5. Furthermore the 5-year survival of those with VI was 74% compared with 91% for those without ($p<0.0001$).

Thus body weight may influence survival in postmenopausal patients with breast cancer, possibly as a result of the presence of unopposed circulating oestrogens at the time of surgery. Oestrogens, by altering cohesiveness of breast cancer cells and modulating secretion of proteases, could influence invasive potential so that excision of tumours in an environment where oestrogens are unopposed could have a deleterious impact on survival.

Previous studies had shown that the effect of timing of surgery in premenopausal patients was present in those with ER-positive and ER-negative tumours, and occurred in those with well-differentiated and poorly differentiated tumours, although to a less significant extent in the latter group. As the phenomenon might result from changes in cell cohesion, and because this could be related to growth rate of tumours, it was of interest to determine whether this was affected by timing of surgery. The most objective way of measuring prolifera-

tion in histopathological material is by flow cytometry, which measures DNA content, and allows calculation of the percentage of cells in S phase. For flow cytometry to be carried out on paraffin-processed tissue, a substantial amount of tissue has to be cut from the block which unfortunately precludes its use on small tumours. Immunohistochemical assessment of proliferative activity has, however, the potential to overcome many of the problems associated with other methods.

The antibody MIB1, which recognizes part of the Ki67 protein in fixed tissue,[31] was used to determine proliferation of breast cancers excised in different phases of the menstrual cycle. Proliferative activity was assessed as the percentage of MIB1-stained cells in the sample. Monoclonal antibody staining was strongly correlated with S-phase fraction ($p<0.001$) and histological grade ($\chi^2 = 18.39$, $p<0.001$), but did not change significantly through the menstrual cycle. Both MIB1 score and time of surgery correlated with overall survival ($\chi^2 = 17.26$, $p<0.01$ and $\chi^2 = 17.45$, $p<0.01$ respectively). The combination of MIB1 score and timing of surgery strongly predicted survival ($\chi^2 = 31.52$, $p<0.01$). Figure 7.6 shows that women with slowly proliferating tumours operated in the

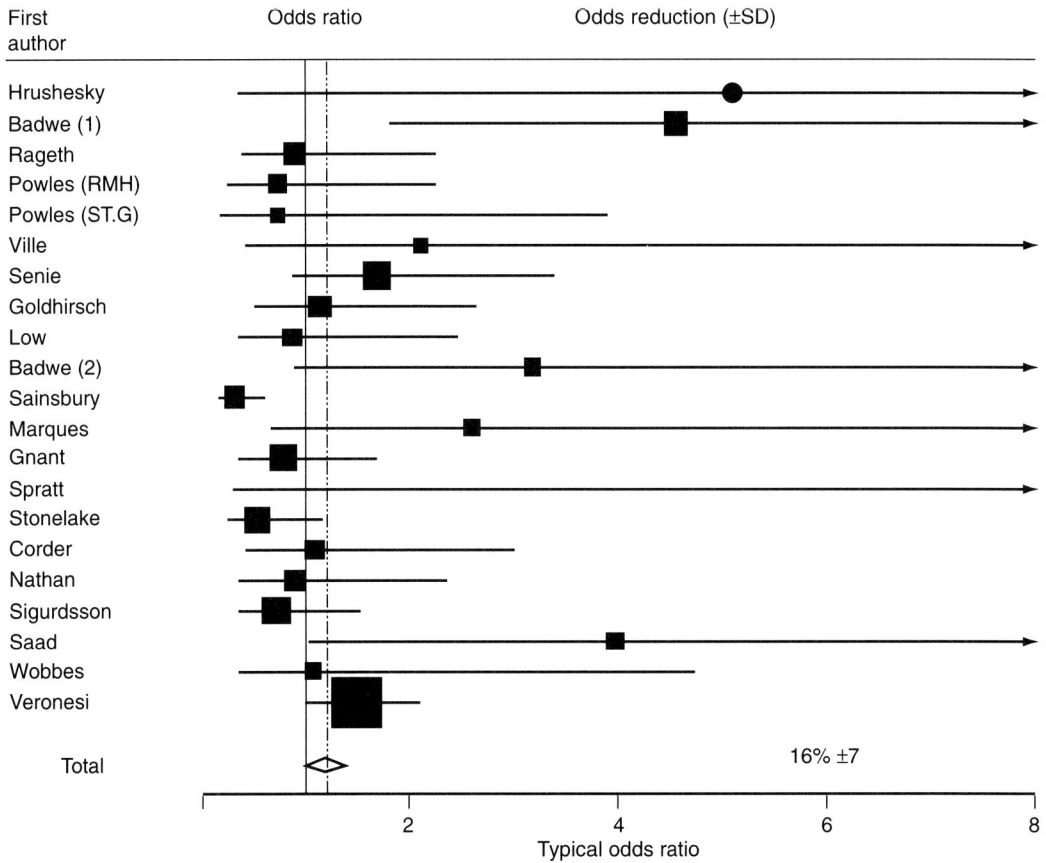

Fig. 7.7 Meta-analysis of 5-year survival rates in published studies on timing of surgery.

luteal phase had the best prognosis, whereas those with rapidly proliferating cancers excised in the follicular phase fared worst. Thus there may be a survival advantage for women with rapidly proliferating cancers who undergo excision during the luteal phase of the menstrual cycle.

META-ANALYSIS

Just as there was a series of contradictory articles after Hruschevsky's first article, there were many gainsayers after the Guy's *Lancet* paper. In 1994, Veronesi et al reported their large series of 1175 premenopausal patients with known date of LMP before surgery.[32] Of

the 525 who underwent surgery in the follicular phase, there were 192 unfavourable events (37%), compared with the 650 who had luteal phase resections and suffered 192 events (30%). In a Cox multivariate analysis, the overall hazard ratio for the entire group was 1.33 ($p = 0.006$), and 1.43 for node-positive cases ($p = 0.03$). There was no significant effect of timing of surgery in node-negative cases.

The article was accompanied by a sceptical editorial, which questioned the reality of the finding and concluded that it was too soon to change policy with regards to timing of surgery.[33] Surgeons were therefore encouraged to maintain the status quo, which could have meant many women suffering relapse as a

Table 7.4 Three-year relapse-free survival in relation to residual carcinoma (RC) at the biopsy site and axillary lymph node status

Nodes	Premenopausal			Postmenopausal		
	RC– (%)	RC+ (%)	p	RC– (%)	RC+ (%)	p
0	86	83	<0.05	79	72	<0.05
1–3	81	59	<0.001	72	68	<0.05
≥ 4	78	37	<0.05	55	41	<0.05

result of follicular phase surgery. For this reason a meta-analysis of the 21 published papers was carried out.[34]

The results are shown in Fig. 7.7, and the overview demonstrated that there was a significant effect of timing of surgery ($p = 0.02$) with a 16% overall reduction in deaths among those who had surgery in the luteal phase. The test for heterogeneity in observed/expected deaths was highly significant ($p = 0.000005$), moreover showing that the scatter of the results was not caused by a normal distribution, and was not the result of chance. It was noted that the large centres reporting positive results (Milan, Sloan-Kettering and Guy's) all had a very structured approach to surgical management which may have enabled the effect to be demonstrated.

PRESENT SITUATION

At Guy's Hospital the policy with regard to timing of surgery was changed in 1991, so that all women over the age of 25 with potentially malignant lesions were offered excision biopsy in the luteal phase. The survival of patients treated since the time of change of policy is shown in Fig. 7.8, with this preliminary result indicating an improved outcome since the re-scheduling of timing of surgery. Very few other centres have adopted such a policy and a study is planned to examine peripheral blood taken during surgery at Guy's Hospital and at another centre where surgery is not timed.

Circulating tumour cells will be sought using polymerase chain reaction (PCR), which will also examine the protease activity of these cells.

Another potentially interesting aspect will be determining the effect of complete versus incomplete excision. The residual tumour cells might be more likely to metastasize during the trauma of subsequent surgery. That this may be the case is suggested by the findings of the Danish Breast Cancer Co-operative Group.[35] A series of 3264 patients with breast cancer were treated by excision biopsy, frozen section and

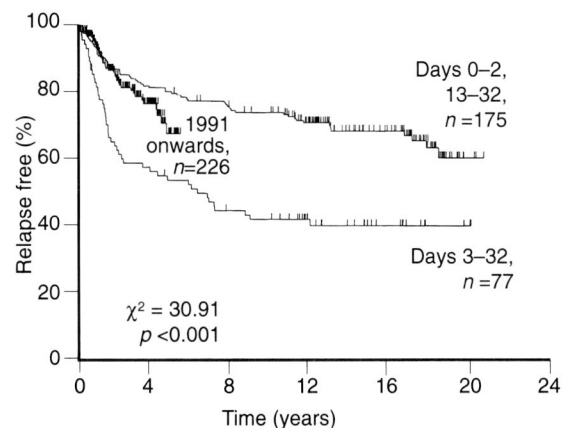

Fig. 7.8 Relapse-free survival of premenopausal patients treated at Guy's Hospital since 1991 compared with those treated 1985–1990.

immediate modified radical mastectomy. Of these 1551 (48%) were found to have residual carcinoma at the biopsy site after histological examination of the mastectomy specimen. Table 7.4 shows the 3-year relapse-free survival percentage of both pre- and postmenopausal patients in relation to residual carcinoma and axillary lymph node status.

Table 7.4 shows that there was a significantly better survival among those who had no residual cancer in the mastectomy and that this occurred in all the subgroups but was most significant in premenopausal women with one to three axillary nodes containing metastases. Thus a situation that exists for only 10–30 minutes (residual cancer while awaiting mastectomy) has a profound impact on prognosis. This suggests that the trauma of cutting through the cancer may enable tumour cells to metastasize.

The simplest way to improve prognosis is to re-schedule surgery for the luteal phase of the cycle, although this may be difficult in some hospitals because of pressure on beds. An alternative approach would be a pharmacological intervention, using a progestin to produce an artificial luteal phase. The efficacy of this approach could be determined by the effect on vascular invasion and subsequently relapse-free survival. Similarly in postmenopausal women an oestrogen/progestin combination could be used, or alternatively first-line tamoxifen before surgery. It is important that in the gadarene rush to test ever more toxic chemotherapy regimens, a simple endocrine approach that can save lives is not neglected. The slow acceptance of the findings on timing of surgery may have already resulted in unnecessary loss of lives.

SYNOPSIS

- The timing of surgery may affect the prognosis in premenopausal breast cancer patients with a significantly better survival in those undergoing luteal phase tumour excision.
- This effect is more pronounced in women with rapidly proliferating cancers, and those with axillary nodal involvement but is independent of the oestrogen receptor status of the tumour.
- Women with blood progesterone levels 4 ng/ml have a significantly better survival than those with progesterone levels of 4 ng/ml or less.
- Tumours excised from premenopausal women during the luteal phase are less likely to show evidence of vascular invasion than those biopsied in the follicular phase.
- Heavier postmenopausal women with breast cancer, who have more endogenous blood oestrogens, are more likely to have tumours with evidence of vascular invasion.

REFERENCES

1. Boyd NF, Campbell JE, Germanson T et al. Body weight and prognosis in breast cancer. *J Natl Cancer Inst* 1981; **67:** 785–9.
2. Mansi JL, Berger U, Eaton D et al. Micrometastases in bone marrow in patients with breast cancer: evaluation as an early predictor of bone marrow metastases. *BMJ* 1987; **295:** 1093–6.
3. Cootie RJR, Rosen PP, Hakes TB et al. Monoclonal antibodies detect occult breast carcinoma metastases in the bone marrow of patients with early disease. *Am J Surg Pathol* 1988; **12:** 333–40.
4. Nissen-Meyer R, Kjellgren K, Malmio K et al. Surgical adjuvant chemotherapy. *Cancer* 1978; **41:** 2088–98.
5. Fentiman IS. Mastalgia mostly merits masterly inactivity. *Br J Clin Pract* 1992; **46:** 158.
6. Goring JJ, Anderson TJ, Battersby S et al. Proliferative and secretory activity in human breast during natural and artificial menstrual cycles. *Am J Pathol* 1988; **130:** 193–204.
7. Ratajzak HV, Sothern RB, Hrushevsky WJM. Estrous influence on surgical cure of breast cancer. *J Exp Med* 1988; **168:** 73–83.

8. Hrushevsky WJM, Bluming AZ, Gruber SA, Sothern RB. Menstrual influence on surgical cure of breast cancer. *Lancet* 1989; **ii:** 949–52.

9. Powles TJ, Jones AL, Ashley S, Tidy A. Menstrual effect on surgical cure of breast cancer. *Lancet* 1989; **ii:** 1343–4.

10. Goldhirsch A, Gelber RD, Forbes J et al. Timing breast cancer surgery. *Lancet* 1991; **338:** 692.

11. Ville Y, Lasry S, Spyratos F et al. Menstrual status and breast cancer surgery. *Breast Cancer Res Treat* 1990; **16:** 119.

12. Beatson CT. On treatment of inoperable cases of carcinoma of the mamma: suggestions for a new method of treatment with illustrative cases. *Lancet* 1896; **ii:** 104–7.

13. Jensen EV, De Sombre ER, Jungblut PW. Estrogen receptors in hormone-responsive tissues and tumors. In: *Endogenous Factors Influencing Host-Tumor Balance*. Wissler RW, Dao TL, Wood S Jr, eds. Chicago: University of Chicago, 1967: 15–30.

14. Rochefort H, Angereau P, Briozzo P et al. Structure, function, regulation and clinical significance of the 52K pro-cathepsin D secretion by breast cancer cells. *Biochimie* 1988; **70:** 43–9.

15. Badwe RA, Gregory WM, Chaudary MA et al. Timing of surgery during menstrual cycle and survival of premenopausal women with operable breast cancer. *Lancet* 1991; **337:** 1261–4.

16. Badwe RA, Richards MA, Fentiman IS et al. Surgical procedures, menstrual cycle phase, and prognosis in operable breast cancer. *Lancet* 1991; **338:** 815–16.

17. Senie RT, Rosen PP, Rhodes P, Lesser ML. Timing of breast cancer excision during the menstrual cycle influences duration of disease-free survival. *Ann Intern Med* 1991; **115:** 337–342.

18. McGuire WL. The optimal timing of surgery: low tide or high tide? *Ann Intern Med* 1991; **115:** 401–3.

19. Gregory WM, Richards MA, Fentiman IS. Optimal timing of initial breast cancer surgery. *Ann Intern Med* 1992; **116:** 268–9.

20. Mohr PE, Wang DY, Gregory WM et al. Serum progesterone and prognosis in operable breast cancer. *Br J Cancer* 1996; **73:** 1552–5.

21. Badwe RA, Bettelheim R, Millis RR, et al. Cyclical tumour variations in premenopausal women with early breast cancer. *Eur J Cancer* 1995; **31A:** 2181–4.

22. Tartter PI, Papatestas AE, Ioannovich J et al. Cholesterol and obesity as prognostic factors in breast cancer. *Cancer* 1981; **47:** 2222–7.

23. Boyd NF, Campbell JE, Germanson T et al. Body weight and prognosis in breast cancer. *J Natl Cancer Inst* 1981; **67:** 785–9.

24. Newman SC, Miller AB, Howe GR. A study of the effect of weight and dietary fat on breast cancer survival time. *Am J Epidemiol* 1986; **123:** 767–73.

25. Tretli S, Haldorsen T, Ottestad L. The effect of pre-morbid height and weight on survival of breast cancer patients. *Br J Cancer* 1990; **62:** 299–303.

26. Vatten LJ, Foss OP, Kvinnsland S. Overall survival of breast cancer patients in relation to preclinically determined total serum cholesterol, BMI, height and cigarette smoking: A population based study. *Eur J Cancer* 1991; **27:** 641–6.

27. Senie RT, Rosen PP, Rhodes P et al. Obesity at diagnosis of breast cancer influences duration of disease free survival. *Ann Intern Med* 1991; **116:** 26–32.

28. Greenberg ER, Vessey MP, McPherson K et al. Body size and survival in premenopausal breast cancer. *Br J Cancer* 1985; **51:** 691–7.

29. Grodin JM, Siiteri PK, MacDonald PC. Source of estrogen production in postmenopausal women. *J Clin Endocrinol Metab* 1973; **36:** 207–14.

30. Badwe RA, Fentiman IS, Millis RR, Gregory WM. Body weight and vascular invasion in postmenopausal women with breast cancer. *Br J Cancer* 1997; **75:** 910–13.

31. Cattoretti G, Becker MHG, Key G et al. Monoclonal antibodies against recombinant parts of the Ki67 antigen (MIB1 and MIB3) detect proliferating cells in microwave-processed formalin fixed paraffin sections. *J Pathol* 1992; **168:** 357–63.

32. Veronesi U, Luini A, Mariani L et al. Effect of menstrual phase on surgical treatment of breast cancer. *Lancet* 1994; **343:** 1544–6.

33. Astrow AB. Timing of breast cancer surgery: nodes hormones and retrospectoscopy. *Lancet* 1994; **343:** 1517.

34. Fentiman IS, Gregory WM, Richards MA. Effect of menstrual cycle phase on surgical treatment of breast cancer. *Lancet* 1994; **344:** 402.

35. Andersen JA, Blichert-Toft M, Jaergaard J et al. Prognostic significance of residual cancer tissue after diagnostic biopsy in breast carcinoma. Three-year short-term results. *Eur J Cancer* 1984; **20:** 765–70.

8

Screening

I could never make out what those damned dots meant.
Lord Randolph Churchill

Evidence of benefit • Disadvantages • Breast self-examination • Compliance • Screening interval • Mammographic views • Histopathology • Assessment

For many years there were fierce arguments between those who knew that mammographic screening was a life-saving exercise and others, more cynical, who maintained that radiographs prolonged lead time but did not have any impact on prognosis. Nowadays even the most sceptical are forced to admit that screening mammography reduces mortality from breast cancer. The debate has now shifted as to the cost–benefit of the exercise and the extent to which public funds should be committed to it. This is a particular concern in Europe because of widely differing incidence rates in the individual states. If scarce health resources are to be invested in mammographic screening, it is most important that maximum use is made of opportunities to educate women about the disease and improve the quality of treatment for early breast cancer.

EVIDENCE OF BENEFIT

Since the original demonstration of reduced breast cancer mortality among screened women who took part in the Hospital Insurance Plan (HIP) trial,[1] there has been a gradual accretion of evidence showing that a significant saving of lives can be achieved. Much of the pioneering work was conducted in Sweden, and data from five randomized trials were analysed in an

Table 8.1 Breast cancer deaths in five Swedish randomized trials of mammographic screening

Centre	Screened	Controls	Relative risk
Malmö	87	108	0.81
Kopparberg	132	91	0.68
Östergötland	119	139	0.82
Stockholm	53	40	0.80
Gothenburg	27	47	0.86
All	**418**	**425**	**0.77**

overview.[2] The trials, conducted in Malmö, Kopparberg, Östergötland, Stockholm and Gothenburg, included a total of 282 777 women followed for 5–13 years. The age at entry was 40–74 and all fatal breast cancer cases were reviewed blindly by an independent end-point committee. As shown in Table 8.1, there was a consistent reduction in deaths from breast cancer in the screened group in all five studies. Overall there were 23% fewer deaths from breast cancer among those randomized to

Table 8.2 Relative risks of breast cancer mortality from a meta-analysis based on age and screening variable

Variable	Women aged 40–49	Women aged 50–74
Case-control study	1.23	0.45
Randomized trial	0.92	0.77
Single-view radiograph	1.02	0.70
Two-view radiograph	0.87	0.83
Interval 12 months	0.99	0.77
Interval 18–33 months	0.88	0.77
Breast examination		
No	0.91	0.76
Yes	0.93	0.80
Follow-up 7–9 years	1.02	0.73
Follow-up 10–12 years	0.83	0.76

From Kerlikowske et al.[3]

screening. The greatest effect was seen in those who were aged 50–69 at the time of randomization (relative risk or RR = 0.71), whereas those aged 40–48 showed a non-significant mortality reduction of 13%. No effect on mortality was seen among those aged 40–48 until 8 years after randomization.

Subsequently a larger meta-analysis was conducted which included these five trials plus four other randomized trials and four case-control studies.[3] Overall the relative risk of death from breast cancer was 0.74 in screened women aged 50–74 but did not differ significantly from unity in those aged 40–49. A subgroup analysis based on age and screening variables is given in Table 8.2. There was a consistent statistically significant reduction in relative risk in all screened women aged 50–74, but no significant effect in any of the subgroups

aged 40–49, except after 10–12 years of follow-up. After that time the relative risk was 0.83, a 17% reduction, but such a benefit could have been achieved by starting screening at age 50.

In the Netherlands, nationwide mammographic screening every 2 years was instigated in 1988. The National Evaluation Team have presented the results up to January 1993.[4] At that time 550 000 women aged 50–69 had been invited and 71% had attended for screening. Breast cancers were detected in 6.8 per 1000 women screened and 36% of the lesions were either ductal carcinoma in situ (DCIS) or invasive and less than 11 mm in diameter. When the cancers detected by screening were compared with those presenting clinically, 20% were over 20 mm in diameter whereas 50% of the symptomatic cases had tumours over 20 mm. These results would support a future mortality reduction among the Dutch population.

DISADVANTAGES

A major concern about mammography was the dose of radiation to which the breasts were exposed. In the HIP study the average skin dose was 80 mGy (8 rad) which would lead to a cumulative exposure of 8 Gy if triennial mammography was performed between ages 45 and 75.[5] This would lead to a doubling in the incidence of breast cancer, as was found in women exposed to multiple fluoroscopies for tuberculosis.[6] Great technical improvements mean, however, that the radiation dosage from each mammogram is now 0.001 Gy (0.1 rad). This dose would lead to an excess of four cancers per million women screened after a 10-year latency period.[7] This is a similar level of risk to taking a 10-mile car journey, smoking one-eighth of a cigarette, or living for 3 minutes at the age of 60.[8]

To obtain good images breast compression is necessary and this can cause discomfort, reported as moderate by 36% and extreme by 9% of women participating in the Canadian National Breast Screening Study.[9] It is possible that this trauma could lead to spread of malignant cells. Van Netten et al hypothesized that, as DCIS may be found in up to 18% of younger women, compression during mammography might lead to rupture of ducts with spillage of malignant cells into surrounding stroma giving them the potential for invasion and distant dissemination. This remains purely speculative because further genetic alterations may be necessary before non-invasive cells acquire an invasive capability.

What is more striking is, however, the difference in breast cancer mortality in screened and non-screened cases in the first 1–2 years after entry to the trial. In all trials there is a small increase in breast cancer deaths in the screened group. A good example of this is provided by the Canadian National Breast Screening Study.[10] In one part of the trial 25 214 women aged 40–49 were offered mammography and clinical examination annually and 25 216 served as unscreened controls. There were 38 deaths from breast cancer in the screened group and 28 in the unscreened group. Within the first 2 years there were 16 screened deaths and 10 unscreened deaths.

Of course these differences are not statistically significant but they are apparent in all screening trials. Thus a few women with breast cancers may suffer an earlier death from breast cancer as a result of screening. It would be of great interest to conduct a multicentre study of tumour histology among women dying of breast cancer within 2 years of screen detection. If there were a higher incidence of vascular invasion this might be used as a selection criterion for adjuvant therapy.

A further disadvantage of screening is that lesions will be detected, excised and found to be benign. Thus the screenee will have had an unnecessary biopsy and suffered anxiety because of suspected malignancy. As with all activities, improvement comes with experience but takes time. Figure 8.1 shows the changes in malignant/benign ratio of biopsies taken by the Epping breast screening service.[11]

There was a gradual improvement over a 4-year period, with the ratio rising from 1.75 at the start to 10.5 by the end of the study. This

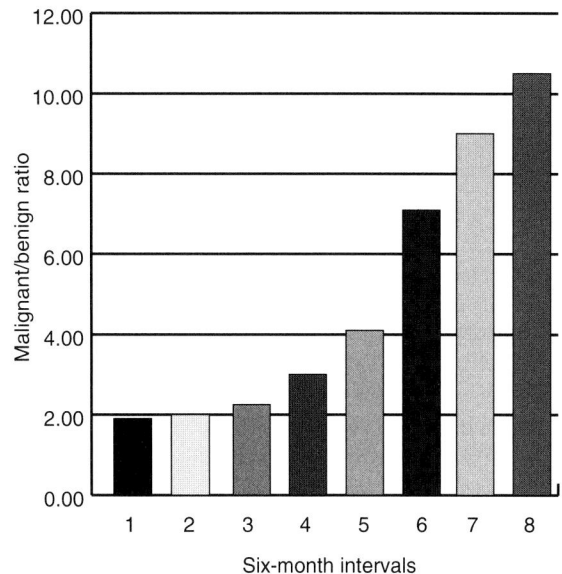

Fig. 8.1 Improvement with time in malignant/benign ratio. (From Warren.[11])

arose partly from increased use of ultrasonography, compression views and fine needle aspiration cytology, but also from greater understanding by the members of the multidisciplinary assessment team about the value and problem areas of others.

This is further illustrated by the results from the first 2 years of nationwide screening in Finland.[12] Of the 112 000 women screened, cancers were found in four per 1000. The detection rate was only 1.6 times that in non-screened women and the false positivity rate of screening was 4% and this varied by region from 1.6–5%. Thus these early results indicated that, although there was high compliance (88%), the specificity was less than that from randomized trials.

Between 10% and 15% of cancers will be undetected on mammograms and these cases may be falsely reassured after screening only to present subsequently with an interval lesion. Although the percentage is related to the interval between screening rounds, the number of views and the number of readers of mammograms, even under the optimal conditions, at least 5% will be missed.

BREAST SELF-EXAMINATION

After enormous expenditure on public education, the accepted view has become that breast self-examination (BSE) has not been demonstrated to reduce mortality from breast cancer in population studies. The situation is complicated by many women being unwilling to examine themselves, some because they find this distasteful, some because it worries them, and others because they have been told by a doctor or nurse that they have 'lumpy breasts'. It has become fashionable to denigrate BSE and encourage 'breast awareness', a distinction that may be lost on many. Women are advised not to examine themselves on a monthly basis but to be aware of changes. This is somewhat optimistic because small breast cancers, although capable of being detected by BSE, are typically asymptomatic; this may prove to be a difficult instruction to follow.

In the UK pilot trial of early detection of breast cancer, BSE was tested in two health districts: Huddersfield and Nottingham. Women were invited to classes where a film was shown followed by a talk. In addition, women attending open-access clinics were instructed by a specially trained nurse.[13] In Nottingham, 28% of women were performing BSE before the study but by one year later this rose to 47% among those who attended.[14] The results, shown in Table 8.3, were conflicting. In Huddersfield the observed mortality rate from breast cancer was less than expected whereas in Nottingham this was reversed. It was concluded that the value of BSE was unproven.

The World Health Organization has sponsored a randomized trial of BSE conducted in Moscow and St Petersburg and started in 1985.[15] A total of 193 000 women, aged 40–64, were randomized to training in BSE or to a control group. The study had sufficient power to detect a 30% reduction in breast cancer mortality, on the assumption that 50–70% of the

Table 8.3 Breast cancer deaths in districts participating in UK trial of BSE			
Centre	Observed	Expected	Relative risk
Huddersfield	91	116	0.78
Nottingham	232	193	1.20

From Ellman et al.[13]

study group continued to practise BSE. After 5 years, in St Petersburg, 190 breast cancers had been found in the BSE group and 192 in the control group, with no differences between the tumours in terms of mean size or incidence of axillary nodal involvement.

By the fourth year after training in BSE only 56% of that group were checking themselves five or more times a year. Of the BSE group 6% referred themselves because of a lump compared with 3% of controls. Significantly more benign breast biopsies were performed in the BSE group (RR = 1.5). These early results therefore suggested that BSE caused more harm than good in Russian women, although it is difficult to decide how much of an impact the political turmoil of the times had on the results. Certainly this trial cannot be taken as incontrovertible proof that BSE is of no value.

In a Japanese survey of BSE in breast cancer patients, it was found that 5% carried out an examination monthly, 35% occasionally and 60% not at all.[16] Of the few who carried out monthly BSE, their tumours were significantly smaller and much less likely to have axillary nodal metastases, as shown in Table 8.4. In addition, none of the monthly BSE group had relapsed. Occasional use of BSE was not associated with a reduced likelihood of having a T0/T1 tumour or of having axillary node negativity. This suggests that the few who carry out regular BSE are both much more likely to

Table 8.4 Relationship of tumour size and nodal status to pattern of BSE

Feature	Monthly BSE	Occasional	Never
Number	12	79	132
T0/T1	10 (83%)	33 (42%)	47 (36%)
Node -negative	11 (92%)	45 (57%)	82 (62%)

From Kurebayashi et al.[16]

detect small breast cancers and have a significantly improved prognosis.

Contrary results were found in a Finnish prospective study of 604 women with breast cancer who were interviewed and asked about BSE practices before diagnosis of disease.[17] Of the 448 who carried out regular BSE, only 34 (8%) had found their tumours as a result of BSE. There was no survival advantage for this small group of individuals.

Although some women will always be unhappy to carry out BSE, the proportion of those able to carry out a check can be improved by education. This was achieved in the Nottingham study,[14] and other experimental approaches may help. Ferris et al determined the baseline BSE rate (49%) in 907 women who were starting, restarting or continuing with oral contraceptives.[18] All the subjects were instructed in BSE and then randomised to receive OCs with a monthly prompt to perform BSE, or prompt-free packets. In a survey conducted after three months 46% of the unprompted group were carrying out monthly BSE, whereas 51% of the prompted group performed BSE once a month.

Clearly the available data do not support extensive commitment of resources to BSE education programmes. Forbidding women to

check themselves could be counterproductive and convince many that the medical profession are discouraging individuals from taking responsibility for their health. Those women who can perform effective BSE may benefit from an earlier diagnosis of a small cancer but this gain for the individual will probably never be detectable as a population mortality reduction.

COMPLIANCE

Premature deaths from breast cancer will not be prevented by screening unless sufficient women at risk attend for regular mammography. Thus it is essential that those in the correct age group are invited and that they are made to feel welcome, treated as healthy sentient beings and not unduly traumatized physically or psychologically by the process. Unless this is achieved regularly, there will be a reduced compliance with an insufficient mortality reduction to justify the expenditure.

Probably the most depressing statistics to emerge from screening trials came from the Edinburgh pilot study.[19] By the third round of screening only 53% of those invited actually took up the offer. Worse than this, of the breast cancers diagnosed subsequently in those who did not attend, 35% were stage III or IV. This implies that some of those who decide not to be re-screened will also deny breast symptoms and present with incurable disease. No matter how good the quality of screening, unless these recalcitrant individuals can be persuaded to participate regularly, lives will be lost unnecessarily.

In Nottingham a sample was taken of 200 women who did not re-attend for screening and compared with 200 who did.[20] Both groups had a similar perception of their risk of breast cancer but those who did not return had less knowledge about the disease. They were more likely to have had an unpleasant experience, at their previous visit, of mammography being painful (41% vs 10%) and worse than expected (32% vs 8%).

To estimate the effect of non-compliance on mortality, Glasziou applied a deattenuation method to a meta-analysis of five screening trials (HIP, Two-county, Malmö, Edinburgh and Stockholm).[21] If 100% compliance had been achieved the predicted reduction in breast cancer mortality was 0.37 (95% confidence interval 0.21, 0.49). As an almost 40% drop in breast cancer deaths is a target to be most ardently pursued, any experimental approaches to improving compliance should be explored no matter how illogical some may seem.

In south-east London 1000 women were sent, with their invitation to attend, a leaflet entitled 'Catch breast cancer in ten minutes'. Their response to the invitation was compared with 1000 controls who received no leaflet. The compliance rates of the two groups were identical. Others have also found that an increased effort does not necessarily lead to a higher compliance rate. Hurley et al assessed three public recruitment methods – community promotion, local media campaigns and propaganda to primary care doctors.[22] In addition, they examined five personal approaches: invitation letters with a specified appointment time or without a definite time, sent once or with a follow-up letter or telephone call to those who did not respond.

Not surprisingly, public strategies were less effective than personal approaches. The most effective was a letter with an appointment and a follow-up letter for non-attenders. This recruited 44% of those invited. However, the most cost-effective approach was an invitation without an appointment time, with a follow-up letter to non-compliers. This recruited 36% of women at a cost of £12.50.

The lack of impact of promotion to general practitioners is almost certainly the result of their pressure of work rather than opposition or lack of interest in screening. In the UK, Northern Ireland has one of the lowest compliance rates. A questionnaire was sent to 173 general practitioners of whom 152 (88%) replied.[23] Although three-quarters believed that screening was worthwhile, only 55% routinely asked their patients to participate, with 56% recording non-attendance in the patient's notes and only 20% contacting non-attenders.

Fletcher et al studied the impact of community-wide intervention in two North Carolina counties in a randomized trial.[24] A telephone survey was conducted before the study and again one year later. Interventions included training sessions for primary care physicians, a media campaign and lectures to community groups. In the experimental community the uptake of mammography rose from 35% to 55%, whereas in the control community it rose from 30% to 40%. An intention to undergo mammography was reported by 30% of the study community and by 17% of the control group.

To try and improve attendance at the second round of screening, a tailored letter, making reference to the prior round of screening was included or not included with the invitation to attend West Glasgow Breast Screening Centre.[25] This did not have any effect on the proportion returning for second round mammography. In another trial, 2368 women were randomized to receive a reminder letter with or without a subsequent letter from their doctor.[26] There was no impact of patient reminders but compliance improved from 22% in the unprompted to 36% in those who received a physician reminder.

There is particular concern that women from ethnic minorities might be disadvantaged by language or cultural barriers and not attend for screening. In particular, studies had shown an uptake of only 30–55% among Asian women compared with non-Asians.[27] After adjustment for socioeconomic status, however, the uptake by Asians and non-Asians did not differ significantly. Another confounding factor is the length of time that the individual has spent in the country. Those Asian women who had been in the UK for 5 years or more had a similar compliance rate to indigenous women.[28] Problems are exacerbated by minority naming systems so that there may be several women with identical names living in the same dwelling.

McAllister and Bowling interviewed 50 Chinese women from Liverpool, 50 Afro-Caribbean women in Camberwell, London and 50 Asian women from Huddersfield, York-

Table 8.5 Proportion of cancers detected at previous screen

Interval (months)	40–49 years (%)	50–59 years (%)	60–69 years (%)
0–11	62	88	85
12–23	32	70	72
24–29	–	54	55

From Tabar et al.[30]

shire.[29] They were aged 50–64 and the majority (95%) had lived in Britain for more than 10 years. All the Afro-Caribbean women had heard of breast cancer compared with 82% of Asians and 76% of the Chinese. In the Afro-Caribbean group, 84% were aware of mammographic screening, compared with 74% of Asians and 56% of the Chinese. Of those who had received an invitation for screening, three-quarters of each of the ethnic groups had attended. Thus, provided that screening invitation and the visit can be made culturally acceptable, there is every reason to expect a good compliance rate in women from ethnic minorities.

SCREENING INTERVAL

The interval between mammographic screens needs to be determined by both breast cancer biology and health economics, together with the age of women being screened. Tabar et al analysed the Swedish two-county study with regards to the time of diagnosis of interval cancers.[30] They compared the observed cancers in the screened group with those developing in the control group, with the ratio between the two representing the proportional incidence of interval cancers. As Table 8.5 shows, a 2-year interval in women aged 40–49 meant that only 32% of cancers were picked up whereas for older women a 2-year interval between screens meant that about 70% of cancers were discov-

ered. Thus if younger women were to be screened this would need to be an annual examination whereas for older women a 2-year interval was appropriate. In Britain the screening interval is 3 years.

This is potentially problematic. Woodman et al reported the interval cancer rate of 137 421 women from Manchester screened between 1988 and 1992.[31] There were 297 interval cancers. Taking the rate of detection as the proportion of the underlying incidence, 31% were diagnosed in the first year after screening, 52% in the second year and 82% in the third year. Thus by the third year the interval cancers were almost the same as would have been expected without screening. When interval cancer rates were compared with the Swedish two-county trial, there was a significantly increased risk in Manchester. In the two-county trial 54% of the underlying cancers were diagnosed as interval cases compared with 82% in Manchester.

In the Malmö trial where the interval between screens was 21 months, the mammograms of 94 interval cases were reviewed by two radiologists.[32] The tumour had been missed in 10 cases (11%), and there were non-specific changes in 22 (22%). There was no abnormality seen in 63 (67%) and these comprised the true interval cancers. Of the 66 cases where the tumour doubling time could be calculated, it was less than 100 days in 27 (41%) so that there was an over-representation of fast-growing cancers among the interval cases. This was reflected in the mortality figures with 20 (21%) dead at the time of reporting. The relative risk of dying was 2.3 for interval cases compared with screen-detected cases.

Although it would appear self-evident that biennial rather than triennial mammography should be offered in national programmes, the priority of this over-extending the age range upwards has yet to be determined. At present, in the UK there are insufficient suitably trained radiologists, but in the meantime the results of a UK Co-ordinating Committee on Cancer Research (UK CCCR) trial comparing 2- and 3-year intervals are awaited.

Table 8.6 Results of UK CCCR trial comparing single and two-view mammography

	Single view	Two view
Number screened	10 058	9982
Recall rate (%)	8.2	7
Prevalence	5.6/1000	6.5/1000

From Wald et al.[35]

MAMMOGRAPHIC VIEWS

The Swedish two-county study used single view oblique mammography and this was used as the basis for breast screening in the UK. With two retrospective studies suggesting that the addition of a craniocaudal view could increase the cancer detection by 9%,[33,34] associated uncertainty prompted the UK Co-ordinating Committee on Cancer Research (UK CCCR) to conduct a randomized trial comparing single view, two-view and two-view with or without double reporting.[35]

There was a significantly lower recall rate in those who had two views as shown in Table 8.6. This was also mirrored in those who were in the trial of double reading where the recall rate was 8.5% after single and 6.3% after two view. One hundred and fourteen cancers were found after two view but in only 92 after single view – an improvement of 24%.

The average cost of screening for breast cancer was calculated at 1992–3 values as £5310 for single view and £5330 for two view. As the calculated marginal cost of the extra cancers diagnosed by two views proved to be £5400, and this was similar to the average cost, it would appear that two-view should replace single view mammographic screening.

Blanks et al compared detection rates of cancers from UK screening centres using single view and two-view mammography in the prevalent round of screening.[36] In centres that used two views there were 3% more non-invasive cancers detected and 7% more invasive cancers measuring 1.5 cm or more. The most major improvement was the detection of small (< 1.5 cm) cancers, of which 42% were picked up by two rather than single view mammograms.

HISTOPATHOLOGY

Now it is accepted that screening reduces mortality, argument persists about the mechanism of the effect. Does mammography just pick up smaller lesions or are they less inherently aggressive, with phenotypic drift making larger lesions less well differentiated? Alternatively are screen-detected lesions mere aberrations which would not have evolved into clinical disease? Certainly the histopathology of screen-detected cancers demonstrates a different profile compared with symptomatic cases, as shown in Table 8.7. Anderson et al reported results from the Edinburgh Randomized Screening Project, with 500 study group cancers and 340 in unscreened controls.[37] There were significantly more cases of DCIS in the screened cases (15% vs 3%). In addition, of the screen-detected invasive cancers, 19% were of special type (tubular, mucoid, medullary papillary lobular and microinvasive).

Table 8.7 Comparative histopathology of screen-detected and symptomatic breast cancers

Screened (%)			Controls (%)			
DCIS	Well differentiated	Node negative	DCIS	Well differentiated	Node negative	Reference
15	19	77	3	9	43	Anderson et al[37]
–	38	83	–	13	57	Klemi et al[38]
16	39	84	3	34	49	Crisp et al[39]
16	–	73	6	–	54	Hakama et al[40]

Less than a quarter of the screen-detected cases had nodal involvement compared with over half the controls. Of those who were invited but did not attend, 44% had larger (>pT2) or inoperable cancers, as did 36% of controls. When the cancers detected at the prevalence screen were compared with those found at the incidence screens, 19% were node positive in the first round and 26% at incidence round. Special type tumours comprised 19% and 18% respectively.

In a study from south-west Finland, Klemi et al compared 126 screen-detected cancers with 125 symptomatic cases.[38] The screen cases had smaller cancers, with more well-differentiated tumours and less frequent axillary nodal metastases. After adjustment for small size, there was still a significantly reduced risk of nodal involvement (odds ratio 0.44) and of having a poorly differentiated cancer (OR = 0.2) in screen-detected cases.

Similar results were obtained by Crisp et al who compared 131 screened with 71 symptomatic cases from north-east England.[39] Of the screen-detected cases 15% were DCIS. Hakama et al reported a similar incidence of DCIS in Finland, comparing 248 screen-detected cancers with 490 symptomatic cases diagnosed before screening was started.[40] More of the screened group had small cancers and less frequent nodal involvement. Ploidy and S-phase fraction (SPF) were also measured in the two groups of patients. Of the prevalence screen cancers, 57% were diploid compared with 77% of incidence round cases. Only 33% of interval cases were diploid, as 25% of non-attenders and 43% of controls. They concluded that, because cancers diagnosed by screening had a low malignant potential, this was an indicator of overdiagnosis or length bias, rather than the result of an early diagnosis.

Review of 2459 cancers diagnosed in the Swedish two-county study suggested that there was a change in grade with increasing size of tumour.[41] This could be interpreted as an indicator of phenotypic drift or as a manifestation of the more rapid growth rate of poorly differentiated cancers. The likelihood is that the answer will be more complex with some tumours remaining well differentiated for their entire clinical course and others becoming more aggressive before clinical presentation, but still being curable if diagnosed mammographically.

ASSESSMENT

Those women found to have a mammographic abnormality may undergo severe distress when recalled for assessment. Indeed the level of anxiety may be higher than in a woman who has found a breast lump. To minimize distress the shortest possible interval should occur between notification of need for assessment and an appointment in the Assessment Clinic.[41]

In 1994–5 1507 605 women were invited and 77% participated in the NHS breast screening programme.[42] Of these 63 925 (5%) were recalled for assessment, and 6500 (10%) were eventually found to have breast cancer. It is those women with false-positive mammographic abnormalities who are the sufferers from screening and, the shorter the time that they spend in a state of suspicion of breast cancer, the more likely they will be to return for subsequent triennial mammography.

In 1995 there were 2000 benign biopsies giving a malignant:benign ratio of 3.25:1. This ratio will rise further as more centres become equipped with and gain experience of stereotactic core needle biopsy. If there is an equivocal clumping of microcalcification, cores containing the microcalcification which are shown to be benign can be taken as reasonable proof that the lesion is non-malignant, and an open biopsy can be avoided.

A small area of trabecular distortion may cause greater difficulty with a differential diagnosis of either a radial scar or a small tubular carcinoma. Frouge et al reported 40 cases with a preoperative diagnosis of a radial scar, of which only 50% proved to be benign.[43] Twelve of the lesions were pure carcinomas and eight were cancers associated with a radial scar. At review there was no discernible difference mammographically between the benign and malignant cases.

Ruiz-Sauri et al applied morphometry and flow cytometry to a series of 17 radial scars and six tubular carcinomas.[44] One case comprised contiguous radial scar and tubular carcinoma. Of the radial scars two were aneuploid on cytophotometry, and 50% of the tubular carcinomas were diploid. Even with sophisticated techniques unable at present to distinguish between the two lesions, women with such mammographic changes will continue to need an open biopsy to confirm the nature of the abnormality.

SYNOPSIS

- Mammography reduces breast cancer mortality by 30% in screened women aged 50 years or more.
- For a few women mammograms may increase the risk of early death from breast cancer.
- Women who carry out regular breast self-examination find smaller tumours but population studies have not shown a survival benefit.
- Compliance can be improved by reminders from general practitioners.
- Two-view mammography is better than single view in terms of improved cancer detection and reduced recall rate.
- Screening may be detecting not only smaller cancers, but also less aggressive lesions which would have changed their biological behaviour after further growth.

REFERENCES

1. Shapiro S. Evidence on screening for breast cancer from a randomised trial. *Cancer* 1977; **Suppl 6**: 2772–82.
2. Nystrom L, Rutqvist LE, Wall S et al. Breast cancer screening with mammography: overview of Swedish randomised trials. *Lancet* 1993; **341**: 973–8.
3. Kerlikowske K, Grady D, Rubin SM et al. Efficacy of screening mammography. A meta-analysis. *JAMA* 1995; **273**: 149–54.
4. De Koning HJ, Fracheboud J, Boer R et al. Nation-wide breast cancer screening in the Netherlands: support for breast cancer mortality reduction. *Int J Cancer* 1995; **60**: 777–80.
5. Strax P, Venet L, Shapiro S. Value of mammography in reduction of mortality from breast cancer in mass screening. *Am J Roentgenol Ther Nucl Med* 1973; **112**: 686–9.
6. Delarue NC, Gale G, Ronald A. Multiple fluoroscopy of the chest: carcinogenicity for the female breast and implications for breast cancer screening programmes. *Can Med Assoc J* 1975; **21**: 1405–13.
7. Feig S. Radiation risk from mammography: is it clinically significant? *AJR* 1984; **143**: 469–75
8. Pochin EE. Why be quantitative about radiation risk estimates? Lecture 2, Lauriston S Taylor

lecture series in radiation protection and measurements. Washington DC: National Council on Radiation Protection and Measurements, 1978.

9. Baines CJ, To T, Wall C. Women's attitudes to screening after participation in the National Breast Screening Study. *Cancer* 1990; **65:** 1663–9

10. Miller AB, Baines CJ, To T, Wall S. Canadian National Breast Screening Study: 1. Breast cancer detection and death rates among women aged 40 to 49 years. *Can Med Assoc J* 1992; **147:** 1459–75.

11. Warren R. Team learning and breast cancer screening. *Lancet* 1991; **338:** 514.

12. Hakama M, Elovainio L, Kajante R, Louhivuori K. Breast cancer screening as public health policy in Finland. *Br J Cancer* 1991; **64:** 962–4.

13. Ellman R, Moss SM, Coleman D, Chamberlain J. Breast self-examination programmes in the trial of early detection of breast cancer: ten year findings. *Br J Cancer* 1993; **68:** 208–12.

14. Calnan MW, Chamberlain J, Moss S. Compliance with a class teaching breast self-examination. *J Epidemiol Community Health* 1983; **37:** 264–70.

15. Semiglazov VF, Moiseyenko VM, Bavli JL et al. The role of breast self-examination in early breast cancer detection (Results of the 5–years USSR/WHO randomised study in Leningrad). *Eur J Epidemiol* 1992; **8:** 498–502.

16. Kurebayashi J, Shimozuma K, Sonoo H. The practice of breast self-examination results in the earlier detection and better clinical course of Japanese women with breast cancer. *Jpn J Surg* 1994; **24:** 337–41.

17. Auvinen A, Elovainio L, Hakama M. Breast self-examination and survival from breast cancer. *Breast Cancer Res Treat* 1996; **38:** 161–8.

18. Ferris DG, Golden NH, Petry J et al. Effectiveness of breast self-examination prompts on oral contraceptive packaging. *J Fam Pract* 1996; **42:** 43–8.

19. Roberts MM, Alexander FE, Anderson TJ et al. Edinburgh trial of screening for breast cancer: mortality at seven years. *Lancet* 1990; **335:** 241–6.

20. Marshall G. A comparative study of re-attenders and non-re-attenders for second triennial National Breast Screening Programme appointments. *J Pub Health Med* 1994; **16:** 79–86.

21. Glasziou PP. Meta-analysis adjusting for compliance: the example of screening for breast cancer. *J Clin Epidemiol* 1992; **45:** 1251–6.

22. Hurley SF, Jolley DJ, Livingston PM et al. Effectiveness, costs and cost-effectiveness of recruitment strategies for a mammographic program to detect breast cancer. *J Natl Cancer Inst* 1992; **84:** 855–63.

23. Kee F. Do general practitioners facilitate the breast screening programme? *Eur J Cancer Prev* 1992; **1:** 231–8.

24. Fletcher SW, Harris RP, Gonzalez JJ et al. Increasing mammography utilization: a controlled study. *J Natl Cancer Inst* 1993; **85:** 112–20.

25. Meldrum P, Turnbull D, Dobson HM et al. Tailored written invitations for second round breast cancer screening: a randomised controlled trial. *J Med Screen* 1994; **1:** 245–8.

26. Burack RC, Gimotty PA, Georger J et al. The effect of patient and physician reminders on use of screening mammography in a Health Maintenance Organisation. *Cancer* 1996; **78:** 1708–21.

27. Hoare T. Breast screening and ethnic minorities. *Br J Cancer* 1996; **74**(suppl XXIX): S38–41.

28. Hoare T, Thomas C, Biggs A et al. Can the uptake of breast cancer screening be increased? A randomised controlled trial of a linkworker intervention. *J Pub Health Med* 1994; **16:** 179–85.

29. McAllister G, Bowling A. Attitudes to mammography among women in ethnic minority groups in three areas of England. *Health Educ J* 1993; **52:** 217–20.

30. Tabar L, Fagerberg G, Day NE, Holmberg L. What is the optimum interval between mammographic screening examinations? An analysis based on the latest results of the Swedish two-county breast cancer screening trial. *Br J Cancer* 1987; **55:** 547–51.

31. Woodman CBJ, Threlfal AG, Boggis CRM, Prior P. Is the three year breast screening interval too long? Occurrence of interval cancers in NHS breast screening programme's north western region. *BMJ* 1995; **310:** 224–6.

32. Ikeda DM, Andersson I, Wattsgard C et al. Interval carcinomas in the Malmö mammographic screening trial. *AJR* 1992; **159:** 287–94.

33. Andersson I. Radiographic screening for breast cancers. III Appearance of carcinoma and number of projections used at screening. *Acta Radiol* 1981; **22:** 407–9.

34. Sickles EA, Weber WN, Galvin HB et al. Baseline screening mammography: one versus two views per breast. *AJR* 1986; **147:** 1149–53

35. Wald NJ, Murphy P, Major P et al. UK CCCR multicentre randomised controlled trial of one and two view mammography in breast cancer screening. *BMJ* 1995; **311:** 1189–93.

36. Blanks RG, Moss SM, Wallis MG. A comparison of two view and one view mammography in the detection of small invasive cancers: results from the National Health Service breast screening programme. *J Med Screen* 1997; **3:** 200–3.

37. Anderson TJ, Lamb J, Donnan P et al. Comparative pathology of breast cancer in a randomised trial of screening. *Br J Cancer* 1991; **64:** 108–13

38. Klemi PJ. Joensuu H, Toikkanen S et al. Aggressiveness of breast cancers found with or without screening. *BMJ* 1992; **304:** 467–9.

39. Crisp WJ, Higgs MJ, Cowan WK et al. Screening for breast cancer detects tumours at an earlier biological stage. *Br J Surg* 1993; **80:** 863–5.

40. Hakama M, Holli K, Isola J et al. Aggressiveness of screen-detected breast cancers. *Lancet* 1993; **345:** 221–4.

41. Tabar L, Fagerberg G, Day N et al. Breast cancer treatment and natural history: new insights from results of screening. *Lancet* 1992; **339:** 412–14.

42. NHS Breast Screening Programme. *NHS Breast Screening Review 1995.*

43. Frouge C, Tristant H, Guinebretiére J-M. Mammographic lesions suggestive of radial scars: microscopic findings in 40 cases. *Radiology* 1995; **195:** 623–5.

44. Ruiz-Sauri A, Almenar-Medina S, Callaghan RC et al. Radial scar versus tubular carcinoma of the breast. *Pathol Res Pract* 1995; **191:** 547–54.

9

Breast conservation

The general trend in cancer is away from the very extensive operations formerly in vogue, and I believe this may be found to be true of future treatment of cancer of the breast.

Geoffrey Keynes (1937)

History • Randomized trials of breast conservation • Is radiotherapy necessary? • Is whole breast irradiation necessary? • Treatment of the axilla • Re-excision

Thankfully, the days have passed when surgeons who performed less than a mastectomy for operable breast cancer were regarded as negligent pariahs who were risking their patients' lives. It could be argued that now the pendulum has swung too far in favour of conservative treatment, so that this is sometimes presented to the patient as an appropriate option under circumstances when a mastectomy would be more likely to reduce the risk of local relapse.

The main reason for the widespread acceptance of breast-conservation therapy has been proof of safety in a series of prospective randomized trials. It must be appreciated that entry criteria were strict, both breast and axillary surgery were optimal and low rates of local relapse occurred only when postoperative radiotherapy was given. Omission of any of these crucial factors should be examined only in the context of randomized trials. Surgeons have not been given a mandate for minimal surgery, even under circumstances of apparently very early breast cancer.

HISTORY

Almost 50 years after William Halsted introduced his radical mastectomy, Geoffrey Keynes, a surgeon at St Bartholomew's Hospital, London, described the results of conservative treatment for operable breast cancer using implanted radium needles.[1] Originally the technique had been employed only in those with inoperable cancers but, after 50 had been treated, with good control of disease, 85 stage I and 91 stage II cases were irradiated. The tumour itself was excised and then radium needles were inserted throughout the breast, axilla, supraclavicular fossa and the upper three intercostal spaces. After 5 years, 71% of the stage I cases survived compared with 29% of those who were stage II. These results appeared to be as good as those after radical mastectomy. As a result of the limited availability of radium, handling problems and subsequent fibrosis as a result of inaccuracies of dosage, radium needles were never used widely to treat breast cancer.

There was scepticism among many surgeons as to whether breast cancer was sensitive to either radium or roentgen rays, but Pfahler was convinced that judicious use of radiotherapy could be as effective as surgery.[2] He reported a series of 1022 patients from Philadelphia with breast cancer given radiation therapy, of whom 53 had early disease. They were treated in this way because either they were too frail or they refused mastectomy. The average duration of symptoms was 16 months. Despite this the 5-year survival was 80%, and stage II cases fared better than surgically treated historical controls.

In Finland Mustakallio used wide excision and postoperative radiation therapy in patients who refused radical surgery and then applied the combined technique to most patients with operable, clinically node-negative disease.[3] The patients received 21 Gy to the breast, axilla and supraclavicular fossa given in six daily fractions of 3.5 Gy. There were 701 patients, of whom 15% were aged 70 years or older and the 10-year survival was 50%.[4] Locoregional relapse occurred in 24%. Mustakallio argued that radical surgery should be abandoned because it was a harmful method that damaged the patient. In addition, he suggested that high dosages of radiation should be avoided because this also had a detrimental effect.

In the 1950s and 1960s the prevailing view of breast cancer was nihilistic with most surgeons and radiotherapists believing that the disease was systemic, rather than localized, at the time of diagnosis. Thus local treatment and local control of breast cancer were unimportant because the prognosis was predetermined and uninfluenced by extent of surgery. In this climate the first randomized controlled trial of breast conservation treatment was started at Guy's Hospital in 1961 by Sir Hedley Atkins.[5] There were 370 patients, aged 50 or more with biopsy-proven operable breast cancer, and they were randomized to either radical mastectomy (188) or wide excision of the cancer (182).

Postoperative radiotherapy was given to both groups, but the techniques differed. The radical mastectomy group were treated with a 300 kV machine and given 25–27 Gy to the supraclavicular triangle, internal mammary chain and axilla. Those treated by wide excision received similar treatment to the gland fields and an additional 35–38 Gy to the breast using a 6 MeV linear accelerator. Thus the radical mastectomy group had an axillary clearance followed by what is now regarded as a low dose of radiotherapy. In contrast the wide-excision cases had

Table 9.1 Local relapse locations in Guy's Hospital breast conservation trial

Site	Wide excision Stage I	Stage II	Radical mastectomy Stage I	Stage II
Axilla	7	13	0	0
Skin	2	8	4	8
Breast	0	3	0	0
SCF	1	1	0	1
Multiple	5	5	0	0
Total	**15**	**30**	**4**	**9**

no axillary surgery followed by inadequate radiotherapy. Of those treated by radical mastectomy, 46% had pathologically involved axillary nodes, and it is likely that there was a similar proportion of stage II cases in the wide excision arm.

As a result, there were significantly more local relapses in the group treated by wide excision and the 10-year results are summarized in Table 9.1. Cases are subdivided on a basis of clinical stage because pathological stage was not available for the wide-excision group. There were significantly more locoregional relapses in the wide-excision group (25% vs 7%), and the main site was the axilla. For the clinical stage I cases the overall survival at 10 years was 80% in both groups, but stage II cases treated by wide excision had a significantly worse survival (30% vs 60%).

Once this significantly increased mortality rate was detected, trial entry was closed to women with stage II disease but continued for clinical stage I cases. Women of any age were entered into the second trial, provided that they were deemed clinically not to have axillary nodal involvement, and between 1971 and 1975 a total of 258 patients was recruited.[6] After a mean follow-up of 9 years, there was a signifi-

Table 9.2 Survival at 16 years in patients with T1 and T2 tumours treated by wide excision or radical mastectomy in Guy's Hospital conservation trials

T classification	Wide excision (%)	Radical mastectomy (%)
T1	40	75
T2	35	40

cantly increased locoregional relapse rate in the wide-excision group (30% vs 8%) and a significantly reduced survival (60% vs 82%). The inescapable conclusion was that this form of breast conservation was inadequate and led to more deaths from breast cancer. In itself this was a very important finding from the first randomized trial of breast conservation because it flew in the face of the popular notion that local treatment had no impact on prognosis. However, there was the paradox that the survival of stage I cases was similar in both treatment arms in the first trial, although not in the subsequent study.

This was resolved by a subsequent re-analysis of the data after a longer follow-up.[7] When cases were subdivided on a basis of T stage it emerged that there were more cases with T1 tumours in the second trial (38% vs 17%). The 16-year survival rates are shown in Table 9.2. For patients with T2 tumours there was no significant difference in survival in those treated by radical mastectomy or wide excision: the surprising finding was that women with T1 tumours fared better when treated by radical mastectomy. Thus it may be particularly important to achieve good control in patients with smaller, better prognosis cancers.

Much of the pioneering work to replace radical surgery with radical radiotherapy was carried out in France. At the Institut Curie, in Paris, Baclesse showed that relatively large cancers could be successfully controlled by giving 66–70 Gy fractionated over a 3-month period.[8] This work was extended by Pierquin et al who used a combination of external radiotherapy and an iridium ([129]Ir) implant (brachytherapy).[9] The technique of iridium implant was introduced to the USA by Hellman et al[10] and this popularized the concept of breast conservation therapy; it was in part responsible for the setting up of several clinical trials.

RANDOMIZED TRIALS OF BREAST CONSERVATION

Milan trials

Between 1973 and 1980 a trial was run at the National Cancer Institute Milan in which 701 patients with breast cancer were randomized to either breast conservation or Halsted mastectomy.[11] Eligible cases had a single tumour measuring up to 2 cm in diameter and were aged less than 70 years. Breast conservation therapy comprised a quadrantectomy (removal of the tumour with at least 2 cm of surrounding normal tissue), axillary clearance and radiotherapy (QUART). Surgery was an *en bloc* resection for upper outer quadrant lesions and separate procedures if the primary was elsewhere in the breast. Postoperatively, the conservation group received 50 Gy to the whole breast and a boost of 10 Gy to the excision site. After 1976, all those with positive axillary nodes received 12 cycles of chemotherapy (cyclophosphamide, methotrexate and 5-fluorouracil, or CMF).

The long-term results after a median follow-up of 16 years are given in Table 9.3.[12] Annual rates of local relapse were very low, being 0.46% after QUART and 0.2% after Halsted mastectomy. There was a relationship between age and local relapse in those treated by QUART. For women aged 45 or younger the annual local relapse rate was 0.91%, compared with 0.29% in those aged 46–55 and 0.19% in women 55 years and older. The overall survival of the two groups was similar, being 66% at 15 years.

Table 9.3 Long-term results in Milan QUART trial of breast conservation

	Breast conservation	Mastectomy
Number	352	349
Surgery	Quadrantectomy, axillary clearance	Halsted
Radiotherapy (Gy)	50 + 10 boost	Nil
Local relapse rate (%)	6	3
Overall survival rate (%)	66	66

Table 9.4 Results of Milan trial comparing QUART with TART

	QUART	TART
Number	360	345
Surgery	Quadrantectomy, axillary clearance	Tumorectomy, axillary clearance
Radiotherapy (Gy)	50 + 10 boost	45 +15 Ir boost
Local relapse rate (%)	5	20
Overall survival rate (%)	85	85

After the successful demonstration of the efficacy of the QUART technique, a second trial was conducted comparing this with a less radical surgical approach in which a tumorectomy and axillary clearance were performed followed by radiotherapy (TART).[13] A total of 705 evaluable cases was entered of whom 345 were treated by TART and 360 by QUART. The aim of the tumorectomy was cytoreductive, with all cases receiving a boost of 15 Gy to the tumour bed 3 weeks postoperatively using interstitial ^{192}Ir.

The results, after a median follow-up of 79 months, are given in Table 9.4.[12] There was a substantially higher local relapse rate in the TART group amounting to 2.45% per year compared with 0.46% in the QUART group, but the overall survival of the two groups was similar. Although this difference was probably the result of more frequent involvement of

excision margins in the TART group, another possible explanation for the increased local recurrence rate was the delay between surgery and implant, making it more difficult to identify the true tumour bed.

NSABP trial B-06

The National Surgical Adjuvant Breast Project (NSABP) recruited 1843 into trial B-06 between 1976 and 1984.[14] The trial aim was to compare breast conservation therapy with mastectomy and to examine the role of breast irradiation. Eligible cases were aged less than 70 and had single breast cancers measuring clinically up to 4 cm in diameter. There were three randomization options: total mastectomy and axillary clearance, segmental mastectomy (wide excision) and axillary clearance, or segmental mastectomy, axillary clearance and external

Table 9.5 NSABP B-06 trial of breast conservation			
	Mastectomy	**Wide excision**	**Wide excision – radiotherapy**
Number	586	632	625
Surgery	Tumorectomy and axillary clearance	Wide excision and axillary clearance	Wide excision and axillary clearance
Radiotherapy (Gy)	Nil	Nil	50 external RT
Local relapse rate (%)	8	22	7
Overall survival rate (%)	63	58	66

From Fisher et al.[15]

radiotherapy (range 50–53 Gy), without a boost. For those randomized to wide excision the margins of the specimen had to be tumour free and, if this was not achieved, a mastectomy was performed. All patients with involved axillary nodes received adjuvant melphalan and fluorouracil.

In 1989, with 1843 evaluable cases, the 8-year results were published and these are summarized in Table 9.5.[15] Of those randomized to wide excision, 10% had positive biopsy margins and were therefore treated by mastectomy. Relapse occurred in 40% of those who were treated by wide excision without radiotherapy compared with only 10% of those who had breast irradiation. This was not accompanied by a significant increase in breast cancer mortality. Nevertheless the high local relapse rate with associated psychological morbidity means that radiotherapy cannot reasonably be avoided in patients with breast cancers up to 4 cm, even when the biopsy margins are ostensibly clear of tumour.

The NSABP B-06 trial had been regarded by many, particularly in North America, as a landmark study and so great consternation and disorientation were caused in 1994 when it became public that one of the investigators had entered falsified data.[16] However, a meta-analysis of major published trials, and a re-analysis

of NSABP B-06 without the cases treated at St Luc Hospital, showed that the odds ratio of death for patients treated by mastectomy rather than conservation therapy was 0.964 (95% confidence interval – 0.804–1.157), suggesting an equivalence of the two methods in terms of mortality.[17]

EORTC trial 10801

The European Organization for Research and Treatment of Cancer (EORTC) ran a multicentre randomized trial between 1980 and 1986 into which 881 eligible breast cancer cases were entered.[18] All were aged 70 years or less and had operable single primary tumours measuring up to 5 cm diameter (T1, T2), and they were randomized to either modified radical mastectomy or breast conservation comprising tumorectomy, axillary clearance and radiotherapy (46–50 Gy to the breast and an interstitial ^{192}Ir boost of 20–25 Gy).

There were 734 patients with stage II disease (81%) and most of the stage I cases were entered from Guy's Hospital. This was because other centres regarded breast conservation therapy as a proven option for such cases. In contrast, the Guy's group were unconvinced because the results of the previous wide-excision trial, which had indicated that patients

Table 9.6 Results of EORTC trial 10801 comparing mastectomy and breast conservation		
	Breast conservation	**Mastectomy**
Number	456	425
Surgery	Tumorectomy, axillary clearance	Modified radical mastectomy
Radiotherapy (Gy)	50 + Ir boost 20	Nil
Local relapse rate (%)	15	9
Overall survival rate (%)	71	73

with T1 cancers had fared better when treated by mastectomy rather than breast conservation.[7] The results, after a median follow-up of 6 years, are given in Table 9.6. There were no significant differences in local relapse or overall survival between those treated by mastectomy and those treated by breast conservation. The local relapse rate in those treated by breast conservation was related to tumour size, being 7% in those with cancers smaller than 2 cm compared with 16% in those with lesions of 2–5 cm.

There were 35 patients who developed local relapse after mastectomy and 19 (54%) developed subsequent relapse after salvage treatment. In the breast conservation group, 50 had local relapse and 21 (42%) had a second relapse after salvage surgery, indicating that the prognosis after local relapse was similar for both forms of treatment. At Guy's Hospital the upper size limit was 4 cm and, once the equivalence of the two techniques became evident, patients whose tumours would have fulfilled entry criteria for the trial were offered breast conservation treatment at the time of diagnosis.

Other trials

Between 1972 and 1980 a small trial was run at the Institute Gustave-Roussy into which patients with tumours measuring up to 2 cm pathologically were randomized to mastectomy (91) or breast conservation (88), comprising tumourectomy, axillary sampling or clearance and radiotherapy (45 Gy with a boost of 15 Gy).[19] All cases had a low axillary dissection, followed by frozen section examination of at least seven nodes. If there was node involvement an axillary clearance was performed. Those node-positive cases then underwent a second randomization to receive or not receive nodal irradiation.

Unfortunately the small size of the trial and multiplicity of treatment options meant that it had insufficient statistical power to confirm the null hypothesis. Despite this the results do at least suggest that patients treated by breast conservation do not fare worse than those who have a mastectomy. Results after a mean follow-up of 14.5 years are given in Table 9.7.[20] There were no significant differences between the two treatment arms in terms of either local relapse or overall survival, although the relative risks were slightly higher in the mastectomy group (1.41 and 1.28). Almost all the relapses occurred in the first 10 years after treatment and were more frequent, there were no differential risk factors for local relapse in the two groups.

The US National Cancer Institute (NCI) ran a randomized trial between 1979 and 1987 into which 237 patients were entered.[21] Although no upper age limit was described, only 25% of cases were aged over 60 years. Patients had operable cancers measuring 5 cm or less and were treated by either modified radical mastectomy (116) or tumorectomy, axillary clearance

Table 9.7 Results of Gustave-Roussy trial comparing mastectomy and breast conservation therapy

	Breast conservation	Mastectomy
Number	88	91
Surgery	Tumorectomy, axillary sample/clearance	Total mastectomy, axillary sample/clearance
Radiotherapy (Gy)	45 + 15 boost	45/no RT
Local relapse rate (%)	9	14
Overall survival rate (%)	73	65

From Arriagada et al.[20]

Table 9.8 NCI trial of breast conservation

	Breast conservation	Mastectomy
Number	121	116
Surgery	Tumorectomy, axillary clearance	Modified radical mastectomy
Radiotherapy (Gy)	45–50	Nil
Local relapse rate (%)	17	9
Overall survival rate (%)	77	75

and radiotherapy (121). The whole breast was irradiated to an isodose of 45–50 Gy and those with positive axillary nodes also received 45–50 Gy to the supraclavicular fossa. Node-positive cases received adjuvant chemotherapy comprising cyclophosphamide and doxorubicin. The results, after a median follow-up of 10 years, are shown in Table 9.8. There were twice as many local relapses in the breast conservation group compared with those who were treated by mastectomy, but the 10-year overall survival of the two groups was similar.

The Danish Breast Cancer Co-operative Group (DBCG) recruited 662 women, aged 69 years or less between 1983 and 1987 from 19 surgical departments.[22] There was no tumour size limit specified but there had to be a possibility of a satisfactory cosmetic result after excision, which could be as much as one-third of the breast tissue. Excision had to achieve gross, rather than microscopical, clearance of tumour. In both breast conservation and mastectomy groups a level I/II axillary dissection was performed. Radiotherapy dose was 50 Gy with an external boost of 10 Gy, which was increased to 25 Gy if the tumorectomy margins were involved.

High-risk patients with tumours bigger than 5 cm, skin or deep fascial invasion, or positive axillary nodes were given adjuvant therapy which was chemotherapy (CMF) in the premenopausal and tamoxifen in the

Table 9.9 Danish Breast Cancer Co-operative Group trial of breast conservation		
	Breast conservation	**Mastectomy**
Number	334	328
Surgery	Tumourectomy, axillary I/II dissection	Total mastectomy, axillary I/II dissection
Radiotherapy (Gy)	50 + 10/25 boost	Nil
Local relapse rate (%)	2	5
Overall survival rate (%)	–	–

postmenopausal. Preliminary results were reported after a median follow-up of 1.75 years and are summarized in Table 9.9. There were more locoregional relapses in the mastectomy group, on both the chest wall and axilla, but this did not reach statistical significance. In one centre 63 patients who had breast conservation treatment were assessed for cosmetic outcome and this was deemed by their oncologist to be either extremely satisfactory or satisfactory in 90%.

The Early Breast Cancer Trialists' Collaborative Group conducted a meta-analysis of randomized trials of radiotherapy and surgery for breast cancer and included an overview of nine studies comparing breast conservation treatment with mastectomy.[23] Overall the total mortality in those treated by mastectomy or breast conservation treatment was the same (23% vs 23%). Recurrence data were available for six trials and this showed fewer relapses after mastectomy (odds ratio = 0.96) but this difference was not statistically significant.

Although there can be no argument about the safety of breast conservation treatment for those treated in controlled trials, there may be doubts concerning the general applicability of breast conservation. Pirtoli et al treated 206 consecutive patients with radiotherapy (45 Gy and 7.5 Gy boost) after breast conserving surgery, and reported an 8-year relapse rate of 12% and overall survival rate of 91% which is similar to that reported in randomized trials.[24] To examine the impact of the publication of results of NSABP B-06 trial, Iscoe et al examined the method of treatment of 37 447 women with breast cancer reported to the Ontario Cancer Registry between 1980 and 1989.[25] As Table 9.10 shows, in 1980 13% of cases had breast conservation treatment and the proportion slowly rose

Table 9.10 Use of breast-conserving surgery in Ontario											
Year	**1980**	**1981**	**1982**	**1983**	**1984**	**1985**	**1986**	**1987**	**1988**	**1989**	**Total**
Percentage	13	17	19	23	28	39	41	41	41	44	32

From Iscoe et al.[25]

Table 9.11 Breast conservation trials comparing radiotherapy with no radiotherapy

Tumour size (cm)	Follow-up (years)	No radiotherapy (%)	Radiotherapy (%)	Reference
≤ 4	8	40	9	Fisher et al[15]
≤ 2	5	18.4	2.3	Liljegren ey al[30]
≤ 4	7.6	35	11	Clark et al[31]
<2.5	3	8.8	0.3	Veronesi et al[32]

until 1985 when there was a sudden increase to 39%, followed by a plateau in use of breast conservation.

It was suggested by the authors that the accelerated use of breast conservation treatment was the result of the publication of results of the B-06 trial.[14] This rather ignores the contemporaneous publication of long-term results from the Milan group.[26,27] That same group compared the outcome of 350 patients treated by QUART in the first Milan trial with that of 1408 subsequently treated outside the trial.[28] Both local relapse rate and all cause mortality were higher in those treated outside the trial. As a result of a relaxation of criteria for breast conservation, the non-trial patients had worse prognostic features. After adjustment for co-variates there was no significant difference in mortality in the two groups. However, the hazard rate for ipsilateral breast relapse was 0.61, indicating that there was a 40% reduction in risk of relapse in the trial cases. Although seemingly this is a major difference, it should be appreciated that the local relapse rate in the trial was only 6% at 16 years so that outside the trial it might be 8%, still representing very good local control.

Voogd et al compared outcome of 464 patients with tumours 3 cm or less undergoing breast conservation treatment, with 459 similar cases treated by mastectomy in community hospitals and reported to the Eindhoven Cancer Registry.[29] After a median follow-up of 6 years the relapse-free and overall survival of the two groups were similar once adjustment had been made for age, tumour size, nodal status and systemic therapy. Thus routine use of breast conservation treatment appears to be the equal of mastectomy, provided that patients are appropriately selected.

IS RADIOTHERAPY NECESSARY?

Radiotherapy involves expensive equipment which, even when used skilfully, may lead to morbidity. Moreover, treatments are time-consuming for patients who may have problems attending for daily fractions. For these reasons it has been questioned whether radiotherapy can be avoided when carrying out breast conservation treatment. As shown in Table 9.11, the first randomized trial to address this question was NSABP B-06 and, by 8 years, 40% of non-irradiated cases had developed a breast relapse even after wide local excision.[15] As patients in that trial had tumours 4 cm or less most subsequent studies included those with smaller cancers.

The Uppsala-Örebro Breast Cancer Study Group started a study, before publication of the NSABP results, in which 381 women with completely excised invasive cancers measuring 2 cm or less (pathologically), and negative nodes after axillary clearance were randomized to postoperative radiotherapy (187) or no further treatment (194).[30] Complete excision was defined as the presence of at least 2 cm of normal tissue around the tumour. The actuarial breast relapse rate at 5 years was 2% in the irradiated group and 18% in the non-irradiated. The relative hazard of breast relapse in the non-irradiated cases increased in the more recently treated cases, being 4.6 in 1984 and 8 in 1988. It was postulated that this was the result of changes in surgical technique and patient selection. There were no differences in distant relapse or overall survival. As part of the study arm morbidity was examined and it was found that radiotherapy had no impact on pain, shoulder mobility or lymphoedema.[33] The major risk factors for postoperative arm morbidity were young age and number of lymph nodes in the axillary dissection. Immediate problems had reduced by almost 50% after 2–3 years of follow-up.

Between 1984 and 1989, the Ontario Clinical Oncology Group (OCOG) ran a trial in which 837 patients, who had tumours sized 4 cm or smaller, clear resection margins and negative nodes after axillary dissection, either had breast irradiation (416) or no radiotherapy (421).[31] Radiotherapy comprised 40 Gy to the entire breast and 12.5 Gy boost to the biopsy site. At a median follow-up of 7.6 years, the breast relapse rate was significantly higher in the non-irradiated group (35% vs 11%). The mortality rate in those who had no radiotherapy was 24% compared with 21% in the other group. Factors predicting for breast relapse were young age (<50 years), tumour size (>2 cm) and high nuclear grade. No group could be identified at very low risk of relapse if not treated with radiotherapy.

At the National Cancer Institute Milan between 1987 and 1989, 567 patients with cancers smaller than 2.5 cm were treated by quadrantectomy and axillary clearance, and then randomized to radiotherapy or no further treatment.[32] After 39 months of median follow-up, breast relapse occurred in 0.3% of those who had received breast irradiation and 8.8% of those who did not. This was age related in that breast recurrence occurred in 16% of those aged 55 or younger but in only 3% of women aged over 55 years.

A non-randomized trial of breast conservation was run at the Joint Center for Radiation

Therapy, Boston between 1986 and 1992 when 87 patients had been enrolled.[34] Eligible cases had invasive breast cancer 2 cm or less in diameter and all had a re-excision of the biopsy site with a 1 cm or more margin of normal breast issue. In addition, all had a histologically negative axilla. The age range was from 27 to 84 years, median 67, and results were reported after a median follow-up of 56 months. By that time breast relapse had occurred in 14 cases (16%), 11 at the tumour site and three in another quadrant. There were no histological features that were peculiar to those who developed breast relapse.

In a randomized trial run at St George's Hospital and the Royal Marsden Hospital, London between 1981 and 1990, 418 women with T1–2 breast cancers were treated by wide excision and level I axillary dissection, and then randomized to receive or not receive radiotherapy.[35] Those with positive nodes were given tamoxifen if the tumour was ER-positive and CMF if ER-negative. After a minimum follow-up of 5 years there had been 13% of local relapses in the irradiated group compared with 35% in the non-irradiated cases. Local relapse rates in relation to excision margins and treatment are given in Table 9.12. This shows the relatively high relapse rate in all groups with 17% of those with involved margins developing relapse after radiotherapy, as well as 12% of

Table 9.12 Local relapse in relation to tumour margins and radiotherapy

Margins	Radiotherapy (%)	No radiotherapy (%)
Clinically clear	15	44
Involved	17	–
Close	8	35
Clear	12	22

From Renton et al.[35]

those with clear margins. It was concluded that radiotherapy could not compensate for inadequate surgery.

The Milan group had the lowest breast relapse rate without radiotherapy, probably as a result of the extent of surgery that was a quadrantectomy. In older women this may be a safe option, particularly when combined with tamoxifen in ER-positive cases. For younger women, even with apparently small tumours, avoidance of radiation has to be regarded as an experimental therapy and should be used only under the controlled circumstances of a randomized trial. At present, in the UK, there is a trial running, BASO II, for patients with similar characteristics to those in the Boston study, with a factorial 2 × 2 design: observation, breast irradiation, tamoxifen and breast irradiation plus tamoxifen. A similar study is being conducted by the EORTC.

It may be possible to select patients for radiotherapy with the use of biomarkers. Silvestrini et al used immunohistochemistry to determine expression of *p53*, *Bcl-2*, and glutathione *S*-transferase-π (*GST*-π) in tumours from 139 patients treated by quadrantectomy and 496 who had both quadrantectomy and radiotherapy.[36] These were chosen as markers of DNA damage repair (*p53*), cellular detoxification (*GST*-π), and control of apoptosis (*p53* and *Bcl-2*). After a median follow-up of 6 years, in the irradiated cases there was no difference in local relapse rates of those with tumours expressing low and high levels of the biomarkers. Among the women who had no breast irradiation, however, those with tumours showing high levels of *p53* and *GST*-π had a threefold increase in breast relapse rate. Low levels of *Bcl-2* were also associated with a slightly increased breast relapse rate.

IS WHOLE BREAST IRRADIATION NECESSARY?

The rationale behind whole breast irradiation is to destroy any residual tumour cells at the biopsy site and eliminate possible undetected multifocal malignancy. However, in NSABP

Table 9.13 Relapse rates in trial comparing tumour bed and whole breast irradiation (RT)

Relapse site	Tumour bed RT	Whole breast RT
Breast	21 (6%)	13 (4%)
Breast and nodes	18 (5%)	5 (1%)
Breast and distant	30 (9%)	17 (5%)
Total	69 (20%)	35 (10%)

From Magee et al.[37]

trial B-06, among those cases who received no radiotherapy after complete local excision, almost all the relapses were in the originally affected quadrant.[14] This would suggest that the main function of radiotherapy is to kill residual cancer cells or possibly prevent progression of peritumoral premalignant tissue. Thus it might be possible to conserve radiotherapeutic resources by concentrating treatment on the affected quadrant only.

A randomized trial was conducted at the Christie Hospital, Manchester, between 1982 and 1987, in which 708 patients with breast cancer sized 4 cm or less received either whole breast and gland field irradiation (355) or tumour bed irradiation (353).[37] Previous surgery comprised gross tumour excision and no axillary surgery. Those who had whole breast irradiation were treated with a tangential pair of 4 MeV beams and received 40 Gy in 15 fractions over 21 days, without a boost. In addition, 40 Gy was delivered to the axillary and supraclavicular gland fields. The patients who received tumour bed irradiation were treated with electrons of beam energy 8–14 MeV, to a dose of 40–42.5 Gy in eight fractions over 10 days to a field of average size 6 × 8 cm.

After a median follow-up of 8 years the overall survival of the two groups was the same (72%). However, as shown in Table 9.13, there were twice as many local relapses in the group treated by tumour bed irradiation (20% vs 10%). The relapse rate in the untreated axilla was 24% compared with 12% in those who had axillary irradiation.

In a multivariate analysis the significant predictors for local relapse were method of treatment, histological grade and vascular invasion. In those who had invasive lobular cancers and tumour bed irradiation, there was a high rate of breast relapse. Thus, if external radiotherapy to the tumour bed is contemplated, patients should have grade I/II cancers completely excised and an axillary dissection.

At Guy's Hospital a different approach was adopted. As iridium implants had been found to give good local control as part of breast conservation treatment, it was considered reasonable to increase the interstitial dosage and omit external radiotherapy. In a pilot study 27 patients with tumours sized 4 cm or less were treated by tumorectomy and axillary clearance followed by a rigid implant, afterloaded with ^{192}Ir to deliver 55 Gy in 5.5 days.[38] The rigid implant was inserted under the same general anaesthetic during which axillary clearance was performed and aimed to encompass a 2 cm margin of normal tissue. After a relatively short follow-up of 27 months, the cosmetic outcome was rated objectively as good or excellent in 80% of cases and subjectively as good/excellent in all but one.

After 6 years of median follow-up, however, relapse within the treated breast had occurred in 10 of 27 (37%).[39] Interestingly, the incidence of distant metastases and overall survival were similar to those for patients treated with iridium implant and external radiotherapy in the EORTC trial 10801.[18] Significant variables predicting for breast relapse were method of treatment, number of involved axillary nodes, menopausal status and tumour type. The results were perplexing because the relapse rate was similar to that in non-irradiated cases in NSABP B-06, even though an apparently adequate dose of 55 Gy had been given.[14] It is possible that there was an over-representation of younger patients with more aggressive tumours. Clearly, a much more selective approach will need to be adopted if tumour bed irradiation is to tested.

TREATMENT OF THE AXILLA

Despite a large body of evidence on the benefits of axillary dissection as part of conservation treatment, this is still one of the most bitterly debated aspects of breast surgery. There was a time when there were many surgeons who had not learned the technique of axillary clearance. Nowadays, as more breast surgery is conducted by those who have had some specialized training, there must be other explanations for the omission of axillary surgery from conservation treatment of invasive cancer. This may stem partly from the increasing proportion of screen-detected cancers that tend to be smaller than symptomatic lesions and less likely to have spread to the axillary nodes. The advantages of axillary clearance need to be re-stated: the procedure leads to good local control, accurate prognostic information and enables the selection of the most effective adjuvant therapy.

The Guy's Hospital wide excision trials indicated that inadequate treatment of the axilla led to more local relapses and more deaths from breast cancer.[5] This was dismissed by many as an egregious result, not in keeping with the prevailing wisdom that breast cancer was a systemic disease whose course was unaffected by local treatment. Since then further evidence has been furnished from a variety of sources.

The Yorkshire Breast Group examined local relapse rates in 960 patients who had a mastectomy together with either axillary sampling (463) or clearance (497).[40] Axillary relapse occurred in 2% of cases who had a clearance but in 7% of those subjected to sampling. In a series of 1624 patients treated at the Joint Center for Radiation Therapy, of those who were not treated with axillary irradiation, 25 developed relapse at that site causing distressing uncontrolled symptoms at death in 24%.[41] Gateley et al reviewed 1681 breast cancer patients of whom 1137 were treated by wide excision or simple mastectomy and 544 treated by Patey

Table 9.14 Danish Breast Cancer Cooperative Group[43] outcome of node-negative breast cancer patients in relation to the number of nodes examined

	1–2	3–4	5–9	≥ 10
Number	1050	3522	1635	938
8-year axillary RFS rate (%)	85	88	91	93
8-year overall survival rate (%)	75	80	80	85

RFS, relapse-free survival.

mastectomy.[42] Uncontrolled axillary relapse occurred in 3% of those who had a Patey operation but in 11% who had no axillary surgery or radiotherapy.

The Danish Breast Cancer Co-operative Group (DBCG) examined the axillary nodal status in 13 851 entered into two trials: DBCG 77 and DBCG 82.[43] There were 7145 (52%) who were pathologically node negative and these patients were followed for a median of 76 months. There was an almost linear relationship between the number of lymph nodes examined by the pathologist and percentage node positivity. Thus, of those cases who had only one node examined, 70% were negative whereas this fell to 45% if 10 or more nodes were examined. This indicates that the fewer nodes removed and examined, the greater the likelihood of understaging disease and leaving residual involved nodes in the axilla. Confirmation of this came from the axillary relapse rates which were significantly elevated in those who had fewer nodes examined, as shown in Table 9.14. Not only were there more axillary relapses but also more overall recurrences and a significantly increased mortality rate in those who had only two lymph nodes examined.

Of course it will be argued that these results were derived from symptomatic cases, screening not being performed in Denmark at that time,

Table 9.15 Axillary nodal status in relation to histological type in Guy's Hospital patients with palpable and impalpable tumours sized 1 cm or less

	Palpable		Impalpable	
	Node negative	Node positive	Node negative	Node positive
Ductal I (%)	75	25	64	36
Ductal II (%)	75	25	72	28
Ductal III (%)	56	44	37	63
Lobular (%)	59	41	82	18
Tubular (%)	75	25	80	20
Total (%)	71	29	67	37

Table 9.16 Five-year relapse-free (RFS) and overall survival (OS) in patients with tumours sized 1 cm or less according to treatment

Treatment	T1a tumours		T1b tumours	
	RFS (%)	OS (%)	RFS (%)	OS (%)
Tumorectomy alone	61	64	67	64
Tumorectomy and axillary clearance	87	94	92	95
Modified radical mastectomy	92	95	83	84

From White et al.[45]

and that the smaller lesions detected mammographically will be less likely to have axillary nodal involvement rendering dissection of the axilla redundant. The extent of axillary involvement in smaller tumours was examined in a series of 336 patients who had invasive cancers sized 1 cm or less treated at Guy's Hospital between 1975 and 1994.[44] The nodal status of patients with palpable and impalpable tumours of different histological types is shown in Table 9.15. Overall, one-third of cases had axillary nodal involvement and the proportions were similar in palpable and impalpable tumours.

Even in those cases with apparently good prognosis tumours (ductal grade I or tubular), a quarter had nodal involvement. This was not just single nodal involvement: 32% had two to three nodes and 24% had four or more nodes containing tumour. For the node-negative cases the 10-year overall survival rate was 90%, whereas it was 68% in node-positive women. Furthermore, there was a significantly better survival for node-positive cases with palpable tumours compared with impalpable node-positive patients (73% vs 43%). This emphasizes the continuing need for axillary surgery in patients with small tumours.

White et al used the Rhode Island State Tumor Registry to assess the value of axillary dissection in 1126 patients with T1 cancers.[45]

Patients were divided into three groups: local excision only (157), local excision and axillary dissection (319), and modified radical mastectomy (650). Choice of treatment was influenced by age of patient: of those who had excision only, 59% were 70 or older, compared with 19% of those undergoing tumourectomy and axillary dissection, and 39% of those treated by modified radical mastectomy. Five-year relapse-free and overall survival of the three groups are given in Table 9.16, subdivided into T1a (≤ 0.5 cm) and T1b (> 0.5, ≥ 1 cm).

This shows that patients treated by tumourectomy alone fared substantially worse than the other two groups, both in terms of relapse-free and overall survival. A similar bad result from undertreatment was seen in those with T1a and T1b lesions, and White et al concluded that axillary dissection should remain as standard surgery for those with invasive breast cancer, regardless of size.

RE-EXCISION

In the randomized trials of breast conservation treatment, the lowest rate of breast relapse was seen in the Milan QUART study, being 6% after 16 years.[12] The probable explanation for this excellent local control was the greater likelihood of complete excision because up to a

Table 9.17 Results of re-excision based on original biopsy margin status

| Positive | | Negative | | Close | | Unknown | | Reference |
No.	(%)	No.	(%)	No.	(%)	No.	(%)	
21/40	(52)	5/19	(26)	9/28	(32)	–		Frazier et al[47]
35/54	(65)	0/7		7/31	(23)	45/100	(45)	Gwin et al[48]
24/54	(44)	0/5		6/24	(25)	12/25	(48)	Pittinger et al[49]
	(54)		**(16)**		**(27)**		**(46)**	**Total**

quarter of the breast tissue was removed in quadrantectomy. To try and achieve equally good results, but with less extensive surgery, a re-excision has been used in many centres when there was margin involvement in the original biopsy or if a postoperative mammogram had shown suspicious residual microcalcification.

One of the main reasons for carrying out a re-excision was because of the unknown margins in patients referred to radiotherapy centres for treatment who had had their original biopsy elsewhere. Under these circumstances, as many as 62% of re-excision specimens showed residual carcinoma, particularly when the first biopsy had shown an extensive intraductal component.[46] If the first biopsy specimen has been handled correctly by the pathologist, the margins are usually reported as being clear, involved or close. When the first biopsy has been performed elsewhere and the margins not inked, even the most experienced pathologist is unable to comment on margin involvement.

Table 9.17 gives the results of re-excision specimens based on the original margin status of the biopsy specimen.[47-49] Overall, when the original specimen was reported as having margin involvement, there was residual tumour in 54% of re-excision specimens, and in 46% of those with unknown margins, compared with 27% of those deemed as having tumour close to the margin.

Re-excision of the original biopsy will reveal residual tumour in up to 50% of cases where there is dubious or definite involvement of specimen margins. This will lead to better local control, sometimes without any cosmetic deficit. If this is not considered reasonable because of the location of the original tumour or the size of the breast, a boost will be necessary, but it is likely that some of these individuals will be at increased risk of breast relapse because of residual invasive or non-invasive cancer.

SYNOPSIS

- Breast conservation is a safe alternative to mastectomy for patients with unifocal breast cancers up to 4 cm in diameter.
- Radiotherapy should be used routinely as part of breast conservation because it substantially reduces the risk of local relapse within the breast.
- Axillary surgery is necessary to improve local control and stage disease and should not be omitted even in patients with tumours sized 1 cm or less.
- More extensive clearance of the tumour will lead to a lower breast relapse rate but may worsen the cosmetic outcome.

REFERENCES

1. Keynes G. Conservative treatment of cancer of the breast. *BMJ* 1937; **ii:** 643–7.
2. Pfahler GE. Results of radiation therapy in 1022 private cases of carcinoma of the breast from 1902 to 1928. *Am J Roentgenol Rad Ther* 1932; **27:** 497–508.
3. Mustakallio S. Uber die Möglichkeiten der Rontgentherapie bei der Behandlung des Bruskrebses. *Acta Radiol* 1945; **26:** 503–11.
4. Mustakallio S. Conservative treatment of breast carcinoma – review of 25 years follow-up. *Clin Radiol* 1972; **23:** 110–16.
5. Atkins HJB, Hayward JL, Klugman DJ, Wayte AB. Treatment of early breast cancer: a report after ten years of a clinical trial. *BMJ* 1972; **2:** 423–9.
6. Hayward JL. The Guy's Hospital trials on breast conservation. In: *Conservative Management of Breast Cancer.* Harris JR, Hellman S, Silen W, eds. Philadelphia: JB Lippincott, 1983: 77–90.
7. Hayward JL, Caleffi M. The significance of local control in the primary treatment of breast cancer. *Arch Surg* 1987; **122:** 1244–7.
8. Baclesse F. Roentgen therapy as the sole method of treatment of cancer of the breast. *Am J Roentgenol Rad Ther* 1949; **62:** 311–18.
9. Pierquin B, Owen R, Maylin C et al. Radical radiation therapy of breast cancer. *Int J Radiat Oncol Biol Phys* 1980; **6:** 17–24.
10. Hellman S, Harris JR, Levene MB. Radiation therapy of early carcinoma of the breast without mastectomy. *Cancer* 1980; **46:** 988–94.
11. Veronesi U, Saccozzi R, Del Vecchio M et al. Comparing radical mastectomy with quadrantectomy, axillary dissection, and radiotherapy in patients with small cancers of the breast. *N Engl J Med* 1981; **305:** 6–11.
12. Veronesi U, Salvadori B, Luini A et al. Breast conservation is a safe method in patients with small cancer of the breast. Long-term results of three randomised trials on 1,973 patients. *Eur J Cancer* 1995; **31A:** 1574–9.
13. Veronesi U, Volterrani F, Luini A et al. Quadrantectomy versus lumpectomy for small size breast cancer. *Eur J Cancer* 1990; **26:** 671–3.
14. Fisher B, Bauer M, Margolese R et al. Five-year results of a randomized clinical trial comparing total mastectomy and segmental mastectomy with or without radiation in the treatment of breast cancer. *N Engl J Med* 1985; **312:** 665–73.
15. Fisher B, Redmond C, Poisson R et al. Eight-year results of a randomized clinical trial comparing total mastectomy and lumpectomy with or without irradiation in the treatment of breast cancer. *N Engl J Med* 1989; **320:** 822–8.
16. National Cancer Institute. NCI issues information on falsified data in NSABP trials. *J Natl Cancer Inst* 1994; **86:** 487–9.
17. National Cancer Institute. Survival after breast-sparing surgery versus mastectomy. *J Natl Cancer Inst* 1994; **86:** 1672–3.
18. Van Dongen JA, Bartelink H, Fentiman IS et al. Factors influencing local relapse and survival and results of salvage treatment after breast-conserving therapy in operable breast cancer: EORTC Trial 10801, breast conservation compared with mastectomy in TNM stage I and II breast cancer. *Eur J Cancer* 1992; **28A:** 801–5.
19. Sarrazin D, Lé M, Rouëssé J et al. Conservative treatment versus mastectomy in breast cancer tumors with macroscopic diameter of 20 millimetres or less. The experience of the Institut Gustave-Roussy. *Cancer* 1984; **53:** 1209–12.
20. Arriagada R, Lé M, Rochard F et al. Conservative treatment versus mastectomy in early breast cancer: patterns of failure with 15 years of follow-up. *J Clin Oncol* 1996; **14:** 1558–64.
21. Jacobson JA, Danforth DN, Cowan KH et al. Ten-year results of a comparison of conservation with mastectomy in the treatment of stage I and II breast cancer. *N Engl J Med* 1995; **332:** 907–11.
22. Blichert-Toft M, Brincker H, Andersen JA et al. A Danish randomized trial comparing breast-preserving therapy with mastectomy in mammary carcinoma. *Acta Oncologica* 1988; **27:** 671–7.
23. Early Breast Cancer Trialists' Collaborative Group. Effects of radiotherapy and surgery in early breast cancer. An overview of the randomized trials. *N Engl J Med* 1995; **333:** 1444–55.
24. Pirtoli L, Belleza A, Pepi F et al. Breast-conserving treatment of early breast cancer. *Acta Oncol* 1993; **32:** 647–51.
25. Iscoe NA, Naylor D, Williams JI et al. Temporal trends in breast cancer surgery in Ontario: can one randomized trial make a difference? *Can Med Assoc J* 1994; **150:** 1109–15.
26. Veronesi U, Zucali R, Luini A. Local control and survival in early breast cancer: the Milan Trial.

Int J Radiation Oncology Biol Phys 1986; **12**: 717–20.

27. Veronesi U, Banfi A, Del Vecchio M et al. Comparison of Halsted mastectomy with quadrantectomy, axillary dissection, and radiotherapy in early breast cancer: long-term results. *Eur J Cancer* 1986; **22**: 1085–9.

28. Marubini E, Mariani L, Salvadori B et al. Results of a breast cancer surgery trial compared with observational data from routine practice. *Lancet* 1996; **347**: 1000–3.

29. Voogd AC, Nab HW, Crommelin MA et al. Comparison of breast-conserving therapy with mastectomy for treatment of early breast cancer in community hospitals. *Eur J Surg Oncol* 1996; **22**: 13–16.

30. Liljegren G, Holmberg L, Adami H-O et al. Sector resection with or without postoperative radiotherapy for stage I breast cancer: five-year results of a randomised trial. *J Natl Cancer Inst* 1994; **86**: 717–22.

31. Clark R, Whelan T, Levine M et al. Randomized clinical trial of breast irradiation following lumpectomy and axillary dissection for node-negative breast cancer: an update. *J Natl Cancer Inst* 1996; **88**: 1659–64.

32. Veronesi U, Luini A, Del Vecchio M et al. Radiotherapy after breast-preserving surgery in women with localized cancer of the breast. *N Engl J Med* 1993; **328**: 1587–91.

33. Liljegren G, Holmberg L, and the Uppsala-Örebro Breast Cancer Study Group. Arm morbidity after sector resection and axillary dissection with or without postoperative radiotherapy in breast cancer Stage I. Results from a randomised trial. *Eur J Cancer* 1997; **33**: 193–9

34. Schnitt SJ, Hayman J, Gelman R et al. A prospective study of conservative surgery alone in the treatment of selected patients with stage I breast cancer. *Cancer* 1996; **77**: 1094–100.

35. Renton SC, Gazet J-C, Ford HT et al. The importance of the resection margin in conservative surgery for breast cancer. *Eur J Surg Oncol* 1996; **22**: 17–22.

36. Silvestrini R, Veronesi S, Benini E et al. Expression of p53. Glutathione *S*-transferase-π, and Bcl-2 proteins and benefit from adjuvant radiotherapy in breast cancer. *J Natl Cancer Inst* 1997; **8**: 639–45.

37. Magee B, Swindell R, Harris M, Banerjee SS. Prognostic factors for breast recurrence after conservative breast surgery and radiotherapy: results from a randomised trial. *Radiother Oncol* 1996; **39**: 223–7.

38. Fentiman IS, Poole C, Tong D et al. Iridium implant treatment without external radiotherapy for operable breast cancer: a pilot study. *Eur J Cancer* 1991; **27**: 447–50.

39. Fentiman IS, Poole C, Tong D et al. Inadequacy of iridium implant as sole radiation treatment for operable breast cancer. *Eur J Cancer* 1996; **32A**: 608–11.

40. Benson EA, Thorogood J. The effect of surgical treatment on local recurrence rates following mastectomy. *Eur J Surg Oncol* 1986; **12**: 267–71.

41. Recht A, Pierce SM, Abner A et al. Regional nodal failure after conservative surgery and radiotherapy for early-stage breast carcinoma. *J Clin Oncol* 1991; **9**: 988–96.

42. Gateley CA, Mansel RE, Owen A et al. Treatment of the axilla in operable breast cancer. *Br J Surg* 1991; **78**: 750.

43. DBCCG, Axelsson CK, Mouridsen HT, et al. Axillary dissection of level I and II lymph nodes is important in breast cancer classification. *Eur J Cancer* 1992; **28A**: 1415–18.

44. Fentiman IS, Hyland D, Chaudary MA, Gregory WM. Prognosis of patients with breast cancers up to 1 cm in diameter. *Eur J Cancer* 1996; **32A**: 417–20.

45. White RE, Vezeridis MP, Konstadoulakis M et al. Therapeutic options and results for the management of minimally invasive carcinoma of the breast: influence of axillary dissection for treatment of T1a and T1b lesions. *J Am Coll Surg* 1996; **183**: 575–82.

46. Schnitt SJ, Connolly JL, Khettry U et al. Pathologic findings on re-excision of the primary tumor site in breast cancer patients considered for treatment by primary radiation therapy. *Cancer* 1987; **59**: 675–81.

47. Frazier TG, Wong RWY, Rose D. Implications of accurate pathologic margins in the treatment of primary breast cancer. *Arch Surg* 1989; **124**: 37–8.

48. Gwin JL, Eisenberg BL, Hoffman JP et al. Incidence of gross and microscopic carcinoma in specimens from patients with breast cancer after re-excision lumpectomy. *Ann Surg* 1993; **218**: 729–34.

49. Pittinger TP, Maronian NC, Poulter CA et al. Importance of margin status in outcome of breast-conserving surgery for carcinoma. *Surgery* 1994; **116**: 605–9.

10

Complications of breast conservation

In nature there are neither rewards nor punishments – there are consequences.

RG Ingersoll

Breast relapse • Poor cosmetic outcome • Evaluation of changes • Angiosarcoma

It is undeniable that safe techniques exist for breast conservation. What is now important is the establishment of the best means of selecting cases with the lowest risk of relapse and of tailoring treatments to individual needs, with minimization of morbidity and optimal cosmetic outcome. This is a pressing need because most cases detected by screening will have small tumours eminently suitable for breast conservation therapy.

BREAST RELAPSE

Patterns of relapse

After optimal conservative surgery and radiotherapy, there is a 1% annual rate of breast relapse.[1] The timing of that recurrence will depend upon the sensitivity of the original tumour to radiotherapy and adjuvant treatment together with the behaviour of premalignant tissue around the tumour or in other quadrants of the breast. Also, the interval between treatment and breast relapse may be of prognostic significance. In a series of 1593 patients with stage I/II treated at the Cancer Institute Marseilles, breast recurrence occurred in 178 (11%).[2] The breast relapse-free survival was 93% at 5 years, 86% at 10 years and 80% at 20

Table 10.1 Location of relapse in relation to disease-free interval

Interval (years)	Original quadrant (%)	Different quadrant (%)
0–2	90	10
3–7	83	17
8–10	68	34
11–15	45	55
≥ 16	0	100

From Kurtz et al.[2]

years. As Table 10.1 shows, most of the relapses within the first 10 years were in the vicinity of the original tumour but subsequently most were in other quadrants. It is the tumours in the original quadrant that are true relapses, most distant lesions being new primary cancers.

Subsequent survival of patients was better for those with a longer disease-free interval. In those relapsing within 2 years, subsequent 5-year overall survival rate was 48%, rising to

61% for those recurring in the third year, 75% for those relapsing in years 4–5, and 84% for patients who relapsed after 5 years. Other than the disease-free interval, other prognostic factors were histological grade and extent of relapse. For those with grade I/II cancers, the 5-year overall survival was 72% compared with 40% in those with grade III tumours. When the recurrence measured 2 cm or less the 5-year survival was 74% and this fell to 42% if the relapse was larger than 2 cm.

Fisher et al re-analysed the data from the NSABP B-06 trial to determine the significance of ipsilateral breast relapse after wide excision, with or without external radiotherapy.[3] After a median follow-up of 9 years, the probability of breast relapse was 12% in the irradiated cases and 43% in the non-irradiated. In the first 3 years after treatment, the annual hazards for breast relapse were 1.4% and 8.5% respectively. Subsequently the hazard for the non-irradiated group fell to 4.6% per year whereas that of the irradiated group remained stable at 1.4%.

In the multivariate analysis for predictors of time to breast relapse, only two factors were significant: use of radiotherapy and pathological tumour size. A second Cox's regression model examined fixed and time-dependent factors for development of distant metastases. Of the fixed co-variates, six were significant: nodal status, poor and intermediate tumour type, nuclear grade, pathological size and age. Combining the fixed and time-dependent co-variates, five were significant predictors for distant metastasis: breast relapse, age, nodal status, tumour types and nuclear grade. This study also showed that early breast relapse was associated with a higher risk of developing distant metastases, as summarized in Table 10.2. Of those relapsing within one year, 76% developed distant metastases compared with only 44% who had a breast relapse more than 12 months after treatment. The probability of distant metastases for those relapsing within 5 years was 57%, but only 18% in those who developed ipsilateral recurrence after 5 years. It was concluded that ipsilateral breast relapse increased the risk of distant metastases and as

Table 10.2 Risk of distant metastases after breast relapse in relation to disease-free interval (DFI)

DFI (years)	Number	Distant metastases (%)
≤ 1	41	76
≤ 2	103	64
≤ 5	191	57
> 5	49	18

From Fisher et al.[3]

a predictive variable was stronger than tumour size.

Veronesi et al examined local relapse and distant metastases in 2233 patients who had been treated by QUART at the Milan Cancer Institute between 1970 and 1987.[4] Within this group of patients, the first event was local relapse in 151 (6%) and distant metastases in 414 (19%). Of those with local relapse, this was deemed to be a new primary in 32 and true local relapse in 119 (79%). During the first year after treatment the probability of breast relapse was more than 1%, but between years 2 and 9, the median annual rate fluctuated around 1.1%. In contrast, the probability of distant metastases rose rapidly to a maximum of 5% at 21 months after surgery and then fell to very low levels by the eighth year, after which it fluctuated haphazardly.

When regression analyses were performed to determine significant predictors of local relapse and distant metastases, interesting differences emerged, as shown in Table 10.3. A significant factor for local relapse was young age with an almost fourfold increase in risk in those aged 35 or less compared with woman over 65, but this had less impact on risk of distant relapse. In terms of size there was a threefold increase in risk of relapse in those with cancers larger than 2 cm compared with those sized 0.5 cm or less, and a quadrupling of risk of distant relapse.

Table 10.3 Risk ratios for local relapse and distant metastases after QUART

Factor	Local relapse	Distant metastases
Age 46–55 vs >65	2.7	0.85
≤ 35 vs >65	3.8	1.9
Size ≥ 2.0 vs 0.5	3.2	4.0
Nodes: 1 vs 0	0.5	1.3
2–3 vs 0	0.5	1.9
≥ 4 vs 0	0.8	4.1
Histology: EIC vs IDC/ILC	1.8	0.9

From Veronesi et al.[4]

When the influence of nodal status was examined, there was a negative relationship between number of nodes involved and risk of breast recurrence, in that those with negative nodes had the highest risk of relapse, possibly because they were more likely to survive long enough for such an event to occur. This was the reverse of the risk for distant metastases which increased directly with regard to number of nodes involved.

The presence of extensive intraductal component led to a doubling in risk of breast relapse compared with those with infiltrating ductal carcinoma (IDC) or infiltrating lobular carcinoma (ILC), but this had no impact on risk of distant metastases. For those patients who developed a breast relapse within the first year of surgery, there was an increased risk of distant relapse (RR = 6.6) compared with those relapsing more than 3 years after surgery.

Histological risk factors for breast relapse

There are some clinical features that are contraindications to breast conservation, such as large or multifocal tumours. Even after excluding such cases there will still be women who will relapse after breast radiotherapy and it would be very useful if these individuals could be identified on a basis of the histological or biological features of the primary tumour. In an attempt to do this, Harris et al conducted a clinicopathological review of 226 patients treated with radiotherapy as part of breast conservation therapy.[5] They sought in particular for three histological features: poorly differentiated nuclei, moderate or marked ductal carcinoma in situ (DCIS) within the primary, and DCIS in surrounding tissue. All three features were present in 53 cases (23%), and ipsilateral breast relapse occurred in 37% of these. Of those with only one feature the 6-year breast relapse rate was 8% and if none was seen there was a zero breast relapse rate. Subsequently Schnitt combined the features of DCIS within the tumour and in the peritumoral tissue as extensive intraductal component (EIC).[6] EIC was defined as being present when more than 25% of the tumour comprised DCIS which was also extended outside the main tumour mass.

Zafrani et al reviewed the histology of 434 patients treated by breast conservation therapy at the Institut Curie, Paris, and related these to risk of breast relapse and survival after a median follow-up of 8.5 years.[7] The most significant pathological indicator of breast relapse was incomplete excision ($p < 0.0001$), followed by lymphatic permeation ($p < 0.02$) and finally EIC ($p < 0.03$). The pathological predictors of breast cancer mortality were lymphatic permeation ($p < 0.0001$), high grade ($p < 0.005$), incomplete surgery ($p < 0.007$), absence of EIC ($p < 0.008$) and tumour size. This suggested that EIC might be a surrogate marker of extent of tumour and likelihood of incomplete excision.

This view was confirmed when Holland et al reviewed pathological material from 214 breast cancer cases treated by mastectomy in Nijmegen.[8] Of the 66 cases with extensive in situ component (EIC+) in the original biopsy, 74% had extensive residual carcinoma compared with 42% of those that had no extensive in situ

Table 10.4 Probability of residual breast carcinoma at a distance from the edge of the biopsy site in patients with and without EIC

	>0.5 cm	>2 cm	>4 cm	>6 cm	>8 cm
Invasive cancer (%)					
EIC+	36	20	12	2	2
EIC–	19	12	7	4	1
DCIS (%)					
EIC+	71	58	32	21	8
EIC–	28	19	5	4	1

From Holland et al.[8]

Table 10.5 Probability of breast relapse in relation to volume of breast tissue excised and presence or absence of EIC

T size	EIC	Small (%)	Medium (%)	Large (%)
T1	EIC+	29	22	10
T1	EIC–	9	2	0
T2	EIC+	36	26	9
T2	EIC–	6	2	3

From Vicini et al.[10]

component (EIC–). The probabilities of finding DCIS and invasive carcinoma at increasing distances from the primary tumour in relation to presence or absence of EIC are given in Table 10.4. Overall, some residual invasive breast cancer or DCIS was present in 74% of those with EIC+, but only 42% of those who were EIC–. Even with a margin of 2 cm from the original biopsy site when EIC was present there was a 20% chance of residual invasive carcinoma within the breast.

Jacquemier et al assessed EIC in specimens from 496 cases treated by breast conservation therapy and found that there was an increased risk of breast relapse (18% vs 8%), but this effect was limited to premenopausal cases.[9] Those with EIC+ were more likely to have had incomplete excision (23% vs 7%), although the relapse rate was high in those who were EIC+, irrespective of margins.

In another study from the Joint Centre for Radiation Therapy, Boston, the originators of EIC, the likelihood of breast relapse in relation to EIC and volume of tissue excised was examined in 507 cases followed for a median of 8 years.[10] On a basis of pathologically measured volume patients were divided into small, intermediate and large biopsies. For those with T1 tumours the volumes were defined as small ($< 13\,\text{cm}^3$), intermediate ($13–48\,\text{cm}^3$), and large ($> 48\,\text{cm}^3$); for T2 tumours, as $< 35\,\text{cm}^3$, $35–74\,\text{cm}^3$ and $> 74\,\text{cm}^3$ respectively. Probabilities of breast relapse are given in Table 10.5, and this clearly shows that the risk of breast relapse in those who are EIC+ is substantially reduced when a larger amount of tissue is removed surgically.

The surrogacy of EIC as a marker of potential residual tumour is important. It should alert the surgeon to carry out a more extensive re-excision, and the pathologist to check the re-excision margins because some of these patients may be better treated by mastectomy and reconstruction rather than breast conservation therapy.

Multifocal disease

Several histopathological studies have shown that breast cancer can be both multifocal and multicentric.[11–14] The two terms have been used interchangeably but have been more clearly defined by Holland.[14] They define multifocality as the presence of in situ disease or lymphatic invasion more than 1 cm from the infiltrating margin, and multicentricity as two areas of cancer separated by normal breast tissue. As such cases are deemed to be at high risk of breast relapse they are usually advised not to undergo breast conservation.[15]

The need for such a rigid approach has been questioned by Kurtz et al who treated 61 patients with more than one macroscopic tumour mass by breast conservation therapy at the Marseilles Cancer Institute.[16] Of these cases, 20 had two or more palpable tumours, two had mammographically detected separate lesions, and 39 were found to have multiple tumours on histological examination of the biopsy specimen. All were treated with 50–60 Gy to the breast and an external boost of 20–25 Gy to the tumour bed. When compared with 525 contemporary cases with unifocal tumours, after a follow-up of 6 years, the breast relapse rate was

11% for unifocal cases, 16% for those with bifocal tumours and 35% in those with three or more separate cancers. Those with clinical or radiological multifocal disease were more likely to relapse than those diagnosed by the pathologist (36% vs 18%). There were 22 cases with negative biopsy margins and one (5%) relapsed whereas, of 39 with involved or indeterminate margins, relapse occurred in 14 (36%).

Hartsell et al reviewed 474 patients treated by breast conservation therapy between 1977 and 1989, of whom 27 had two or more tumour masses.[17] Although all had macroscopically clear margins, four (15%) were found to have microscopic disease at the margin. Postoperative radiotherapy was given to a dose of 45–54 Gy and 11 received an electron boost of 6–20 Gy. After a median follow-up of 4.5 years, one breast relapse occurred in a patient with dubious margins, who also had synchronous distant metastases.

These results suggest that multicentric disease need not be an absolute contraindication to breast conservation but only if pathological confirmation of clear margins has been obtained for each tumour. In addition, a postoperative mammogram should be taken to exclude the presence of residual microcalcification. Even with these precautions, such cases are at increased risk of recurrence and, if mastectomy is not going to be performed, they should be warned accordingly.

Invasive lobular carcinoma

Invasive lobular carcinoma can be difficult to diagnose and the extent of disease may be indeterminate because of the Indian-file pattern of infiltration. In a histological study of mastectomy specimens from patients with ILC, Gump et al found that separate foci were present in 50% compared with 19% in those with invasive ductal cancers.[18] This would suggest a greater likelihood of residual disease after gross tumour excision, but possibly the diffuse distribution of the tumour cells might make them more susceptible to whole breast irradiation.

This is suggested by the results of the Christie Hospital trial comparing tumour bed irradiation with whole breast irradiation in which the relapse rate for ILC treated by local radiation was higher than after whole breast irradiation.[19]

Schnitt et al reported 49 cases of ILC treated with tumour excision and breast radiation with a median follow-up of 6 years.[20] Relapse occurred in 12% as compared with 11% in contemporaneously treated cases with IDC. When those with IDC were divided on a basis of presence or absence of EIC, the breast relapse rates were 23% and 5% respectively. Hence, ILC itself was not associated with a high risk of relapse. Almost all relapses in those with ILC were next to the original tumour site.

Kurtz et al reported a series of 861 breast cancer cases treated by breast conservation therapy, of whom 67 (8%) had ILC.[21] There was a 14% breast relapse rate for ILC after breast conservation, compared with 9% in those with invasive ductal carcinoma, and those with ILC were more likely to recur in a different quadrant. Both of these series were reported from radiotherapy centres where the previous surgery had been of variable extent. In the trials such as NSABP B-06, where wide local excision was performed, with histologically clear margins, ILC was not associated with any increased risk of breast relapse.[22]

Young age

As discussed in Chapter 18, young women (aged $\leq$ 35) are at increased risk of breast relapse after breast conservation, partly because they are more likely to have poorly differentiated cancers and also because those tumours are extensive (as indicated by presence of EIC). Greater care must be exercised in advising breast conservation in younger women even though there may be great pressure from the patient to avoid a mastectomy. Provided that the patient has a well-differentiated operable cancer that has been completely excised (in the luteal phase), and an axillary dissection is performed, young women can be safely treated by conservation therapy.

Salvage treatment

If a patient develops an operable breast relapse after breast conservation therapy, it is customary to exclude distant metastatic disease and, having done this, to advise a salvage mastectomy, with or without immediate reconstruction. Considering that this might be overtreatment, Kurtz et al postulated that wide excision alone might be feasible for patients who relapsed at the original tumour site.[23] In a series of 1245 cases treated by breast conservation therapy, 118 (9%) developed an isolated breast relapse of whom 52 (44%) were treated by wide excision, with an additional axillary dissection in 18. With a median follow-up of 6 years after salvage surgery, a second locoregional relapse occurred in 12 (23%), whereas two patients developed recurrence in a previously undissected axilla. The second relapse was operable in 10 patients (83%). The survival rate after first salvage operation was 79% at 5 years and 64% at 10 years.

In a subsequent study of prognostic factors for successful breast-conserving salvage surgery, Kurtz et al analysed results at a median follow-up of 51 months after salvage surgery, by which time second breast relapse had occurred in 16/50 (32%).[24] A Cox multivariate analysis was conducted and the two independent prognostic variables were disease-free interval and the margins on the salvage resection specimen. For those who relapsed within 5 years of first treatment, second relapse occurred in 15 of 32 (47%) compared with one of 18 (6%) in those who relapsed more than 5 years after breast conservation. When the resection margins were positive or indeterminate, a second breast recurrence occurred in 8 of 17 (47%) compared with 8 of 28 (24%) of those with clearly negative margins.

In EORTC trial 10801, the survival after salvage treatment was similar in those who were originally treated by either breast conservation therapy or modified radical mastectomy.[25] Fifty per cent of both groups were alive 4 years after local relapse treated by salvage mastectomy or excision and radiotherapy. Wide local excision of an isolated breast recurrence does appear to be a reasonable option for patients who develop a second cancer in the treated breast more than 5 years after first being treated. For those relapsing earlier, unless it can be shown unequivocally to be a new primary by virtue of different tumour grade or the presence of DCIS, salvage mastectomy should be advised. Recurrent disease should be treated radically because some patients can still be cured of their disease by effective ablative surgery.

A review was conducted at Guy's Hospital of 448 patients treated by tumourectomy, axillary clearance and breast irradiation, of whom 67 (15%) developed an ipsilateral breast relapse after a median follow-up of 64 months.[26] The median interval between breast conservation therapy and relapse was 31 months and, after re-staging, 22 proved to have metastatic disease. The relapse was detected clinically in 24 (54%) and mammographically in 21 (46%), and 41 (91%) were of similar histology to the original carcinoma. Of the 45 with isolated breast relapse, 75% were true or marginal relapses, 12% were in another quadrant and 13% were diffuse, with 37 (82%) of the recurrences being operable.

All the operable cases had salvage surgery (total mastectomy) and 51% were still alive 5 years later. The later that breast relapse occurred after breast conservation therapy, the better the prognosis. Of those who relapsed within 2 years, 79% had either extensive local relapse or distant metastases compared with only 26% of those relapsing after 2 years ($p = 0.0004$). Further local relapse after salvage surgery occurred in 11 (29%), which was controlled by further surgery or radiotherapy in nine but the other two cases had uncontrolled local disease.

To compare the outcome after salvage surgery for locoregional relapse after either breast conservation or mastectomy, van Tienhoven et al reviewed 1807 patients treated in EORTC 10801 and DBCG 82-TM.[27] Locoregional relapse without distant metastases occurred in 133, of whom 67 were originally treated by modified radical mastectomy and 66 by breast conservation therapy. The 5-year survival rates after

salvage surgery were 58% and 57% respectively. In a multivariate analysis, the significant prognostic factors for survival after relapse were the histological node status and vascular invasion. When potential factors predicting for time to second locoregional relapse were examined, three emerged as significant: extent of local relapse, time to first relapse and the histological node status. For those treated by breast conservation therapy, disease-free interval and extent of relapse were the only significant variables predicting for length of subsequent disease-free interval after first relapse. Optimum therapy after relapse needs to be determined by multicentre randomized trials, taking into account the disease-free interval and histology of the original and subsequent tumours.

POOR COSMETIC OUTCOME

The aim of breast conservation is to obtain disease control as effectively as mastectomy but with preservation of normal body image. The former objective has been achieved but sometimes at the cost of an impaired cosmetic outcome. Quadrantectomy gives good local control but may be associated with a major tissue deficit. Higher dosages of radiation will reduce relapse at the expense of skin telangiectases and breast fibrosis. A lot of effort has been put into devising sometimes complex methods of objectively assessing cosmetic outcome, in order that different techniques can be compared. This is the logical approach but what really matters is whether the patient is satisfied with the result.

Radiotherapy and cosmetic outcome

Standard treatment from a 4–6 MeV linear accelerator is a dosage of 45–50 Gy delivered in 23–25 fractions over 5–6 weeks, and this is skin sparing and without undue associated fibrosis. A boost is given particularly when there are positive biopsy margins, but the value of this has not yet been determined. A boost may lead to skin pigmentation when given as electrons, or to breast fibrosis if an implant is used.

To assess the contribution of a boost to local control, the EORTC has conducted trial 10882 in which patients with tumours sized 5 cm or less were treated by wide excision and axillary clearance, followed by breast irradiation (50 Gy).[28] Those with negative tumour margins were randomized to no boost or an interstitial (15 Gy) or external (16 Gy) boost. For cases with involved margins a randomized boost of 10 or 25 Gy was given. Between 1987 and 1992, 1458 cases were entered but no results are yet available.

McRae et al examined the dose volume in 11 patients treated with an iridium implant and compared these in five cases who developed severe breast fibrosis or fat necrosis with 51 who had no severe complications.[29] A minimum tumour volume dose of 20 Gy was specified. The mean volumes of the implants were significantly greater in all those who developed complications.

In a subset of 51 patients who were treated by breast conservation therapy at Guy's Hospital as part of EORTC 10801, cosmetic outcome was examined in relation to skin dose of radiation.[30] All had a flexible implant inserted at the time of axillary clearance and were afterloaded with iridium-92 (^{192}Ir) to deliver 20 Gy in 2 days. Skin doses were measured during both the implant and subsequent external radiotherapy (46 Gy), using lithium fluoride microrods. There was no relationship between skin dose and skin pigmentation, oedema or fibrosis. However, those with larger breasts and with tumours in the lower half of the breast were more likely to receive skin doses of more than 50 Gy which led to development of telangiectases and a worse cosmetic outcome. This was probably caused by changes in posture changing the interstitial dose distribution.

It may take up to 5 years for radiation-induced changes to manifest and so it is important that cosmetic outcome is not assessed too soon after surgery and radiotherapy. Rose et al evaluated cosmetic outcome in 593 patients treated by breast conservation therapy at the Joint Center for Radiation Therapy, Boston, using objective criteria, after a median follow-up of 6 years.[31] The features sought were breast oedema, retraction, fibrosis, telangiectases and arm oedema. For each a score of none, minimal, moderate or severe was assigned: 'normal' being no radiation change, 'minimal' a change perceptible only to the trained observer, 'moderate' an obvious change or defect and 'severe' a major deformity or functional impairment. Cases were evaluated every 6 months.

At 3 years, 65% had an excellent result, 25% good, 7% fair and 3% poor, and this was maintained subsequently with 94% of those deemed to have an excellent result being similarly assessed at 7 years. Adjuvant chemotherapy had an impact on cosmetic outcome with only 40% of those so treated having an excellent result compared with 71% of non-treated cases. Patients with smaller lesions also fared better, with 73% of those with T1 tumours rated excellent against 55% of those with T2 cancers.

Paradoxically, although patients with large breasts may undergo extensive surgical resection, without any apparent tissue deficit, subsequent response to radiotherapy can lead to a poor cosmetic outcome. Pezner et al examined predictive factors for breast oedema after breast conservation therapy in 47 cases.[32] Surgery comprised wide excision and axillary clearance or sampling in 87% and radiotherapy was delivered by cobalt-60 telotherapy in 94% to a dosage of 45–51 Gy. An iridium boost was given to 40% and an external boost to 23%, with a total boost dose of 15–25 Gy. Breast oedema was defined as the presence of one of the following: breast enlargement with or without pain, peau d'orange, diffuse skin erythema and diffuse hyperpigmented skin pores. By these criteria, skin oedema occurred in 16 cases (34%). Breast oedema was noted more frequently in those cases that had a full axillary clearance, but this was not statistically significant. The only significant predictor was breast size measured by bra cup. Oedema occurred in 15% of those with bra cup size A and B compared with 48% of those taking C/D/DD.

At Guy's Hospital, a measure of cosmetic outcome based on breast compliance was devel-

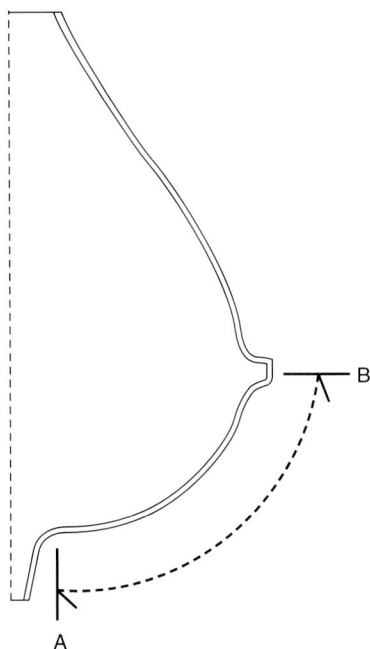

Fig. 10.1 Sagittal section through the breast showing distance from (A) inframammary fold and (B) midpoint of nipple.

Table 10.6 Radiation effect in relation to breast size

Breast size	None/mild (%)	Moderate (%)	Severe (%)
Small	98	2	0
Medium	85	11	4
Large	70	20	10

From Moody et al.[34]

those who had a satisfactory outcome was 1.5 cm compared with 0.8 cm in the unsatisfactory outcome group ($p < 0.001$). Thus a simple measurement may be useful as a method of evaluating cosmetic outcome in an objective manner.

Moody et al analysed late radiation effects in a prospective study of 559 women who had breast cancer treated by tumorectomy and radiotherapy.[34] These patients were participants in a randomized trial comparing three different fractionation schedules: 50 Gy in 25 fractions, 42.9 Gy in 13 fractions and 39 Gy in 13 fractions. Cosmetic outcome was determined from serial photographs taken annually and subsequently scored blindly by two male doctors and a female senior nurse. Intraobserver variation was good (84–88%) for both breast size (small medium or large) and change in breast appearance. Ratings of radiation effect and breast size are given in Table 10.6. No patients with small breasts developed severe radiation effects but this occurred in 4% of those with medium and 10% of those with large-sized breasts. Among those women with large breasts a moderate or severe change was found in 30%.

Surgery and cosmetic outcome

As part of the Milan trial which compared QUART (quadrantectomy, axillary clearance and radiotherapy) with TART (tumorectomy,

oped.[33] Compliance was the difference between the anterior breast surface distance from the inframammary fold to the nipple with the patient in the erect and supine positions, as shown in Fig. 10.1. In a series of 100 normal controls the mean difference was 1.8 cm. Compliance was also measured in 51 women who had undergone breast conservation within EORTC trial 10801.[25] Cosmetic outcome was rated by two clinicians using the criteria of the JCRT: excellent, good, fair and poor.[31] The first two were combined as satisfactory and the latter two as unsatisfactory. In addition, the patients were asked to rate their cosmetic result as satisfactory or unsatisfactory. The clinical rating was that 11 (15%) had an unsatisfactory and 40 (85%) a satisfactory result. All patients in the satisfactory group were also in agreement with this. The mean compliance difference in

Table 10.7 Computer-assessed comparison of QUART and TART cases

Difference in measurement	TART (%)	QUART (%)
Nipple height > 3 cm	7	21
Inferior profile > 3 cm	3	11
Midline–nipple > 1.5 cm	5	17

From Veronesi et al.[35]

axillary clearance and radiotherapy), the cosmetic outcome was assessed in 148 consecutive cases.[35] Frontal photographs were taken 18–24 months after treatment and computer analysed to determine difference in height of the nipples, difference in height of inferior breast profile, and difference in distance between midline and nipples. As Table 10.7 shows, the group treated by QUART (75) had a worse computer-assessed cosmetic outcome than the 73 cases treated by TART. There was a difference of more than 3 cm in nipple height between treated and untreated breast in 21% of QUART cases compared with 7% of TART cases. When patients were asked to rate their cosmetic outcome, 75% of those treated by QUART considered it to be good/excellent, compared with 90% of the TART group.[36]

In EORTC 10801 trial the cosmetic outcome in those treated by breast conservation therapy was rated by doctor and patient every year and three photographs were taken after 2 and 4 years, which were rated by a panel.[37] Evaluation of cosmesis by clinicians one year after treatment was good/excellent in 79% but this fell to 69% at the last evaluation. After one year 87% of patients rated their cosmetic result as good or excellent compared with 78% at their final evaluation.

Christie et al compared live assessment with photography in 24 patients who underwent breast conservation and adjuvant chemotherapy

with 23 who had breast conservation therapy without chemotherapy.[38] All had local or wide excision and most (96%) had a level II axillary clearance. Whole breast irradiation (44 Gy) with an electron boost (20 Gy) was used in 24 whereas 23 had 50 Gy to the breast and a 10 Gy boost with electrons. Cosmesis was assessed by patient and spouse as excellent, good, fair or poor, and bra cup size before and after treatment was recorded. Live assessment was conducted a minimum of 18 months after irradiation by a radiation oncologist and a research nurse who were not involved in treatment of the patient. Included in the assessment were breast size, skin pigmentation, telangiectases, breast oedema, arm diameter, arm power and arm function. In addition, upward and lateral retraction of the nipple were recorded using Pezner's method.[32] At the same visit photographs were taken for subsequent evaluation.

Of all the features studied, changes in nipple height were the most consistent determinant of both objective and subjective assessment of cosmetic outcome and this could be readily determined from photographs. Thus for simplicity in studies of cosmetic outcome after breast conservation therapy, photographs should be taken on an annual basis and final conclusions drawn only after a minimum of 5 years of follow-up after surgery and radiotherapy.

A new approach to the problem of tissue deficit after wide excision is replacement of volume loss by latissimus dorsi miniflap.[39] A series of 20 patients had a wide excision and axillary dissection performed through a lateral inframammary incision. After this, a portion of latissimus dorsi was harvested which was equivalent to the wide excision volume. This was achieved by dividing the muscle tendon and fascia between the muscle fibres and teres major, after which the muscle belly was incised along the inferior and posterior margins, leaving the neuromuscular bundle intact. The flap was then displaced laterally into the wide excision site.

When cosmetic results were compared with 38 cases who had wide excision without tissue replacement, breast retraction leading to an unsatisfactory result occurred in 34% of those who had wide excision alone but in only 10% of those who had wide excision and miniflap. Use of the miniflap allowed a larger resection with 57% of specimens weighing more than 150 g whereas of the wide excision specimens 13% were over 150 g. After wide excision alone 37% had involved margins compared with only 10% of those who had a miniflap.

EVALUATION OF CHANGES

A substantial amount of the morbidity associated with breast conservation is the result of uncertainty in the clinician's mind about the significance of changes in the breast. Consequent investigations may also greatly distress the patient who has fears about recurrence. Clinical evaluation of the irradiated breast can be extremely difficult and it may not be possible to determine clinically whether a lump or an area of thickening is caused by fibrosis, fat necrosis or tumour relapse. It does not matter if follow-up is conducted by radiation oncologist, medical oncologist or surgeon, provided that the clinician is experienced in the assessment of the conserved breast.

It has been customary for patients to be reviewed every 3–4 months for the first 3 years after treatment, 6-monthly for a further 2 years, and thereafter annually. Pressure is mounting from purchasers of health care to reduce costs and so follow-up visits may be either reduced or abolished. This will be an adverse step because cases treated by breast conservation therapy will benefit from annual mammography and detection of relapse may be facilitated by expert clinical evaluation.

In a series of 214 patients treated by breast conservation at Guy's Hospital, after a mean follow-up of 26 months a new lump had developed in 17 cases (8%).[40] All of these lumps were biopsied proving seven to be malignant and ten benign. Most of the benign lumps were caused by fat necrosis. There were no clinical features that could distinguish between benign and malignant lumps but mammography was more

Table 10.8 Clinical, mammographic and histological findings in patients with breast lumps after breast conservation therapy

Clinical lump	X-ray opacity	Micro-calcification	Malignant (%)
+	−	−	28
+	+	−	67
+	−	+	100
−	−	+	68
−	+	+	62

From Solin et al.[43]

likely to show a mass or microcalcification in malignant lumps.

As a result of the uncertainties of clinical examination and the reluctance to over-expose the breast to ionizing radiation, attempts have been made to use alternative imaging techniques for assessment of the treated breast. Ulmer et al carried out a prospective study of the use of thermography in 309 women who had breast cancers treated by wide excision and radiotherapy.[41] Breast relapse occurred in 17 but the thermographic pattern after breast conservation was so variable that there were no detectable thermographic differences between those that recurred and those without relapse. A similar lack of efficacy of thermography in detection of locally recurrent and contralateral breast cancers was reported by Mahoney.[42]

In a series of 145 breast biopsies performed on women who had previously undergone breast conservation, Solin et al compared clinical findings, mammographic appearance and eventual histology.[43] Results are given in Table 10.8, which shows that a lump without a mammographic abnormality was malignant in only 27%, whereas if both a mammographic mass and microcalcification were seen, the lump was invariably a relapse.

Fine needle aspiration of suspected lumps although carrying a much lower morbidity than excision biopsy does carry the risk of an inadequate sample leading to a false-negative diagnosis. A core needle biopsy is more accurate. In Solin's series the positive core needle biopsy rate was 94% compared with 25% for fine needle aspiration cytology (FNAC). Hence, unless FNAC gives an unequivocal diagnosis of fat necrosis, a negative result should be regarded as an indication for core biopsy or an open procedure.

Cox et al carried out regular follow-up on 123 patients treated by breast conservation therapy to determine the timescale for development of stable clinical and radiological findings after surgery and radiotherapy.[44] The mean size of the mammographic scar was 3.5 cm at 6 months after surgery, and this decreased to a stable 2 cm by 2 years. No scar was seen in 27% but in the remainder it was stellate in shape and subsequently disappeared in 16%. This suggests that any increase in scar size is an indication for obtaining a histological or cytological diagnosis.

When there is a radiological suspicion of relapse, magnetic resonance imaging (MRI), with gadolinium enhancement, can be a useful additional investigation.[45] If the MRI scan shows enhancement after injection of contrast, this is strongly suggestive of recurrence and a biopsy is required (if necessary after MRI localization with placement of a non-ferrous marker).

ANGIOSARCOMA

An increasing number of angiosarcomas in irradiated breast skin have been reported and details of these are given in Chapter 22. The mean interval between original radiotherapy and diagnosis of sarcoma was 6 years and average age at diagnosis of angiosarcoma was 63 years (range 47–83). These tumours usually present as a red, blue or violet lump, sometimes with ecchymosis, in oedematous skin. Most were treated by total mastectomy.

After relatively short follow-up 18 (53%) were alive and well without recurrence. The average survival after diagnosis of angiosarcoma was 13.5 months. The incidence among women who have had radiotherapy as part of breast conservation is very low. The three cases from the Istituto Tumori Milan were derived from a total of 3295 patients treated over a 17-year period, representing an incidence of 0.09%.[46] The small but definite risk underlines the need both to monitor most carefully irradiated patients and to biopsy pigmented lesions developing within the irradiated field.

SYNOPSIS

- Ipsilateral breast relapse occurs annually in 1% of cases treated by breast conservation and within the first 5 years is likely to be a true recurrence, whereas after this time it is usually a new primary.
- There are no absolute histological contraindications to breast conservation therapy but extensive intraductal component is an indicator of extensive tumour so that wide excision is necessary.
- Young women (aged ≤ 35) are at increased risk of relapse because of more frequent extensive disease and poorly differentiated cancers.
- Standard salvage treatment after relapse is mastectomy but selected cases with completely excised recurrence may be observed.
- Cosmetic outcome after breast conservation is determined by extent of surgery and breast size with a worse outcome in those with larger breasts.
- Follow-up after breast conservation therapy should be conducted by experienced clinicians with annual mammography to exclude ipsilateral relapse and contralateral new primaries.

REFERENCES

1. Sarrazin D, Dewar JA, Arriagada R et al. Conservative management of breast cancer. *Br J Surg* 1986; **73**: 604–6.
2. Kurtz JM, Amalric R, Brandone H et al. Local recurrence after breast-conserving surgery and radiotherapy. Frequency, time course, and prognosis. *Cancer* 1989; **63**: 1912–17.
3. Fisher B, Anderson S, Fisher ER et al. Significance of ipsilateral breast tumour recurrence after lumpectomy. *Lancet* 1991; **338**: 327–31.
4. Veronesi U, Marubini E, Del Vecchio M et al. Local recurrences and distant metastases after conservative breast cancer treatments: partly independent events. *J Natl Cancer Inst* 1995; **87**: 19–27.
5. Harris JR, Connolly JL, Schnitt SJ et al. The use of pathologic features in selecting the extent of surgical resection necessary for breast cancer patients treated by primary radiation therapy. *Ann Surg* 1984; **201**: 164–9.
6. Schnitt SJ, Connolly JL, Harris JR et al. Pathologic predictors of early local recurrence in stage I and II breast cancer treated by primary radiation therapy. *Cancer* 1984; **53**: 1049–57.
7. Zafrani B, Vielh P, Forquet A et al. Conservative treatment of early breast: prognostic value of the ductal in situ component and other pathological variables on local control and survival. *Eur J Cancer* 1989; **25**: 1645–50.
8. Holland R, Connolly JL, Gelman R et al. The presence of an extensive intraductal component following limited excision correlates with prominent residual disease in the remainder of the breast. *J Clin Oncol* 1990; **8**: 113–18.
9. Jacquemier J, Kurtz JM, Amalric R et al. An assessment of extensive intraductal component as a risk factor for local recurrence after breast-conserving therapy. *Br J Cancer* 1990; **61**: 873–6.
10. Vicini FA, Eberlein TJ, Connolly JL et al. The optimal extent of resection for patients with stages I or II breast cancer treated with conservative surgery and radiotherapy. *Ann Surg* 1991; **214**: 200–5.
11. Rosen PP, Fracchia AA, Urban JA. 'Residual' mammary carcinoma following simulated partial mastectomy. *Cancer* 1975; **35**: 739–47.
12. Schwartz GF, Patchefsky AS, Feig SA et al. Multicentricity of non-palpable breast cancer. *Cancer* 1980; **45**: 2913–16.
13. Lagios MD, Westdahl PR, Rose MR. The concept and implications of multicentricity in breast carcinoma. *Pathol Ann* 1981; **16**: 83–102.
14. Holland R, Velig SHJ, Mrvrunac M et al. Histologic multifocality of TIS, T1–2 breast carcinomas. *Cancer* 1985; **56**: 979–90.
15. Danoff BF, Haller DG, Glick JH, Goodman RL. Conservative surgery and irradiation in the treatment of early breast cancer. *Ann Intern Med* 1985; **102**: 634–42.
16. Kurtz JM, Jacquemier J, Amalric R et al. Breast-conserving therapy for macroscopically multiple cancers. *Ann Surg* 1990; **212**: 38–44.
17. Hartsell WF, Recine DC, Griem KL et al. Should multicentric disease be an absolute contraindication to the use of breast-conserving therapy? *Int J Radiat Oncol Biol Phys* 1994; **30**: 49–53.
18. Gump FE, Habif DV, Logerfo P et al. The extent and distribution of cancer in breasts with palpable primary tumors. *Ann Surg* 1986; **204**: 384–90.
19. Magee B, Swindell R, Harris M, Banerjee SS. Prognostic factors for breast recurrence after conservative breast surgery and radiotherapy: results from a randomised trial. *Radiother Oncol* 1996; **39**: 223–7.
20. Schnitt SJ, Connolly JL, Recht A et al. Influence of infiltrating lobular histology on local tumor control in breast cancer patients treated with conservative surgery and radiotherapy. *Cancer* 1989; **64**: 448–54.
21. Kurtz JM, Jacquemier J, Torhorst J et al. Conservation therapy for breast cancers other than infiltrating ductal carcinoma. *Cancer* 1989; **63**: 1630–5.
22. Fisher ER, Sass R, Fisher B et al. Pathologic findings from the National Surgical Adjuvant breast project (protocol 6): II. relation of breast recurrence to multicentricity. *Cancer* 1986; **57**: 1717–24.
23. Kurtz JM, Amalric R, Brandone H et al. Results of wide excision for mammary recurrence after breast-conserving therapy. *Cancer* 1988; **61**: 1969–72.
24. Kurtz JM, Jacquemier J, Amalric R et al. Is breast conservation after local recurrence feasible? *Eur J Cancer* 1991; **27**: 240–4.
25. Van Dongen JA, Bartelink H, Fentiman IS et al. Factors influencing local relapse and survival and results of salvage treatment after breast-conserving therapy in operable breast cancer:

EORTC Trial 10801, breast conservation compared with mastectomy in TNM stage I and II breast cancer. *Eur J Cancer* 1992; **28A:** 801–5.

26. Chaudary MA, Nagadowska M, Smith P et al. Local relapse after breast conservation treatment: outcome following salvage mastectomy. *Breast* 1998; in press.

27. van Tienhoven G, Voogd AC, Paterse HL et al. Prognosis after salvage treatment for loco-regional recurrence after mastectomy or breast conserving therapy in two randomized trials (EORTC 10801 and DBCG-82TM). *Eur J Cancer* 1998; in press.

28. Ptaszynski A, Van den Bogaert W, Van Glabbeke M et al. Patient population analysis in EORTC Trial 22881/10882 on the role of a booster dose in breast-conserving therapy. *Eur J Cancer* 1994; **30A:** 2073–81.

29. McRae D, Rodgers J, Dritschilo A. Dose-volume and complication in interstitial implants for breast carcinoma. *Int J Radiation Oncol* 1987; **13:** 525–9.

30. Habibollahi F, Mayles HMO, Mayles WPM et al. Assessment of skin dose and its relation to cosmesis in the conservative treatment of early breast cancer. *Int J Radiat Oncol Biol Phys* 1987; **14:** 291–6.

31. Rose MA, Olivotto I, Cady B et al. Conservative surgery and radiation therapy for early breast cancer. *Arch Surg* 1989; **124:** 153–7.

32. Pezner RD, Patterson MP, Hill LR et al. Breast edema in patients treated conservatively for stage I and II breast cancer. *Int J Radiat Oncol Biol Phys* 1985; **11:** 1765–8.

33. Tsouskas LI, Fentiman IS. Breast compliance: a new method for evaluation of cosmetic outcome after conservative treatment of breast cancer. *Breast Cancer Res Treat* 1990; **15:** 185–90.

34. Moody AM, Mayles WPM, Bliss JM et al. The influence of breast size on late radiation effects and association with radiotherapy dose inhomogeneity. *Radiother Oncol* 1994; **33:** 106–112.

35. Veronesi U, Volterrani F, Luini A et al. Quadrantectomy versus lumpectomy for small size breast cancer. *Eur J Cancer* 1990; **26:** 671–3.

36. Sacchini V, Luini A, Tana S et al. Quantitative and qualitative cosmetic evaluation after conservative treatment for breast cancer. *Eur J Cancer* 1991; **27:** 1395–1400.

37. Van Dongen JA, Bartelink H, Fentiman IS et al. Randomized clinical trial to assess the value of breast-conserving therapy in stage I and II breast cancer, EORTC 10801 trial. *J Natl Cancer Inst Monogr* 1992; **11:** 15–18.

38. Christie DRH, OíBrien MY, Christie JA et al. A comparison of methods of cosmetic assessment in breast conservation treatment. *The Breast* 1996; **5:** 358–67.

39. Raja MAK, Straker VF, Rainsbury RM. Extending the role of breast-conserving surgery by immediate volume replacement. *Br J Surg* 1997; **84:** 101–5.

40. Chaudary MA, Girling A, Girling S et al. New lumps in the breast following conservation treatment for early breast cancer. *Breast Cancer Res Treat* 1988; **11:** 51–8.

41. Ulmer HU, Brinkmann M, Frischbier H-J. Thermography in the follow-up of breast cancer patients after breast-conserving treatment by tumorectomy and radiation therapy. *Cancer* 1990; **65:** 2676–80.

42. Mahoney L. Methods for detecting locally recurrent and contralateral second primary breast cancer. *Can J Surg* 1986; **29:** 372–3.

43. Solin LJ, Fowble BL, Schultz DJ et al. The detection of local recurrence after definitive irradiation for early stage carcinoma of the breast. *Cancer* 1990; **65:** 2497–2502.

44. Cox CE, Greenberg H, Fleisher D et al. Natural history and clinical evaluation of the lumpectomy scar. *Am Surg* 1993; **59:** 55–9.

45. Cohen EK, Leonhardt CM, Shumak RS et al. Magnetic resonance imaging in potential postsurgical recurrence of breast cancer: pitfalls and limitations. *Can Assoc Radiol* 1996; **47:** 171–6.

46. Zucali R, Merson M, Placucci M et al. Soft tissue sarcoma of the breast after conservative surgery and irradiation for early mammary cancer. *Radiat Oncol* 1994; **30:** 271–3.

11

The role of mastectomy

What though the field is lost, all is not lost.

John Milton

History • Clinical trials • Prophylactic antibiotics • Suction drains • Indications for mastectomy

The object of surgical treatment of breast cancer is to prevent local recurrence, obtain accurate prognostic information and maximize the chances of cure. For a variety of reasons, in some patients the best way to achieve this is by performing a mastectomy. There is a common misconception that mastectomy is a redundant procedure which has been superseded by first-line systemic therapy followed by radiotherapy, with or without local surgery. There is still a substantial proportion of patients who have multifocal disease, large primary tumours or an aversion to breast conservation, for whom a mastectomy is necessary. If a mastectomy is being considered for a patient with invasive breast cancer, the aim should be to maximize local control. This means that the axilla does need to be dissected, particularly if the indication for mastectomy is a large primary tumour.

Table 11.1 Local control after mastectomies performed by Halsted and his peers

Surgeon	Number	Local relapse-free rate (%)
Bergmann	114	45
Billroth	170	18
Czerny	102	38
Fischer	147	25
Gussenbauer	151	36
König	152	40
Kuster	228	40
Lucke	110	34
Volkmann	131	40
Halsted	50	84

HISTORY

It is now over 100 years since William Halsted of Johns Hopkins Hospital published the results of his complete method of mastectomy.[1] Before this the local control after mastectomy was poor and Halsted realized that, unless a radical approach was adopted, tumour could be present at the margins of excision and therefore inevitably local relapse would follow. Halsted carried out an *en bloc* resection of breast axilla, pectoral muscles and supraclavicular nodes. He reviewed the previous publications, mostly emanating from the Austro-Hungarian empire and these are summarized in Table 11.1.[2] The list, which looks like a Who was Who of nineteenth century surgery, shows that Halsted achieved an astonishing 84% local control rate whereas other surgeons had a local control rate of 18–45%. This was all the more remarkable because three-quarters of the patients had stage III disease. Many of the patients had advanced disease caused not only by late presentation, but also because physicians were reluctant to refer cases for surgery as they regarded the condition as untreatable and incurable. One hundred years later this nihilism still persists in some unenlightened doctors and patients.

Only a few months later Willy Meyer published 'An improved method of the radical operation for carcinoma of the breast'.[3] As he was concerned that handling of the tumour by the surgeon and assistant might lead to dissemination via the lymphatics, he first removed the axillary contents followed by the breast and pectoral muscles. This was performed through an oblique elliptical incision whereas Halsted used a vertical mirror image 6 incision. Meyer had conceived the operation independently of Halsted and concluded 'further experience must show whether Halsted's or my plan of operating deserves preference'. Ironically the operation now known as Halsted's procedure is closer to that devised by Willy Meyer. Radical mastectomy became the accepted operation for breast cancer for over 50 years until challenged by McWhirter.[4] This Scottish radiotherapist irradiated the axilla after simple (total) mastectomy and achieved results which were similar to those following radical mastectomy.

As a different approach, Patey argued that local spread was most likely to be lymphatic and that fascia might be a barrier at an early stage of the disease. He therefore modified the radical mastectomy to remove the pectoralis minor but leave the pectoralis major intact.[5] In a comparison of 42 patients treated by radical mastectomy and 40 treated by modified radical mastectomy the local relapse-free survival of the two groups was 76% and 82% respectively. As well as achieving good local control the Patey operation avoided the chest wall indentation that occurred after the Halsted procedure. The procedure was modified further by Madden who performed a mastectomy and

axillary clearance but without removal of either the major or minor pectoral muscle.[6]

At this time Handley demonstrated that lymphatic spread from the breast occurred not only laterally into the axilla, but also medially to the internal mammary nodes.[7] This meant that in some cases there would be residual cancer even after Halsted's operation and so Urban designed the extended radical mastectomy, the acme of radical surgery, which aimed to extirpate all locoregional malignancy with an *en bloc* resection of breast, axillary nodes, ribs, costal cartilages and internal mammary nodes.[8]

Gradually it became apparent that these major surgical procedures were having little impact on long-term survival with, at best, only one in five patients alive 20 years after surgery, even when there had been no local relapse of the disease. This suggested that breast cancer was more likely to have undetectable micrometastases at the time of treatment for which systemic rather than radical local treatment would be necessary in order to reduce mortality.

CLINICAL TRIALS

Multiple trials have been conducted, many of which compared radical with modified radical mastectomy, total mastectomy with or without radiotherapy, or radical against extended radical surgery. Although many are now of historic interest only, they do form a basis for selecting the most appropriate method of mastectomy. They do not support the notion that total mastectomy is the best method of achieving local control in patients with invasive disease.

Total versus radical mastectomy

In 1968 a randomized trial started at Groote Schuur Hospital, Capetown in which patients with stage I and II breast cancer were treated by either total or radical mastectomy.[9] Those in the total mastectomy group with palpable nodes had these singly resected (cherry-picking) and tumour deposits were found in 16

Table 11.2 Locoregional relapse at 40 months in trial comparing total and radical mastectomy

	Total mastectomy	Radical mastectomy
Number of cases	51	44
Flap relapse	7 (14)	1 (2)
Axillary relapse	5 (10)	0
Total	**12 (24)**	**1 (2)**

Values in parentheses are percentages.
From Helman et al.[9]

Table 11.3 Ten-year results of NSABP B-04 comparing radical and total mastectomy with or without radiotherapy in clinically node-negative cases

	Radical	Total + radio-therapy	Total
Number	362	352	365
Axilla relapse	5 (1)	11 (3)	65 (18)
SCF relapse	4 (1)	1 (0.3)	11 (3)
10-year survival rate (%)	46	48	41

Values in parentheses are percentages.
From Fisher et al.[11]

of 25 (64%) compared with 22 of 53 (40%) of the radical mastectomy group. When the trial had been in progress for 40 months and 95 patients had been entered, a preliminary analysis was performed. Results are given in Table 11.2. There was a high rate of skin flap and axillary relapse in the total mastectomy group and so the trial was prematurely terminated.

Subsequently the long-term results were reported after 25 years of follow-up.[10] By this time 30% of the radical mastectomy group had died of breast cancer compared with 42% of the total mastectomy cases. This did not achieve statistical significance, probably as a result of the relatively small number of cases in the study because it had stopped accrual too early. Overall, 26% of the radical group developed local relapse against 37% of the total mastectomy group.

In NSABP trial B-04, there was a three-way randomization for patients with clinically negative axillary nodes: radical mastectomy, total mastectomy with axillary irradiation and total mastectomy without irradiation. If there were clinically suspicious nodes these were resected and, if positive, patients were randomized to modified radical mastectomy or total mastectomy with axillary irradiation. The 10-year results are given in Table 11.3,[11] which shows a significantly higher relapse rate (18%) within the group who had no treatment to the axilla. This did not translate into a statistically significant effect on mortality although fewer of this group survived 10 years. In all, over 20% of the total mastectomy group relapsed which is an unacceptable rate of local treatment failure.

A clinical trial was started in 1967 in Cardiff and London in which 230 patients with clinically negative axillae were randomized to treatment by either a total or radical mastectomy.[12] The total mastectomy group had an axillary sample and, if there was nodal involvement in the sample or clearance specimen, the axilla was irradiated. There were 66 patients who had radical mastectomy alone and 64 who had total mastectomy without radiotherapy and their outcome is summarized in Table 11.4. There were more axillary relapses in the total mastectomy group (19% vs 2%). There were fewer survivors at 10 years in the total mastectomy group but, again, this did not achieve statistical significance.

In the Malmö trial, which ran between 1969 and 1974, 195 women with breast cancers sized

Table 11.4 Results of Cardiff trial comparing radical mastectomy with total mastectomy

	Radical mastectomy	Total mastectomy
Number	66	64
Axillary relapse	1 (2)	12 (19)
Scar relapse	10 (15)	9 (13)
10-year survival rate (%)	66	58

Values in parentheses are percentages.

5 cm or less were randomized to either radical mastectomy and postoperative radiotherapy (97) or total mastectomy alone (98).[13] After a mean follow-up of 5.5 years, axillary relapse had occurred in 28 (29%) of the total mastectomy group. After 20 years of follow-up the overall survival of the group treated by radical mastectomy and radiotherapy was worse than the total mastectomy cases (45% vs 40%) and, although this was not statistically significant, it might have resulted from long-term morbidity of radiotherapy.

Radical versus total mastectomy and radiotherapy

Both the NSABP B-04 and Cardiff trials had an option for patients with clinically positive axillary nodes of randomization to radical mastectomy, or total mastectomy followed by gland field irradiation; the results of these two trials are shown in Table 11.5, together with those from the south-east Scotland and Manchester studies.[11,12,14,15] The dosage of radiotherapy in NSABP B-04 was 45 Gy to the axilla, supraclavicular fossa and internal mammary chain compared with 40 Gy in the Cardiff study. Local relapse rates were similar in both arms of NSABP B-06 but in the Cardiff trial there was a higher rate of local relapse in those treated by total mastectomy and radiotherapy.

The south-east Scotland trial was a multicentre study for women aged 35–69 with operable breast cancer and, after a follow-up of 12 years, there were significantly more local relapses and a poorer overall survival in those treated by

Table 11.5 Outcome in trials comparing radical mastectomy with total mastectomy and axillary irradiation

Trial	Follow up (years)	Total mastectomy + radiotherapy			Radical mastectomy			Reference
		No.	LR (%)	OS (%)	No.	LR (%)	OS (%)	
NSABP	10	294	13	26	292	15	30	Fisher et al[11]
Cardiff	10	39	31	38	31	9	41	Roberts et al[12]
SE Scotland	12	242	17	50	256	12	55	Langlands et al[14]
Manchester	10	159	38	31	149	39	35	Lythgoe et al[15]

LR, local relapse; OS, overall survival.

Table 11.6 Outcome in trials comparing total mastectomy with total mastectomy and axillary irradiation

Trial	Follow-up (years)	No radiotherapy			Radiotherapy			Reference
		No. (%)	Axillary relapse (%)	OS	No. (%)	Axillary relapse (%)	OS	
Southampton	3	76	28	81	74	9	78	Turnbull et al[16]
CRC	10	1140	10	70	1103	2	73	CRC[17]
Manchester	10	359	37	55	355	19	62	Lythgoe et al[15]
NSABP	10	365	18	41	352	3	48	Fisher et al[11]

total mastectomy and radiotherapy.[13] The Manchester regional trial reported no significant differences in either local relapse or overall survival at 10 years.[15] In all of these studies the survival of the radical mastectomy group was better than that of those treated by total mastectomy and radiotherapy, although only in the south-east Scotland study did this achieve statistical significance.

Total mastectomy with or without axillary radiation

In the Southampton study 150 patients aged under 70 years, with stage I/II disease, were treated by total mastectomy and an axillary node sample, after which they were all randomized to receive axillary irradiation or to be observed.[16] Results are given in Table 11.6, which shows that after a relatively short follow-up of 3 years there were substantially more axillary relapses in those who had no axillary irradiation (28% vs 9%), but at that time no effect on overall survival. A trial, which started as the King's/Cambridge study and became the Cancer Research Campaign (CRC) trial, compared immediate axillary irradiation with a watch and wait policy in 2243 women with stage I/II breast cancer.[17,18] Of the participants 25% had stage II, far fewer cases than would have been expected, suggesting that there was

some selectivity of entry to the study. Despite this, there were significantly more axillary relapses in the watch and wait group (10% vs 2%). There were slightly more deaths in the non-irradiated group but this was not statistically significant.

The Manchester study had a high rate of axillary relapse after irradiation (19%) but an even higher rate in the group with non-treated axillas.[15] There was no significant effect on survival, nor was there in NSABP B-04,[11] although in all the studies the patients with non-treated axillae fared slightly worse.

Of course, the old arguments about the axilla have become largely redundant because it is now understood that the major prognostic factor in early breast cancer is the extent of involvement of the axillary nodes. This has to be determined by the pathologist on an adequate sample (≥ 10 nodes) removed by the surgeon. There is also a greater appreciation of the profound psychological impact of local relapse of disease on the patient and therefore the need to maximize local control at the time of first treatment.

Modified versus radical mastectomy

Nowadays most mastectomy procedures are either a Patey or a Madden operation, and it is assumed that these are the equal of Halsted's

Table 11.7 Outcome in trials comparing modified and radical mastectomy

Number	Follow-up (years)	Local RFS (%)		Overall survival (%)		Reference
		MRM	RM	MRM	RM	
534	5	78	75	78	85	Turner et al[19]
311	10	89	94	64	71	Maddox et al[20]

RM, radical mastectomy; MRM, modified radical mastectomy.

operation. There is some support for this view from clinical trials which have compared modified with radical mastectomy. Turner et al conducted a prospective trial between 1969 and 1976 into which 534 patients with stage I/II disease were randomized to radical mastectomy (278) or modified radical mastectomy (256).[19] The results are given in Table 11.7, which indicates that the relapse-free survival of the two groups was the same but with a trend towards better overall survival in the radical mastectomy group. In those patients with larger tumours, but without axillary nodal involvement, there was a better overall survival at 5 years among those treated by Halsted's operation (85% vs 78%).

In the Alabama Breast Cancer project 311 cases were treated by either radical (136) or modified radical mastectomy (175), and if found to have involved axillary nodes were given adjuvant chemotherapy.[20] There was no statistically significant difference in relapse-free or overall survival of the two groups but there were fewer relapses and deaths in those treated by radical mastectomy. In the subset of patients with T2/T3 tumours and involved axillary, there was a statistically better survival in those treated by radical mastectomy (59% vs 38%). Hence, if primary or salvage surgery is contemplated for a large tumour there will be a better chance of ablating local disease by Halsted's operation.

Radical versus extended radical mastectomy

As a result of the Sixth International Cancer Congress held in Moscow in 1962, an international cooperative study was set up to compare radical mastectomy with extended radical mastectomy in five cancer centres: Lima, Milan, Villejuif, Rome and Warsaw.[21] Results are given in Table 11.8. Between 1963 and 1968, 1580 patients with T1, T2 and T3 tumours were entered and, after 10 years, there were no significant differences between survival in the two groups.

Meier argued that the *en bloc* resection described by Urban was not performed in the international cooperative study and therefore set up another trial at the University of Chicago to compare Urban's operation with Halsted's procedure.[22] There were 123 patients recruited all with stage I/II invasive cancers, of whom one was lost to follow-up. Overall there was no significantly different survival in the two groups, but of the subgroup with medial or central cancers there was a significantly better 10-year survival for the extended radical mastectomy group (86% vs 60%).

A multicentre study was conducted in 11 hospitals in the Shikoku District of Japan which had similar randomization options; 192 women with stage II breast cancer were entered.[23] After 5 years of follow-up there was no difference in

Table 11.8 Outcome of trials comparing extended and radical mastectomy

| Trial | Follow-up (years) | Extended radical | | Radical | | Reference |
		No.	OS (%)	No.	OS (%)	
International Cooperative	10	703	56	750	53	Lacour et al[21]
University of Chicago	10	56	70	56	82	Meier et al[22]
Shikoku	5	96	92	96	93	Morimoto et al[23]

overall survival or rate of local relapse. It is difficult to justify any role for extended radical mastectomy, even for patients with medial or central tumours. For such cases internal mammary lymphoscintigraphy may be of value to delineate the internal mammary chain so that radiotherapy can be more accurately directed to potential sites of residual disease in the anterior mediastinum.

PROPHYLACTIC ANTIBIOTICS

Apart from the unusual circumstances of salvage procedures for fungating infected tumours, mastectomy is usually regarded as a clean operation but an incidence of postoperative infections in 4–18% has been variously reported.[24-28] To determine whether prophylactic antibiotics could reduce postoperative wound infections, Platt et al ran a trial in which 606 women undergoing breast surgery were randomized to receive either a single injection of cefonicid (1 g intravenously), 30 minutes preoperatively or no antibiotic prophylaxis.[29] Of the cefonicid-treated and control groups, 36% had a modified radical mastectomy. A definite wound infection was detected in 11 (4%) of the cefonicid group and 18 (6%) of the control group and probable infections in 6 (2%) and 8 (3%) respectively. Thus overall, there was a 35% reduction in wound infections in those treated with prophylactic antibiotics.

Wagman et al randomized 118 women undergoing mastectomy to either cefazolin (25 mg/kg) intravenously half an hour before surgery or a placebo injection.[30] In this double-blind trial there were three infections in the treated group and five in the controls and this did not amount to a significant difference. Chen et al reviewed 144 patients treated by mastectomy between 1970 and 1976 and 225 who underwent the same procedure between 1980 and 1986.[31] In the first time period, of those who underwent a single-stage procedure, 6% developed a wound infection compared with 11% of those who had a biopsy followed some days later by mastectomy. In the second time period the infection rate for one stage procedures was 3% and for two-stage operations 8%. Almost all the infections were caused by *Staphylococcus aureus*.

As a result of the uncertainty about the efficacy of antibiotic prophylaxis, Platt et al carried out a meta-analysis of published randomized trials and observational data.[32] Information was available concerning 1287 breast operations and the overall infection rate was 4%. In 44% of the cases prophylactic antibiotics had been used and these were responsible for a 38% reduction in infection, regardless of operation type . Procedures taking more than 2 hours were at highest risk of subsequent infection and the data suggested that antibiotics would prevent one infection for every 40 operations.

SUCTION DRAINS

In the USA it has been customary to discharge patients from hospital with their drains in situ, but in Europe they stayed in hospital longer and used not to be sent home until the drainage was less than 25 ml/24 hours, which meant that some were inpatients for up to 3 weeks. As resources became more scarce such a protracted stay became economically untenable. Some balance has had to be achieved between bed utilization and postoperative support for patients who may be feeling very vulnerable. To address this question a trial was conducted at Guy's Hospital, in which 100 patients undergoing modified radical mastectomy were randomized to have their suction drains removed 3 or 6 days postoperatively.[33]

There were 98 evaluable cases and the two groups were similar in terms of age, weight, tumour size, nodes removed and nodal involvement. A wound infection was noted in two patients whose drains were removed after 3 days and one case who had drains removed after 6 days. After discharge, patients were reviewed in the clinic and any wound seroma was drained externally using pre-vacuumed tubes. Those discharged after 3 days had an average of three external aspirations (volume 685 ml) compared with two aspirations in the 6-day group (mean volume 958 ml). Shoulder movement was normal in both groups. This suggests that early drain removal after mastectomy is not associated with excess morbidity and allows more efficient use of hospital beds.

INDICATIONS FOR MASTECTOMY

The change in nomenclature of simple mastectomy being called total mastectomy gives the erroneous impression that this is a sufficient procedure for the treatment of invasive breast cancer. It is an inadequate operation for accurate staging of breast cancer and carries the risk of leaving disease in the axilla which, if untreated, will at very least lead to relapse and morbidity and possibly give rise to distant metastases and premature death.

The indications for total mastectomy are: extensive ductal carcinoma in situ, sarcoma and salvage surgery for patients who have relapsed after breast conservation therapy that included axillary clearance. Total mastectomy should not be used as the standard treatment of breast cancer in elderly women until such time as randomized trials have shown that a sufficiently low incidence of axillary relapse can be achieved with tamoxifen.

Modified radical mastectomy is indicated in women with cancers over 4 cm in size who do not wish to try primary chemotherapy, or those whose tumours fail to shrink with such treatment. In addition, patients with multifocal invasive disease are best served by a modified radical mastectomy. Peau d'orange is usually regarded as a contraindication to mastectomy, but if this lies over the tumour and is of smaller dimension than the cancer, the disease can be regarded as locally advanced but operable. The same is true when there is a small area of skin infiltration or ulceration over the cancer.

Despite the proof of safety of breast conservation there are still many women, some of them medical, who prefer to have the 'complete' operation and will feel secure only if a modified radical mastectomy has been performed. Some older women may decide that they would prefer the relative simplicity of surgery rather than the logistic complexity of multiple radiotherapy visits for treatment. This decision should rest with the patient, rather than as a deliberate suggestion from the surgeon, because many older women will be not wish to undergo a major change in body image.

SYNOPSIS

- The function of mastectomy is to maximize local control, determine prognostic markers, and sometimes cure patients with larger breast cancers.
- To achieve this aim an axillary dissection is necessary which forms part of a Patey or Madden mastectomy.
- Patients with very large cancers may need

a radical rather than a modified radical mastectomy to achieve local control.

* Total mastectomy should be reserved for

patients with extensive DCIS, sarcoma or salvage surgery for relapse after breast conservation therapy.

REFERENCES

1. Halsted WS. The results of operations for the cure of cancer of the breast performed at the Johns Hopkins Hospital from June 1889 to January 1894. *Arch Surg* 1894; **20**: 497–501.
2. Halsted WS. The results of operations for the cure of cancer of the breast performed at the Johns Hopkins Hospital from June 1989 to January 1894. *Johns Hopkins Hosp Rep* 1895; **4**: 297–349.
3. Meyer W. An improved method of the radical operation for carcinoma of the breast. *Med Rec* 1894; **46**: 746–51.
4. McWhirter R. The value of simple mastectomy and radiotherapy in the treatment of cancer of the breast. *Br J Radiol* 1948; **21**: 599–605.
5. Patey DH, Dyson WH. The prognosis of carcinoma of the breast in relation to the type of operation performed. *Br J Cancer* 1948; **2**: 7–13.
6. Madden JL, Kandalaft S, Bourque R. Modified radical mastectomy. *Ann Surg* 1972; **175**: 624–34.
7. Handley RS, Thackray AC. Invasion of the internal mammary lymph glands in carcinoma of the breast. *Br J Cancer* 1947; **1**: 15–20.
8. Urban JA. Radical excision of the chest wall for operable breast cancer. *Cancer* 1951; **4**: 15–20.
9. Helman P, Bennett MB, Louw JH et al. Interim report on trial of treatment for operable breast cancer. *S Afr Med J* 1972; **46**: 1374–5.
10. Dent DM, Gudgeon CA, Murray EM. Mastectomy with axillary clearance versus mastectomy without it. *S Afr Med J* 1996; **86**: 670–1.
11. Fisher B, Redmond C, Fisher ER et al. Ten-year results of a randomized clinical trial comparing radical mastectomy with or without radiation. *N Engl J Med* 1985; **312**: 674–81.
12. Roberts MM, Forrest APM, Blumgart LH et al. Simple versus radical mastectomy. *Lancet* 1973; **i**: 1073–6.
13. Borgström S, Linell F, Tennvall-Nittby L, Ranstam J. Mastectomy only versus radical mastectomy and postoperative radiotherapy in node negative resectable breast cancer. A randomised trial. *Acta Oncol* 1994; **33**: 557–60.
14. Langlands AO, Prescott RJ, Hamilton T. A clinical trial in the management of operable cancer of the breast. *Br J Surg* 1980; **67**: 170–4.
15. Lythgoe JP, Palmer MK. Manchester regional breast study – 5 and 10 year results. *Br J Surg* 1982; **69**: 693–6.
16. Turnbull AR, Turner DTL, Chant ADB et al. Treatment of early breast cancer. *Lancet* 1978; **ii**: 7–9.
17. Cancer Research Campaign Working Party. Management of early cancer of the breast. Report on a multicentre trial supported by the CRC. *BMJ* 1976; **i**: 1035–8.
18. Cancer Research Campaign Working Party. Cancer Research Campaign (King's/Cambridge) trial for early breast cancer. A detailed update at the tenth year. *Lancet* 1980; **ii**: 55–60.
19. Turner L, Swindell R, Bell WGT et al. Radical versus modified radical mastectomy. *Ann R Coll Surg Engl* 1981; **63**: 239–43.
20. Maddox WA, Carpenter JT, Laws HT et al. Does radical mastectomy still have a place in the treatment of primary operable breast cancer? *Arch Surg* 1987; **122**: 1317–20.
21. Lacour J, Le M, Caceres E et al. Radical mastectomy versus radical mastectomy plus radical internal mammary dissection. Ten year results of an international co-operative trial in breast cancer. *Cancer* 1983; **51**: 1941–3.
22. Meier P, Ferguson DJ, Karrison T. A controlled trial of extended radical versus radical mastectomy. *Cancer* 1989; **63**: 188–95.
23. Morimoto T, Monden Y, Takashma S et al. Five-year results of a randomized clinical trial comparing modified radical mastectomy and extended radical mastectomy for stage II breast cancer. *Surg Today* 1994; **24**: 210–14.
24. Beatty JD, Robinson GV, Zaia JA et al. A prospective analysis of nosocomial wound infection after mastectomy. *Arch Surg* 1983; **118**: 1421–4.
25. Hayes JA, Bryan RM. Wound infection following mastectomy. *Aust N Z J Surg* 1984; **54**: 25–7.
26. Say CC, Donegan WA. A biostatistical evalua-

tion of complications from mastectomy. *Surg Gynecol Obstet* 1974; **138:** 370–6.

27. Tejler G, Aspegren K. Complications and hospital stay after surgery for breast cancer: a prospective review of 385 patients. *Br J Surg* 1985; **72:** 542–4.

28. Zintel HA, Nay HR. Postoperative complications of radical mastectomy. *Surg Clin North Am* 1964; **44:** 313–23.

29. Platt R, Zaleznik DF, Hopkins CC et al. Perioperative antibiotic prophylaxis for herniorrhaphy and breast surgery. *N Engl J Med* 1990; **322:** 153–60.

30. Wagman LD, Tegtmeier B, Beatty JD et al. A prospective randomized double-blind study of the use of antibiotics at the time of mastectomy. *Surg Gynecol Obstet* 1990; **170:** 12–16.

31. Chen J, Gutkin Z, Bawnik J. Postoperative infections in breast surgery. *J Hosp Infect* 1991; **17:** 61–5.

32. Platt R, Zucker JR, Zaleznik DF et al. Perioperative antibiotic prophylaxis and wound infection following breast surgery. *J Antimicrob Chemother* 1993; **31:** 43–8.

33. Parikh H, Badwe RA, Ash CM et al. Early drain removal following modified radical mastectomy: a randomized trial. *J Surg Oncol* 1992; **51:** 266–9.

12

Breast reconstruction

Be not the first by whom the new are tried
Nor yet the last to lay the old aside.

Alexander Pope

Immediate versus delayed reconstruction • Safety of silicone implants • Complications of implants • Type of flap • Nipple reconstruction

There are still many breast cancer patients for whom the best first-line treatment is a mastectomy, and others for whom this becomes necessary as a result of relapse after conservation treatment. For these individuals, breast reconstruction may help to maintain or restore body image and, as a result of the ingenuity of plastic surgeons, a plethora of techniques is available. In most specialized breast units immediate or delayed reconstruction is available and the close cooperation of surgical oncologists and plastic surgeons can lead to both good local control and a satisfactory aesthetic outcome for the patient.

It is important that the patient is aware of what can be achieved by plastic surgery but also understands that, although the breast shape is being rebuilt, this will not have the same sensation, nor necessarily the same size, as preoperatively. In addition, whenever possible photographs of the range of results of reconstruction should be available. If 4 cm is taken as the upper size limit for breast conservation therapy, most patients will not need a mastectomy so that, even if the cosmetic result is suboptimal objectively, many will still be pleased with an intact body image and relatively normal nipple and skin sensation. Many centres have an upper tumour size limit

of 2 cm, however, with the result that many more of their patients will need breast reconstruction.

IMMEDIATE VERSUS DELAYED RECONSTRUCTION

As breast reconstructive procedures became available they were generally used to rebuild a breast mound some time after radical surgery because of worries that an immediate operation might increase the risk of local relapse and mask subsequent relapse. The situation became complicated by the acceptance of breast conservation for patients with single smaller cancers, which meant that mastectomy came to be used mainly for patients with larger or multifocal cancers with an increased risk of local relapse. For many, particularly older, surgeons this reinforced concern that immediate reconstruction might not be safe.

Webster et al reviewed results of immediate reconstruction after radical mastectomy in 85 patients and conducted a case-control study to compare outcome with patients having mastectomy without reconstruction.[1] The controls were matched for age, TNM stage, axillary nodal status and type of operation and all had at least 5 cm skin clearance on the mastectomy specimen. There were 33 patients who underwent latissimus dorsi flap, 35 who had TRAM flaps and 17 subpectoral implants. In terms of local relapse, distant recurrence and overall survival, there were no differences between the reconstructed cases and unreconstructed controls, suggesting that immediate reconstruction was safe. After 10 years of follow-up there had been local relapse in 11% of the reconstructed group and 14% of the mastectomy cases.[2] Death from breast cancer occurred in 38% and 36% respectively and this similarity in outcome indicated that reconstruction was unlikely to affect a patient's prognosis.

In Edinburgh, Scotland a randomized trial was conducted comparing immediate and delayed reconstruction with psychosocial morbidity being measured in both groups.[3] For those who had immediate reconstruction there were significant advantages in terms of return to work, freedom with dress and self-image. Wellisch et al found similar approval of cosmetic outcome in women undergoing immediate and delayed procedures, implying that it was unnecessary for a patient to experience post-mastectomy deformity before accepting the results of reconstruction.[4]

Johnson et al reported results from the Mayo Clinic on 118 patients treated by immediate reconstruction using subpectoral implants and found that the 5-year survival was 81%, compared with 87% for those treated by radical mastectomy alone, indicating no major worsening of prognosis in the reconstructed cases.[5] Wound complications in 395 breast cancer cases were examined by Vinton et al who reviewed 90 patients undergoing immediate breast reconstruction after mastectomy and 305 who had mastectomy alone.[6] Taking a definition of obesity as body mass index 27.3 or over, the reconstruction group, being younger, contained fewer obese individuals (25% vs 35%). Results are shown in Table 12.1, and it may be seen that there were more complications in those who underwent mastectomy without reconstruction (48% vs 31%). Seromas were less frequent and the duration of axillary drainage was shorter in the reconstruction group, although the number

Table 12.1 Comparison of complications after mastectomy and mastectomy with immediate reconstruction

Complication	Mastectomy	Mastectomy + reconstruction
Wound infection (%)	13	13
Seroma (%)	30	13
Axillary drainage (days)	11	8
Flap drainage (days)	7	10
Haematoma	5	2
Skin necrosis	18	16
Any complications (%)	48	31

From Vinton et al.[6]

of days of drainage from the wound flap drain was greater. As the major risk factor for postoperative complications was obesity this would have biased the results in favour of the reconstruction group, but nevertheless this does not indicate that reconstruction itself leads to more wound problems.

O'Brien examined both the early complications of mastectomy with or without reconstruction and reported outcome after 20 months of follow-up in 402 patients, of whom 113 had mastectomy with immediate reconstruction and 289 were treated by mastectomy alone.[7] Most patients (83%) had a subpectoral tissue expander or permanent prosthesis inserted, 14% had a transverse rectus abdominis myocutaneous (TRAM) flap and three cases had a latissimus dorsi flap. The postoperative complications of both groups are given in Table 12.2. There were more seromas after mastectomy alone and slightly more wound infections. Prosthesis-specific problems in the reconstruc-

Table 12.2 Comparison of complications after mastectomy and mastectomy with immediate reconstruction

Complication	Mastectomy	Mastectomy + reconstruction
Wound infection (%)	5	3
Seroma (%)	19	3
Haematoma (%)	0.3	2
Skin necrosis (%)	2	5
Prosthesis (%)	–	14
Any complications (%)	28	31

From O'Brien et al.[7]

tion group were infection (8), exposure (2), migration (3), leakage (1) and capsule formation (1). Local relapse occurred in 6% of those who had mastectomy alone and 1% of the reconstruction group ($p < 0.05$).

Hence, although there are no results from randomized trials, these data all support the safety of immediate reconstruction in patients undergoing mastectomy.

SAFETY OF SILICONE IMPLANTS

In most breast reconstruction procedures, an implant is placed subcutaneously or submuscularly and most are made of silicone (polydimethylsiloxane), because this material was always regarded as biologically inert. This now appears to be an oversimplification. Prostheses comprise an outer Silastic envelope filled either with saline or silicone gel (10% cross-linked polymer retaining silicone oil). The outer silicone elastomer is a cross-linked polymer, compounded with fumed silica for strength, but nevertheless semipermeable, allowing diffusion of the inner gel (silicone bleed).

Teuber et al measured serum silicon levels in 72 women with silicone implants and 55 age-matched controls using inductively coupled plasma atomic emission spectroscopy and found significantly elevated levels in the patients (0.28 vs 0.13 mg/l).[8] In a series of patients who had undergone augmentation mammoplasty with silicone implants, Truong et al found that silicon was present in excised axillary lymph nodes using energy dispersive X-ray elemental analysis.[9] These studies revealed that silicon was bleeding from the prosthesis but did not analyse the chemical form in which it was present. Pfleiderer and Garrido quantified silicone concentrations in the liver of 15 women with implants and eight volunteers, using ^{1}H NMR localized spectroscopy.[10] Silicone was detectable in all the patients who had implants in situ for 3–4 years, but there was no direct relationship between time of implantation and silicone concentration, whereas in one patient who had had the implants removed 14 months previously, no silicone was detectable. Silicone concentrations in the liver were higher in women with ruptured, compared with intact, prostheses.

Rupture of a prosthesis may occur in up to 5% of cases and this may be associated with localized inflammatory changes: rubor, dolor, calor and tumor.[11] At a histological level there is an increased deposition of fibrous connective tissue, granulomata and foreign body giant cells.[7] Clinically this may induce capsule formation leading to a significant worsening of cosmetic result and even more seriously might lead to development of autoimmune disease. Miyoshi et al described a polyarthritis which occurred after paraffin and silicone injections for breast enlargement which they dubbed 'human adjuvant disease'.[12] In 1982, Van Nuven et al reported three cases of connective tissue disease in women with silicone implants: rheumatoid arthritis, systemic lupus erythematosus (SLE) and one with mixed connective tissue disease.[13] After this first intimation of a problem, the trickle became a torrent.

Table 12.3 Cohort studies of connective tissue disease giving relative risks in women with implants

Patients	Controls	Rheumatoid arthritis	Systemic sclerosis	SLE	Reference
102	102	1	1	1	Teich et al[16]
222	80	1.2	1	1	Wells et al[17]
749	1498	0 vs 2	0 vs 1	0 vs 0	Gabriel et al[18]
500	Population	0.2 vs 1%	0.2 vs 0.01%	0.4 vs 0.2%	Peters et al[19]
824	Population	1.4	–	–	McLaughlin et al[20,21]
235	210	0.65	–	–	Giltay et al[22]
1 183	86 318	0.4	0 vs 14	0 vs 96	Sanchez-Guerrero et al[23]
10 830	384 713	1.2	1.5	1.2	Hennekens et al[24]

There is evidence that silicone acts as a potent immunological stimulus, akin to Freund's adjuvant, in rats given bovine serum albumin as a test antigen.[14] Vojdani et al measured antibodies in the blood of 520 women with silicone implants and possible immunological disorders who were complaining of myalgia or arthralgia, fatigue, or generalized pain and compared these with blood from 520 women without implants.[15] Overall, silicone-specific antibodies were significantly elevated in women with implants and the percentage of patients with silicone antibodies varied with the specialty of the referring doctor. Antibodies were found in 52% of those from general practice, 59% of rheumatology clinic cases and 83% of those referred by plastic surgeons.

To determine whether there was a true association between silicone implants and human connective tissue disease a series of cohort and case-control studies have been conducted. Eight cohort studies have examined this question.[16–24] These are summarized in Table 12.3 and indicate the limitations of this type of approach for studying rare diseases. In most studies, there were insufficient cases among the women with implants to draw any reasonable conditions, particularly when the

incidence of disease was based on self-report rather than definite diagnosis. In the most recent report, from the Women's Health Study, there was an overall significant increase in connective tissue disease among those who reported breast implants (RR = 1.24, p = 0.0015).[24] This was only of borderline significance for any of the individual diseases, and there were no significant trends with regards to duration of implant.

Case-control studies, in contrast, with patients identified through rheumatology departments were better able to analyse the association between connective tissue disease and silicone implants,[25–31] and these were subsequently subjected to a meta-analysis by Wong.[32] The studies looked at rheumatoid arthritis, systemic sclerosis (scleroderma) and systemic lupus erythematosus. Results are given in Table 12.4. Wong calculated that the relative risk of rheumatoid arthritis in women with implants compared with controls was 0.85 (0.48–1.51), scleroderma, 0.94 (0.50–1.35), and SLE, 0.33 (0.06–2.03).[33] As all are less than unity, with relatively narrow 95% confidence intervals, this does not support a linkage between the presence of a silicone implant and increased risk of connective tissue disease.

Table 12.4 Case-control studies of rheumatoid arthritis (RA), scleroderma (SS) and SLE in women with silicone implants

| Cases | Controls | Relative risks of connective tissue disease | | | Reference |
		RA	SS	SLE	
300	1456	0.41	–	–	Hochberg et al[27]
794	4289	0.76	–	0.36	Burns[28]
869	2061	–	1.25	–	Englert and Brooks[29]
274	1184	–	0.35	–	Wigley et al[30]
251	289	–	0.89	–	Wolfe[31]
741	741	–	0.5	–	Wigley et al[30]
637	1134	–	1.35	–	Wolfe[31]
Meta-analysis		0.85	0.94	0.33	Wong[32]

As well as rheumatological diseases, there have also been reports of neurological conditions in women with silicone implants and these have included motor neuron disease,[33] multiple sclerosis-like syndrome,[34] peripheral neuropathy[35] and memory impairment.[36] All of these observations emanated from one group and so Rosenberg analysed medical records, clinical evaluations and laboratory tests derived from 131 patients who were deemed to have a silicone implant-related neurological disease.[37] There was confirmation of neurological symptoms in 82% of those with fatigue, 76% of those with cognitive impairment or memory loss and 66% of those with myalgia, but 66% of patients had no detectable abnormality on neurological examination. There was no pattern of laboratory tests or of abnormalities and no neurological diagnosis could be made in 82% of cases. Rosenberg concluded that there was no evidence that silicone implants were causally related to development of any neurological disease.

A further concern with silicone implants is of a possible increase in risk of cancer in women who had had augmentation mammoplasty, or a later diagnosis of cancers caused by the implant masking clinical and radiological signs. To examine the influence of implants on stage at diagnosis, Clark et al studied 1768 women with breast cancer of whom 33 had prior implants and 1735 had not had previous breast augmentation.[38] As Table 12.5 shows, fewer of those with implants had mammographically detected cancers but palpable tumours in the implant group were significantly smaller than those without implants.

This was associated with an overall significant reduction in percentage of cases with histologically involved axillary nodes (19% vs 41%). This was even more marked among those with palpable tumours (22% vs 58%). These data suggest a better rather than a worse prognosis for cancers in women with silicone implants, possibly because of increased breast self-examination or greater frequency of clinical examinations.

Further support for the safety of implants came from a study conducted in Los Angeles in which 3111 women with implants were followed for a median of 10.6 years during which time 21 had developed breast cancer.[39] The stage at diagnosis of malignancy was similar to that of other women living in Los Angeles. In another cohort study of 11 676

Table 12.5 Comparative features at diagnosis of breast cancer in women with and without silicone implants

Feature	Implant	No implant
Number	33	1735
Radiography detected (%)	24	46
Tumour < 2 cm (%)	82	63
Positive nodes (%)	19	41
Palpable node positive (%)	22	58
Radiologically node positive (%)	13	15

From Clark et al.[38]

Table 12.6 Cumulative incidence of complications after implants, according to indication

Reason for implant	60 days	270 days	5 years
Cosmetic (%)	4	6	12
Cancer (%)	4	20	34
Prophylactic (%)	3	16	30

From Gabriel et al.[42]

women living in Alberta, Canada, who had breast implants, there were 41 subsequent breast cancer cases.[40] The survival after diagnosis of these women was similar to that of other non-implanted patients.

Both the Los Angeles and Alberta studies had shown a lower than expected incidence of cancer in women with implants: in Los Angeles there were 21 cases and 32 were expected,[39] in Alberta the respective figures were 41 and 86.[40] Brinton et al examined risk in a population-based case-control study of 2174 women, aged less than 55 with breast cancer and 2009 age-matched controls.[41] A prior breast implant was reported by 36 cases and 44 controls. After adjustment for risk factors such as family history, body size and frequency of screening, the relative risk of breast cancer was 0.6. Taking all these results together there is no evidence that silicone implants lead to an increased risk of breast cancer.

COMPLICATIONS OF IMPLANTS

To quantify the surgical complications after an implant for reconstruction or augmentation,

Gabriel et al reviewed the case-notes of 749 women who had implants at the Mayo Clinic, Minnesota.[42] After a mean follow-up of 7.8 years, 178 (24%) cases had surgery for complications which included capsule contraction (17%), implant rupture (6%), haematoma (6%) and wound infection (3%). The indication for implant was cosmetic in 532 (71%), mastectomy for cancer 125 (17%) and prophylactic mastectomy 92 (12%). As is shown in Table 12.6, there was a significantly increased cumulative risk of complications in those who had an implant as part of reconstruction.

By 5 years, further surgery was necessary in 34% of those who had reconstruction for cancer but in only 12% of those who had augmentation mammoplasty. These data underline the fact that patients with breast cancer who are going to have reconstruction should be aware of the relatively high rate of complications, in order that they are not unduly alarmed by the unexpected.

TYPE OF FLAP

Decisions about the type of reconstruction offered should be based upon the physical characteristics of the patient together with a knowledge of her psychosocial needs. In reality the procedure offered depends upon the experience and training of the breast surgeon and the availability or unavailability of a plastic surgeon. Reconstruction enables the breast surgeon to extend the repertoire of operations performed and this is to be encouraged, provided that appropriate training has been given and a sufficient volume of work is available to maintain competence.

Tissue expander

Technically the simplest and therefore most ubiquitous procedure is insertion of a subpectoral tissue expander which is subsequently slowly inflated to produce a skin mound slightly larger than required, after which the permanent implant is inserted. Such procedures are suitable only for women with small or medium-sized breasts who have not had prior skin irradiation. Modena et al reviewed 88 cases who had a Madden mastectomy with immediate reconstruction which was a latissimus dorsi flap in 26, a simple prosthesis in four and a tissue expander in 58.[43]

All the patients who had a latissimus dorsi flap had a good cosmetic result and none had any complications. In contrast only 62.5% of those who had a tissue expander had a good cosmetic result and complications occurred in 43%. The most common problem was capsule formation (20%), followed by infection (15%), expander rupture (5%) and skin necrosis (3%). If the patient is to have the best chance of a good cosmetic result, and the least risk of complications, a latissimus dorsi flap will be more likely to achieve this than a tissue expander.

Instead of placing the implant submuscularly it may be inserted into the original biopsy cavity after wide excision in order to try and improve the cosmetic outcome. Thomas et al reported a series of 59 patients in whom this procedure had been performed, followed by radiotherapy to the breast and axilla in node-positive cases.[44] After 12 months only 39% had a satisfactory cosmetic result. Furthermore, 19% of implants had to be removed because of wound breakdown, infection or capsule formation. Thus the combination of subcutaneous siting of a prosthesis and external radiotherapy can be problematic.

Latissimus dorsi flap

The latissimus dorsi myocutaneous flap has justifiably been the workhorse of breast reconstruction since it enables the placement of healthy skin on the anterior chest wall with a very low (1%) risk of flap necrosis. It is particularly useful when reconstruction is being performed after salvage mastectomy in patients who have had radiotherapy as part of breast conservation therapy. It does not carry enough tissue bulk so that in most cases an implant is necessary. To avoid lateral dislocation into the axilla the lateral aspect of the submuscular pocket has to be secured. There is some associated shoulder weakness and occasional long-term pain associated with the donor site scar. Despite these potential problems, the latissimus dorsi flap remains the simplest and most effective method of carrying out successful breast reconstruction.

Transverse rectus abdominis (TRAM) flap

Prior ablative surgery may result in the thoracodorsal pedicle being damaged or excised thus negating a latissimus dorsi flap, resulting from muscle atrophy and dubious flap viability. As a result of this Hartrampf et al devised the TRAM flap, taking a transverse ellipse of infraumbilical skin, fat and one rectus abdominis muscle with the superior epigastric vascular pedicle.[45] The TRAM flap has the additional advantage of providing sufficient bulk of tissue making a silicone prosthesis unnecessary. The surface area of skin carried is about four times greater than the area of muscle and depends upon a blood supply from communications between superior and inferior deep epigastric vessels together with anastomoses between the deep and superficial systems across the midline.

In an early series of 60 patients who had 65 TRAM flap procedures, Scheflan and Dinner reported flap necrosis in 12%, abdominal hernia in 8%, fat necrosis in one case, myalgia paraesthetica in one and abdominal wall seroma in

Table 12.7 Early complications of 122 rectus abdominis flaps

Complication	Percentage
Flap site discharge	25
Partial flap necrosis	23
Total flap necrosis	2
Seroma	9
Haematoma	9
Delayed wound healing	21
Donor site infection	6

From Shrotria et al.[47]

another.[46] They suggested that TRAM flap was indicated in patients needing additional soft tissue on the chest wall who had moderately excessive lower abdominal fat, and who wanted autogenous tissue rather than a silicone implant. In addition, it could be useful in those who had previously had a failed latissimus dorsi flap or multiple implant failures. Contraindications to the operation were gross obesity, heavy smoking, prior lower abdominal surgery and advanced age.

After performing 122 TRAM flaps for reconstruction mastectomy (106) or chest wall cover after salvage surgery (16), the Cardiff group assessed the short- and long-term complications of the procedure.[47] In the majority (72%), a vertical flap was taken, in 6% the vertical flap was folded to form a cone (Drever procedure[48]), and a transverse flap was used in 22% with a combined vertical and transverse flap in 3%. Complications were least common after cosmetic vertical flaps (12.5%), more frequent after Drever operations (29%) and most often occurred after transverse flaps (43%). The early complications are summarized in Table 12.7, and the most frequent was discharge from the site of the flap. Partial skin or skin and fat necrosis was seen in 23% and total flap necrosis was rare and occurred in only two cases.

Late complications occurring between 2 and 6 months after surgery were flap discharge (4%) and asymmetry (25%). An abdominal incisional hernia occurred in 5% and there was altered abdominal hernia in 7%. Thus, although rectus abdominis flaps are not without complications, most of these are minor if the procedure is performed by experienced surgeons.

Free flaps

Using microsurgical techniques, free flaps can be used to re-fashion a breast mound with the most frequently used being the free TRAM flap. Although the free TRAM flap carries similar complications to the standard TRAM flap, less rectus abdominis muscle needs to be taken and the medial contour of the breast looks better because a tunnel for the vascular pedicle is unnecessary.[49] Provided that the surgeon has experience in microvascular procedures the free flap takes a similar time to a standard TRAM flap, with possibly better skin viability as a result of the relatively large donor vessels.

NIPPLE RECONSTRUCTION

It is customary to perform nipple reconstruction as a second procedure after either latissimus dorsi or TRAM flap. Several techniques may be used including labial grafts, contralateral areola or tattooing. In addition, stick-on plastic nipples are available. Decisions on nipple reconstruction will depend largely upon the individual patient, her social background and marital status. Many patients will regard nipple reconstruction as unnecessary because their main aim is to replace an external prosthesis with an internal volume replacement.

SYNOPSIS

- The best cosmetic and tactile outcome for breast cancer patients occurs after breast conservation therapy rather than mastectomy and breast reconstruction.
- Many cases will need mastectomy as a result of the size of the primary tumour but

reconstruction can be carried out as either an immediate or delayed procedure with no effect on prognosis.

- Silicone implants are safe after mastectomy with no increased risk of relapse, or of connective tissue or neurological disease.
- In women who have had augmentation mammoplasty, implants do not delay detection of breast cancer.
- Although tissue expanders can be useful in women with small or medium-sized breasts, they do not achieve as good a cosmetic outcome as latissimus dorsi flaps, which can also be used when the chest wall has been irradiated.
- Rectus abdominis flaps, either transverse or vertical, replace lost breast tissue without need for a prosthesis but with more potential complications than latissimus dorsi flaps.

REFERENCES

1. Webster DJT, Mansel RE, Hughes LE. Immediate reconstruction of the breast after mastectomy. Is it safe? *Cancer* 1984; **53:** 1416–19.
2. Patel RT, Webster DJT, Mansel RE, Hughes LE. Is immediate postmastectomy reconstruction safe in the long-term? *Eur J Surg Oncol* 1993; **19:** 372–5.
3. Dean C, Chetty U, Forrest APM. Effects of immediate breast reconstruction on psychosocial morbidity after mastectomy. *Lancet* 1983; **i:** 459–62.
4. Wellisch DK, Schain WS, Noone RB, Little JW. Psychosocial correlates of immediate versus delayed reconstruction of the breast. *Plast Reconstr Surg* 1985; **76:** 713–18.
5. Johnson CH, van Heerden JA, Donohue JH et al. Oncological aspects of immediate breast reconstruction following mastectomy for malignancy. *Arch Surg* 1989; **124:** 819–24.
6. Vinton AL, Traverso LW, Zehring RD. Immediate breast reconstruction following mastectomy is as safe as mastectomy alone. *Arch Surg* 1990; **125:** 1303–8.
7. O'Brien W, Hasselgren P-O, Hummel RP et al. Comparison of postoperative wound complications and early cancer recurrence between patients undergoing mastectomy with or without immediate breast reconstruction. *Am J Surg* 1993; **166:** 1–5.
8. Teuber SS, Saunders RL, Halpern GM et al. Elevated serum silicon levels in women with silicone gel implants. *Biol Trace Elemental Res* 1995; **48:** 121–30.
9. Truong LD, Cartwright J, Goodman MD et al. Silicone lymphadenopathy associated with augmentation mammoplasty. *Am J Surg Pathol* 1988; **12:** 484–91.
10. Pfleiderer B, Garrido L. Migration and accumulation of silicone in the liver of women with silicone gel-filled breast implants. *Magn Reson Med* 1995; **33:** 8–17.
11. Kessler DA. The basis of the FDA's decision on breast implants. *N Engl J Med* 1992; **18:** 1713–15.
12. Miyoshi K, Miyramura T, Kobayashi Y et al. Hypergammaglobulinaemia by prolonged adjuvanticity in man. Disorders developed after augmentation mammoplasty. *Jpn J Med* 1964; **2122:** 9–14.
13. Van Nuven SA, Gatenby PA, Basten A. Post-mammoplasty connective tissue disease. *Arthritis Rheum* 1982; **25:** 694–7.
14. Naim JO, Lanzafame RJ. The adjuvant effect of silicone gel breast on antibody formation in rats. *Immun Invest* 1993; **22:** 151–4.
15. Vojdani A, Brautbar N, Campbell AW. Antibody to silicone and native macromolecules in women with silicone implants. *Immunopharmacol Immunotoxicol* 1994; **16:** 497–503.
16. Teich Alasia S, Ambroggio GP, Di Vittoria S et al. Autoimmune connective tissue disease and silicone implants. *International Confederation for Plastic and Reconstructive Surgery*, 7th Congress, Berlin, Germany, June 2–6, 1993.
17. Wells KE, Cruse W, Baker JL et al. The health status of women following cosmetic surgery. *Plast Reconstr Surg* 1994; **93:** 907–12.
18. Gabriel SE, O'Fallon WM, Kurland LT et al. Risk of connective tissue diseases and other disorders after breast implantation. *N Engl J Med* 1994; **330:** 1697–702.

19. Peters W, Keystone E, Lee P et al. Silicone gel implants and connective tissue disease: an analysis of 500 consecutive patients. *Plastic Surgical Forum.* Annual Scientific Meeting, New Orleans, 1993.

20. McLaughlin JK, Fraumeni JF, Olsen J, Mellemkjaer L. Breast implants, cancer, and systemic sclerosis. *J Natl Cancer Inst* 1994; **86:** 1424.

21. McLaughlin JK, Olsen J, Friis S, Mellemkjaer L. Re: breast implants, cancer, and systemic Sclerosis. *J Natl Cancer Inst* 1995; **87:** 1415–16.

22. Giltay E, Moens HJB, Riley AH, Tan RG. Silicone breast prostheses and rheumatic symptoms: a retrospective follow-up study. *Ann Rheum Dis* 1994; **53:** 194–6.

23. Sanchez-Guerrero J, Colditz GA, Karlson EW et al. Silicone breast implants and the risk of connective-tissue diseases and symptoms. *N Engl J Med* 1995; **332:** 1666–70.

24. Hennekens CH, Lee I-M, Cook NR et al. Self-reported breast implants and connective-tissue diseases in female health professionals. *JAMA* 1996; **275:** 616–21.

25. Dugowson CE, Daling J, Koepsell TD et al. Silicone breast implants and risk of rheumatoid arthritis. *Arthritis Rheum* 1992; **35:** S66.

26. Goldman JA, Greenblatt J, Joines R et al. Breast implants, rheumatoid arthritis, and connective tissue disease in a clinical practice. *J Clin Epidemiol* 1995; **48:** 571–82.

27. Hochberg MC, Perlmutter DL, White B et al. The association of augmentation mammoplasty with systemic sclerosis: results from a multi-center case-control study. *58th Annual Meeting of the American College of Rheumatology.* Minneapolis. October 23–27, 1994.

28. Burns CG. The epidemiology of systemic sclerosis: a population based case-control study. Doctoral thesis. University of Michigan, 1994.

29. Englert HJ, Brooks P. Scleroderma and augmentation mammoplasty – a causal relationship? *Aust N Z J Med* 1994; **24:** 74–80.

30. Wigley FM, Miller R, Hochberg MC, Steen V. Augmentation mammoplasty in patients with systemic sclerosis: data from the Baltimore Scleroderma Research Center and Pittsburgh Scleroderma Data Bank. *Arthritis Rheum* 1992; **35:** S46.

31. Wolfe F. Silicone breast implants and the risk of fibromyalgia and rheumatoid arthritis. *59th National Scientific Meeting of the American College of Rheumatology.* San Francisco, October 21–26, 1995.

32. Wong O. A critical assessment of the relationship between silicone breast implants and connective tissue diseases. *Reg Toxicol Pharmacol* 1996; **23:** 74–85.

33. Ostermeyer-Shoaib B, Patten BM, Ashizawa T. Motor neuron disease after silicone breast implants and silicone injections into the face [Abstr]. *Ann Neurol* 1992; **32:** 254.

34. Ostermeyer-Shoaib B, Patten BM. A multiple-sclerosis-like syndrome in women with breast implants or silicone fluid injections into breasts [Abstr]. *Neurology* 1994; **44**(suppl 2): A158.

35. Ostermeyer-Shoaib B, Patten BM. Silicone adjuvant disease: more neurological cases [Abstr]. *Ann Neurol* 1992; **32:** 254.

36. Brown S, Patten BM, Cooke N et al. Silicone breast implants: association with abnormal SPECT scans and memory defects [Abstr]. *Can J Neurol Sci* 1993; **Suppl 4:** S177.

37. Rosenberg N. The neuromythology of silicone breast implants. *Neurology* 1996; **46:** 308–14.

38. Clark CP, Peters GN, O'Brien KM. Cancer in the augmented breast. *Cancer* 1993; **72:** 2170–4.

39. Deapen DM, Brody GS. Augmentation mammoplasty and breast cancer: a five year update of the Los Angeles study. *Plast Reconstr Surg* 1992; **89:** 660–5.

40. Berkel H, Birdsell DC, Jenkins H. Breast augmentation: a risk factor for breast cancer? *N Engl J Med* 1992; **326:** 1649–53.

41. Brinton LA, Malone KE, Coates RJ et al. Breast enlargement and reduction: results from a breast cancer case-control study. *Plast Reconstr Surg* 1996; **97:** 269–75.

42. Gabriel SE, Woods JE, O'Fallon WM et al. Complications leading to surgery after breast implantation. *N Engl J Med* 1997; **336:** 677–82.

43. Modena S, Benasutti C, Marchiori L et al. Mastectomy and immediate breast reconstruction: oncological considerations and evaluation of two different methods relating to 88 cases. *Eur J Surg Oncol* 1995; **21:** 36–41.

44. Thomas PRS, Ford HT, Gazet J-C. Use of silicone implants after wide local excision of the breast. *Br J Surg* 1993; **80:** 868–70.

45. Hartrampf CR, Scheflan M, Black PW. Breast reconstruction with a transverse abdominal island flap. *Plast Reconstr Surg* 1982; **69:** 216–24.

46. Scheflan M, Dinner MI. The transverse abdominal island flap: Part 1. Indications, contraindications, results, and complications. *Ann Plast Surg* 1983; **10:** 24–35.

47. Shrotria S, Webster DJT, Mansel RE, Hughes LE. Complications of rectus abdominis myocutaneous flaps in breast surgery. *Eur J Surg Oncol* 1993; **19**: 80–3.

48. Drever JM, Hodson-Walker NJ. Immediate breast reconstruction after mastectomy using a rectus abdominis myodermal flap without an implant. *Can J Surg* 1982; **25**: 429–31.

49. Grotting JC, Urist MM, Maddox WA, Vasconez LO. Conventional TRAM flap versus free microsurgical TRAM flap for immediate breast reconstruction. *Plast Reconstr Surg* 1989; **83**: 828–41.

13

First-line systemic treatment

To dream of new dimensions.

Robert Graves

Background • Primary chemotherapy for operable disease • Relapse after treatment • Acceptability of primary chemotherapy • Tumour features and response to chemotherapy • Randomized trials • Primary endocrine therapy • Surgical problems

There has been an insidious encroachment of medical oncologists into areas once regarded as the preserve of the surgeon. As it became evident that chemotherapy could palliate the symptoms of advanced disease, and indeed achieve a complete remission in some patients with inoperable cancers, so cytotoxic attention became focused on operable breast cancer. Confirmation of the efficacy of adjuvant cytotoxic chemotherapy was the removal of the last barrier keeping oncologists away from surgically untreated patients, opening the floodgates of primary treatment with chemotherapy (neoadjuvant therapy) in women with operable breast cancer.

The rationale for use of first-line chemotherapy was threefold. First, it was hoped that early systemic therapy might destroy micrometastatic disease present at the time of diagnosis. Second, as breast conservation came to be recognized as a safe option for patients with single breast cancers up to 4 cm in diameter, so some women with larger tumours were seeking to avoid mastectomy (which might be possible if shrinkage of the primary tumour could be achieved). Finally, rather than all deaths from breast cancer being the result of growth of pre-existing micrometastases, some might result

from dissemination of viable tumour cells during the act of surgery, and this could be reduced by tumour shrinkage or ablation by chemotherapy.

BACKGROUND

Using an experimental rodent model, Fisher showed that removal of a mammary primary led to increased proliferation of distant metastases within 24 hours, probably as a result of dormant cells in G0 converting to a cycling state.[1] The maximum reduction in growth of metastases was seen when cyclophosphamide was given preoperatively. Other work had shown that the extent of metastatic disease was directly related to size of primary tumour, and that cure rates were higher in animals with smaller tumours.[2]

Angiogenesis is a necessary requirement for growth of secondary tumours, being observed in animal model pulmonary metastases within 5 days of tumour excision, but not occurring in controls who had not undergone surgery.[3] It was hypothesized that there is secretion by the primary tumour of an angiogenesis inhibitor which maintained the balance between proliferation and apoptosis in metastases. This

Table 13.1 Non-randomized studies of primary chemotherapy in patients with inoperable breast cancer

No.	Chemotherapy	CR	PR	SD	PD	Reference
31	FAC × 2	0	24 (77)	7 (23)	0	Morrow et al[4]
71	CAMFTP	37 (52)	29 (41)	5 (7)	0	Swain et al[5]
90	CMFT × 3	0	63 (70)	27 (30)	0	Schwartz et al[6]
174	FAC × 2	29 (17)	123 (71)	22 (12)	0	Hortobagyi et al[7]
87	CAFVPr × 3	19 (22)	48 (55)	20 (23)	0	Perloff et al[8]
54	CAMFPT × 7	13 (24)	36 (67)	5 (9)	0	Danforth et al[9]
160	CMFVP	15 (9)	116 (73)	29 (18)	0	Luboinski et al[10]
125	FAC × 3	12 (10)	69 (55)	40 (32)	4 (3)	Gardin et al[11]
792		**125 (16)**	**508 (64)**	**155 (20)**	**4**	

F, fluorouracil; A, doxorubicin (Adriamycin); C, cyclophosphamide; M, methotrexate; T, tamoxifen; P, premarin; V, vincristine; Pr, prednisone. CR, complete remission; PR, partial response; SD, static disease; PD, progressive disease. Numbers in parentheses are percentages.

balance could be disturbed by attempted removal of the primary tumour and restored by preoperative systemic therapy.

As a result of the relatively poor results after irradiation of stage III inoperable breast cancers, primary chemotherapy was introduced in an attempt to improve local control by cytoreduction, and possibly to improve survival by attacking distant micrometastatic disease. Non-randomized series of cases with stage IIIa and IIIb are outlined in Table 13.1. Morrow et al used a combination of fluorouracil, doxorubicin (Adriamycin), cyclophosphamide (FAC) and tamoxifen, given for two cycles and achieved a partial response in 24, and sufficient shrinkage to allow mastectomy in five others.[4] No patient developed progressive disease while on chemotherapy.

Swain et al used a combination of chemotherapy, cyclophosphamide, doxorubicin, methotrexate and fluorouracil, together with attempted oestrogenic synchronization using tamoxifen and premarin (CAMFTP).[5] This was given until maximum tumour response was seen: the median number of courses to complete remission (CR) being five, to partial response (PR) three and to static disease (SD) five. A combination of cyclophosphamide, methotrexate, fluorouracil and tamoxifen (CMFT) was given for three cycles by Schwartz et al who induced a partial remission in 70%.[6]

Other regimens achieved a 9–22% complete response,[7–11] but in only one series was there any progression of disease while chemotherapy was being given.[11] Overall the response rate (CR + PR), using heterogeneous treatments, was 80%. Among those cases treated by mastectomy there was no residual malignancy in 5% of those given two or three cycles,[7,11] but there was in 36% of those who received chemotherapy until maximum response was achieved.[9]

A small randomized trial was conducted at Guy's Hospital in which 24 women with locally advanced breast cancer were randomized to chemotherapy followed by radiotherapy, or primary radiotherapy and subsequent chemotherapy.[12] This comprised four cycles of doxorubicin (Adriamycin) and vincristine (AV),

Table 13.2 Response of operable breast cancers to first-line chemotherapy

No.	Chemotherapy	CR	PR	Pathological CR	BCT	Reference
33	CMF × 3	5	18			Bonadonna et al[13]
33	CMF × 4	4	21			
33	FAC × 3	6	23			
33	FAC × 4	5	20			
33	FEC × 3	7	18			
165	**Total**	**27 (17)**	**100 (61)**	**7 (5)**	**142 (88)**	
192	VTMF × 4	60 (31)	82 (43)	–	192 (100)	Jacquillat et al[14]
126	AVCF × 6	41 (33)	64 (51)	1 (1)	107 (85)	Belembaogo et al[15]
158	MxVCF × 3	32 (20)	64 (41)	0	77 (49)	Calais et al[16]
50	ECisF × 6	33 (66)	16 (32)	11 (22)	47 (94)	Smith et al[17]
50	THPNCF	26 (52)	18 (36)	11 (22)	39 (78)	Chollet et al[18]

A, doxorubicin (Adriamycin); C, cyclophosphamide; Cis, cisplatin; E, epirubicin; F, fluorouracil; M, methotrexate; Mx, mitozantrone; N, vinorelbine; T, thiotepa; THP, pirarubicin; V, vinblastine.

CR, complete remission; PR, partial response; Path CR, pathological complete response; BCT, breast conservation therapy. Numbers in parentheses are percentages.

then radiotherapy followed by eight cycles of cyclophosphamide, methotrexate and fluorouracil (CMF), or radiotherapy followed by four cycles of AV and then eight cycles of CMF. The objective regression rate was 83% in those who had AV–radiotherapy (AV-RT) and 92% in those who had radiotherapy–AV (RT-AV). The median duration of response in the RT-AV group was 10.5 months compared with 33 months for those who had first-line chemotherapy. With this high response rate in patients with a large tumour burden, the prospects for shrinking smaller operable cancers looked encouraging.

PRIMARY CHEMOTHERAPY FOR OPERABLE DISEASE

A series of 165 patients with breast cancers measuring 3 cm or greater were treated with first-line chemotherapy at the Istituto Nazionale Tumori, Milan.[13] They comprised five sequential groups of 33 patients, given various chemotherapy regimens, and the results are shown in Table 13.2. Response rates ranged from 70% to 87%, with the best response being seen after three cycles of FAC. Breast conservation therapy was enabled in 88% of cases. There were 75% complete pathological responses, with no residual malignancy in the tumorectomy and axillary clearance specimens.

Using a combination of neoadjuvant and consolidation therapy, Jacquillat et al treated 250 patients of whom 192 had operable disease.[14] Treatment comprised vinblastine, thiotepa, methotrexate and fluorouracil (VTMF), with tamoxifen in most cases. Radiotherapy was given to all cases and none was treated by mastectomy.

Belembaogo et al used a more prolonged regimen of six cycles of doxorubicin (Adriamycin), vincristine, cyclophosphamide and fluorouracil (AVCF) in 66 operable breast

Table 13.3 Toxicity of first-line chemotherapy regimens

Chemo-therapy	Haemo-globin	Leuko-cytes (%)	Platelets (%)	Nausea vomiting (%)	Liver function (%)	Hair loss (%)	Reference
CMF	0	8	2	26	15	17	Bonadonna et al[13]
FAC	0	8	2	50	8	100	Bonadonna et al[13]
FEC	0	18	0	100	0	100	Bonadonna et al[13]
VTMF	0	9	0	96	0	45	Jacquillat et al[14]
AVCF	0	0	0	23	0	99	Belembaogo et al[15]
EVCF	2	12	4	28	0	33	Calais et al[16]
NVCF	2	10	6	14	0	14	Calais et al[16]
ECisF	2	2		20		28	Smith et al[17]
THPNCF	25	81	20			100	Chollet et al[18]

See Table 13.2 for type of chemotherapy.

cancer cases, with added methotrexate (AVCFM) in another 80 patients.[15] Despite this more aggressive approach the rate of tumour shrinkage and breast conservation was similar to that reported from Milan. In only one case was there complete histological disappearance of tumour. In a series of 77 patients reported from the Centre Hospitalier et Universitaire, Tours, after three cycles of mitozantrone, vincristine, cyclophosphamide and fluorouracil, only 77 (49%) were deemed to have had sufficient tumour shrinkage for them to be treated by breast conservation.[16]

Smith et al used a more aggressive regimen, giving continuous infusion of fluorouracil, via an ambulatory pump, together with 3-weekly epirubicin and cisplatin.[17] This achieved a 98% CR/PR rate, with 22% of cases having no pathological evidence of residual tumour. In this study there was no relationship between size of the original tumour and response to treatment, nor in that of Calais et al,[16] whereas Bonadonna et al found that the size reduction was inversely proportional to the original tumour diameter.[13]

Very similar results were reported by Chollet et al who used a combination of THP–doxorubicin, vinorelbine, cyclophosphamide and fluorouracil in 50 patients with tumours sized over 3 cm of whom 38 (76%) received granulocyte colony-stimulating factor (G-CSF) or granulocyte–macrophage CSF (GM-CSF) support.[18] Treatment was given every 3 weeks for four to six cycles. There was a clinical complete response in 52% and a pathological complete remission in 22%.

The side effects of each of the above chemotherapy regimens are given in Table 13.3. This shows that WHO grade 3 or 4 toxicity leukopenia and anaemia were uncommon with any of the treatments, except THPNCF which induced severe myelotoxicity.[18] Most of the anthracycline-containing regimens produced alopecia, requiring a wig in almost all patients. The exception to this was the series of Smith et al in which, as a result of scalp cooling, only 28% developed alopecia. FEC gave rise to protracted vomiting in all treated patients.

Table 13.4 Local and distant relapse after primary chemotherapy			
Follow-up (months)	Breast relapse No. (%)	Distant relapse No. (%)	Reference
12	2/83 (2)	11/83 (13)	Bonadonna et al[13]
62	20/192 (10)	26/192 (14)	Jacquillat et al[14]
30	2/126 (2)	12/126 (10)	Belembaogo et al[15]
38	11/158 (7)	38/158 (24)	Calais et al[16]
15	2/50 (4)	4/50 (6)	Smith et al[17]
31	4/50 (8)	4/50 (8)	Chollet et al[18]

RELAPSE AFTER TREATMENT

Short-term follow-up relapse rates are shown in Table 13.4. After a minimum follow-up of 12 months there had been a breast recurrence in two of Bonadonna's patients, one treated by breast conservation, the other by mastectomy.[13] In a multivariate analysis of predictive factors for relapse Jacquillat et al reported that tumour size, grade, and regression of tumour were significant independent variables.[14] Belembaogo et al reported no breast relapses in those treated by breast conservation, but 3/41 (7%) of those receiving radiotherapy alone and 2/19 (11%) of those who were treated by modified radical mastectomy when their tumours failed to shrink sufficiently.[15] There were similar local relapse rates in those treated by breast conservation, 6/77 (8%), and mastectomy, 5/81 (6%), in the study of Calais et al.[16] In Smith's cases there were only two breast relapses, one in a patient who had only one course of treatment.[17] After 31 months follow-up there had been locoregional relapse in 16% of Chollet's cases and 6% had died of metastatic disease.[18]

ACCEPTABILITY OF PRIMARY CHEMOTHERAPY

At Guy's Hospital Breast Unit, a pilot study was conducted to determine the applicability of first-line chemotherapy for patients with large primary tumours that measured clinically over 4 cm.[19] During a 16-month period, 82 patients were seen with large breast cancers of whom 40 were inoperable and 42 had operable tumours. Eleven were deemed unsuitable: six because of suspected extensive or multifocal disease and five because of severe co-morbidity. In all cases a core needle biopsy was performed at the first clinic visit, and the patient was then seen in the surgical results clinic. The surgeon gave an explanation of the treatment options available, together with an indication that mastectomy might be necessary if the chemotherapy failed to shrink the tumour.

Interviews were taped and subsequently rated independently to determine whether the patient had been given adequate information according to pre-agreed criteria. Those expressing an interest in neoadjuvant therapy were seen subsequently by a medical oncologist and a radiotherapist, who gave further information that was also recorded and independently rated.

The planned chemotherapy was mitozantrone and mitomycin (MM) given intravenously every 3 weeks for two to four cycles, although because of low efficacy this was subsequently changed to epirubicin, fluorouracil and cyclophosphamide (EFC). Those who became suitable for breast conservation were treated by

Table 13.5 Features of women with larger tumours opting for first line chemotherapy or mastectomy

Feature	Primary chemotherapy	Mastectomy	p
Age (median) (years)	44.5	64	0.007
Postmenopausal*	7 (44)	10 (78)	0.07
Symptom duration (median) (weeks)	4	6	0.42
Tumour size (median) (cm)	5.25	4.5	0.11

* Values in parentheses are percentages.

tumorectomy, axillary clearance and breast irradiation.

Of the 30 women who were asked to participate, 14 (47%) chose mastectomy and 16 (53%) opted for first-line chemotherapy. The characteristics of these two groups of women are shown in Table 13.5. The most striking difference was that those choosing mastectomy were significantly older and hence more likely to be postmenopausal. Neither duration of symptoms nor clinical tumour size had any significant effect on their choice. This does indicate, however, that, after a full explanation of the treatment involved, its toxicity and the uncertainty with regard to outcome, about half of those women with larger tumours will opt for a mastectomy. The acceptability of first-line chemotherapy would probably be increased if it were possible to predict those individuals most likely to respond.

TUMOUR FEATURES AND RESPONSE TO CHEMOTHERAPY

As most cytotoxic agents are most effective against actively proliferating cancers, Remvikos et al measured S-phase fraction (SPF) of tumour cells obtained cytologically from premenopausal women and compared this with response to FAC.[20] Of those with an SPF of less than 5%, only 46% had a complete or partial

response, whereas in 84% of those with an SPF of 5–10% the CR/PR was 84%, rising to 100% in those with SPF over 10%.

Spyratos et al carried out sequential cytopunctures on 35 women receiving preoperative chemotherapy (CMFAV).[21] Of the 35 tumours, 10 were diploid and 25 aneuploid. Regression was seen in only one (10%) of the diploid tumours but in 15 (60%) of the aneuploid lesions. There was a change in DNA content of 10 (40%) of the aneuploid tumours and regression occurred in 9 (90%) of these. Subsequent relapse of disease occurred in 11 of 25 (44%) of those with aneuploid tumours and one of 10 (10%) of the diploid cancers.

In a series of 20 patients with locally advanced disease undergoing first-line chemotherapy, O'Reilly et al took cytological specimens before and during treatment, to measure DNA flow cytometry.[22] DNA ploidy could be estimated in 16 of 20 of which four were diploid and none had a CR (2 PR, 2 SD). Of the 12 aneuploid cancers, all responded (5 CR, 7 PR).

Gardin et al measured thymidine labelling index (TLI) in 36 patients with locally advanced disease who had three courses of FAC followed by a mastectomy.[23] TLI was evaluated before treatment and in the final mastectomy specimen. Of those with a high pre-treatment TLI (>1.4%), regression occurred in 15 of 18 (83%), but in only 10 of 18 (56%) of those with low TLI.

Table 13.6 Randomized trials comparing neoadjuvant and adjuvant chemotherapy in operable breast cancer

Trial design	Follow-up (months)	5-year LRFS (%)	5-year OS (%)	Reference
EVM × 3, MTV × 3, Surg (n = 134)	34	75	94	Mauriac et al[26]
Surg, EVM × 3, MTV × 3 (n = 138)		75	85	
ACF × 4, local therapy (n = 200)	54	73	86	Scholl et al[27]
Surg, ACF × 4 (n = 190)		81	78	
TMF × 2, RT, Mast, TMF × 4 (n = 137)	53	86	81	Semiglazov et al[28]
RT, Mast, TMF × 6 (n = 134)		78	71	
Mt × 4, Surg, MT × 4 (n = 101)	28	99	87	Powles et al[29]
Surg, MT × 8 (n = 99)		97	91	

LRFS, local relapse-free survival; OS, overall survival.

There were five cases with a high TLI in the mastectomy specimen and only one relapsed at 2 years compared with 42% of the others. Paradoxically, patients with the most rapidly proliferating tumours, whose growth rate was least affected by chemotherapy, appeared to have the lowest relapse rate.

In a different approach to prediction of response, MacGrogan et al conducted an immunohistochemical study of core biopsies taken from 128 patients before chemotherapy comprising three cycles of epirubicin, vincristine and methotrexate (EVM), followed by three cycles of mitomycin C, thiotepa and vindesine (MTV).[24] In a multivariate analysis of predictive factors for response to chemotherapy, the most significant was primary tumour size (<4 cm), followed by oestrogen receptor-negative status (<10%), and cell proliferation (MIB1 >40%). In terms of overall survival and metastasis-free survival, the major predictor for both was *c-erbB-2*. There were 97 cases with *c-erbB-2*-negative tumours and their overall survival was 83% whereas, of the 28 *c-erbB-2*-positive cases, only 64% survived.

RANDOMIZED TRIALS

Scholl et al conducted a clinical trial at the Institute Curie in which 196 women with operable breast cancer were randomized to receive either neoadjuvant therapy for two preoperative cycles and then four postoperative courses, compared with six postoperative adjuvant cycles of the same agents.[25] Chemotherapy comprised doxorubicin (Adriamycin), cyclophosphamide and fluorouracil (ACF). In the neoadjuvant group, those with static or progressive disease after two cycles were given doxorubicin (Adriamycin), methotrexate, vindesine and thiotepa (AMVT) for four cycles.

At the time that the trial was set up, there was no convincing proof of benefit for node-negative women given adjuvant chemotherapy, and so those in the surgery group who were found to be in this category were not given postoperative chemotherapy. In the neoadjuvant group, because of tumour shrinkage, only 22 (22%) required mastectomy, compared with 31 (32%) in the adjuvant arm. After a median follow-up of 54 months, the neoadjuvant group had a slightly better survival, as a result of the exclusion of the better prognosis node-negative cases from the adjuvant group. When compared as originally randomized there was no difference in survival of the two groups.

At the Fondation Bergonie in Bordeaux, Mauriac et al entered 272 premenopausal women with tumours measuring more than 3 cm into a trial comparing three cycles of neoadjuvant epirubicin, vincristine and methotrexate (EVM) followed by three cycles of mitomycin C, thiotepa and vindesine (MTV), or mastectomy followed by the same regimen as adjuvant therapy.[26] As Table 13.6 shows, after a median follow-up of 34 months, the local relapse rate was similar in both groups but there was a small but significant benefit for the group given first-line chemotherapy. Scholl et al used doxorubicin, cyclophosphamide and fluorouracil as either preoperative or postoperative adjuvant therapy and reported a 5-year survival advantage for the neoadjuvant group (85% vs 78%).[27]

In St Petersburg, Russia, Semiglazov et al compared a combination of neoadjuvant chemotherapy (thiotepa, methotrexate and fluorouracil, TMF) plus preoperative radiotherapy with radiotherapy alone in patients with stage IIb/IIa disease.[28] All cases underwent mastectomy with axillary clearance, and received either four or six cycles of postoperative TMF, so that both groups had the same dosages of chemotherapy. Both disease-free and overall survival was better in the neoadjuvant group (81% vs 72% and 86% vs 78% respectively).

Powles et al randomized between adjuvant and neoadjuvant therapy, using either methotrexate, mitozantrone and mitomycin C (3M) or methotrexate and mitozantrone (2M) together with tamoxifen.[29] Early in the trial patients were given 3M plus tamoxifen but, because an interaction between mitomycin and tamoxifen caused haemolytic uraemic syndrome, subsequent cases were given 2M and tamoxifen.

Diagnosis of malignancy was made by either core needle biopsy or fine needle aspiration cytology. In the adjuvant group who had surgery first, there were four cases of ductal

carcinoma in situ (DCIS) and so it is likely that a similar number were in the neoadjuvant arm and would therefore have received unnecessary chemotherapy. This illustrates the need to obtain a histological core needle biopsy before instigating chemotherapy. Use of first-line chemotherapy downstaged many tumours so that mastectomy was performed in only 13% compared with 28% of those who had primary surgery. In terms of completeness of excision at the time of tumourectomy, margins were involved in 18 of 71 (25%) of those given postoperative chemotherapy and 28 of 88 (32%) of the neoadjuvant group.

PRIMARY ENDOCRINE THERAPY

As an alternative to cytotoxic chemotherapy, endocrine therapy has been widely used in treatment of advanced and early breast cancer, both as adjuvant treatment and as sole therapy for elderly women with operable disease. Mansi et al treated 42 patients with large but operable breast cancers.[30] A complete remission was seen in one case and 19 (45%) had a partial response, with progressive disease occurring in two (5%). Median time to maximum response was 4 months and the median duration of therapy was 9 months.

Anderson et al gave endocrine treatment to 61 patients with tumours over 4 cm in size and achieved a CR/PR in 24 (39%).[31] For premenopausal cases therapy comprised ovarian ablation and goserelin, and postmenopausal women were given tamoxifen or aminoglutethimide. Taking oestrogen receptor negativity as being less than 20 fmol/mg cytosol protein, 15 (25%) were oestrogen receptor (ER) and none of these cases responded to treatment whereas, of the ER-positive patients, CR/PR was seen in 24 (52%).

In an attempt to select those patients who would be most likely to respond to tamoxifen, Soubeyran et al carried out an immunohistochemical study on core biopsies taken from 208 postmenopausal patients before starting treatment.[32] Of the potential markers, pS2 protein (derived from oestrogenic stimulation of breast

Table 13.7 Markers of response to first-line tamoxifen

Marker	Patients		Responders (CR/PR)	
	No.	**(%)**	**No.**	**(%)**
pS2-negative	55	(26)	20	(36)
pS2-positive	153	(74)	90	(52)
ER-negative	36	(17)	12	(33)
ER-positive	172	(83)	98	(57)

From Soubeyran et al.[32]

tumour cells in vitro) and ER status were the only significant predictors, as shown in Table 13.7. Taking pS2 negativity as being less than 3% of cells staining, there was only a 36% response rate in this group compared with 52% in pS2-positive cases. Only one third of ER-negative cases responded compared with 57% of ER-positive cases.

SURGICAL PROBLEMS

To examine the surgical morbidity after primary systemic therapy, Forouhi et al randomized 79 patients to undergo modified radical mastectomy (n = 39) or systemic treatment followed by mastectomy (n = 40).[33] In the group undergoing immediate mastectomy, there were 14 minor and 7 major complications and after systemic first-line therapy there were 11 minor and 6 major complications. The major complications after immediate surgery were prolonged seromas (two), major wound infections (three) and extensive wound necrosis (two), which after first-line systemic therapy were one, four and two, respectively. In a multivariate analysis, the only independent predictor of postoperative complications was obesity.

In terms of breast conservation therapy after neoadjuvant treatment, Zurrida et al analysed 226 cases who presented with tumours over

3 cm and were given first-line chemotherapy.[34] The site and size of the cancer were tattooed before starting a variety of chemotherapy regimens.[13] Patients were assessed surgically 3 weeks after the final cycle of chemotherapy and, if the tumour measured less than 3 cm, breast conservation treatment was planned. An attempted wide local excision (quadrantectomy) was performed and the specimen margins examined by frozen section. If tumour extended to the resection margin, another wider excision was performed, and if this showed incomplete excision, a mastectomy was carried out. All cases had an axillary clearance whether undergoing breast conservation therapy or mastectomy. All patients treated by breast conservation therapy received postoperative breast irradiation. A major indicator of likelihood of breast conservation therapy was the size of the cancer at presentation, as shown in Table 13.8.

Risk of local relapse after surgery was largely determined by lack of response to chemotherapy. Of those with tumours over 3 cm after neoadjuvant therapy who were treated by mastectomy, local relapse occurred in 22% compared with 5% in those undergoing breast conservation therapy. Furthermore, the mastectomy cases were more likely to have axillary nodal involvement (83% vs 58%). Nodal status was also an indicator of risk of local relapse

Table 13.8 Surgical treatment after first-line chemotherapy and size of tumour at presentation

Tumour size (cm)	Number	Breast conservation therapy No. (%)	Mastectomy No. (%)
3–4	141	138 (98)	3 (2)
4.1–5	56	45 (80)	11 (20)
>5	29	20 (69)	9 (31)

which occurred in 13 of 136 (10%) of node-positive cases and 4 of 90 (4%) of those who were node negative.

Both clinical and radiological assessment of response of the primary tumour and lymph nodes are less accurate than pathological evaluation of operative specimens. Although some have hailed neoadjuvant treatment as the death knell of breast surgery, the reports of mortality may be premature. Surgery still plays an important role in determining response to first-line systemic therapy, and subsequent prognosis. Close attention to surgical technique is necessary to select those cases suitable for breast conservation therapy and the smaller proportion who will need mastectomy, probably followed by radiotherapy, to minimize the risk of local relapse.

SYNOPSIS

- First-line chemotherapy can achieve sufficient tumour shrinkage to enable breast conservation in about 80% of patients with operable cancers sized over 3 cm.
- The subsequent rate of breast relapse after primary chemotherapy followed by radiotherapy is 2% per year.
- After a full explanation of treatment and likelihood of response only 50% of patients may opt for first-line chemotherapy.
- Patients with more rapidly proliferating tumours, as measured by thymidine labelling index, S-phase fraction or MIB1 positivity, are most likely to respond to chemotherapy.
- Clinical trials comparing primary chemotherapy with postoperative chemotherapy have shown a small but significant benefit in terms of both relapse-free and overall survival in those given neoadjuvant therapy.
- Primary tamoxifen may provide a less toxic treatment for some patients with ER-positive breast cancers.

REFERENCES

1. Fisher B, Gunduz N, Saffer EA et al. Influence of the interval between primary tumor removal and chemotherapy on kinetics and growth of metastases. *Cancer Res* 1983; **43:** 1488–92.
2. Gunduz N, Fisher B, Saffer EA. Effect of surgical removal on the growth and kinetics of residual tumor. *Cancer Res* 1989; **x:** 3861–5.
3. Holmgren L, O'Reilly MS, Falkman J. Dormancy of micrometastases: balanced proliferation and apoptosis in the presence of angiogenesis suppression. *Nature Med* 1995; **1:** 149–53.
4. Morrow M, Braverman A, Thelmo W et al. Multimodal therapy for locally advanced breast cancer. *Arch Surg* 1986; **121:** 1291–6.

5. Swain SM, Sorace RA, Bagley CS et al. Neo-adjuvant chemotherapy in the combined modality approach of locally advanced nonmetastatic breast cancer. *Cancer Res* 1987; **47:** 3889–94.

6. Schwartz GE, Cantor RI, Biermann WA. Neoadjuvant chemotherapy before definitive treatment for stage III carcinoma of the breast. *Arch Surg* 1987; **122:** 1430–4.

7. Hortobagyi GN, Ames FC, Buzdar AU et al. Management of stage III primary breast cancer with primary chemotherapy, surgery and radiation therapy. *Cancer* 1988; **62:** 2507–16.

8. Perloff M, Lesnick GJ, Korzun A et al. Combination chemotherapy with mastectomy or radiotherapy for stage III breast carcinoma: a Cancer and Leukemia Group B study. *J Clin Oncol* 1988; **6:** 261–9.

9. Danforth DN, Lippman ME, McDonald H et al. Effect of preoperative chemotherapy on mastectomy for locally advanced breast cancer. *Am Surg* 1990; **56:** 6–11.

10. Luboinski G, Nagadowska M, Pienkowski T. Preoperative chemotherapy inoperable cancer of the breast. *Eur J Surg Oncol* 1991; **17:** 603–7.

11. Gardin G, Rosso R, Campora E et al. Locally advanced non-metastatic breast cancer: analysis of prognostic factors in 125 patients homogenously treated with a combined modality approach. *Eur J Cancer* 1995; **31A:** 1428–33.

12. Rubens RD, Sexton S, Tong D et al. Combined chemotherapy and radiotherapy for locally advanced breast cancer. *Eur J Cancer* 1980; **16:** 351–6.

13. Bonadonna G, Veronesi U, Brambilla C et al. Primary chemotherapy to avoid mastectomy in tumors with diameters of three centimeters or more. *J Natl Cancer Inst* 1990; **82:** 1539–45.

14. Jacquillat C, Weil M, Baillet F et al. Results of neoadjuvant chemotherapy and radiation therapy in the breast-conserving treatment of 250 patients with all stages of infiltrative breast cancer. *Cancer* 1990; **66:** 119–29.

15. Belembaogo E, Feillel V, Chollet P et al. Neoadjuvant chemotherapy in 126 operable breast cancer. *Eur J Cancer* 1992; **28A:** 896–900.

16. Calais G, Berger C, Descamps P et al. Conservative treatment feasibility with induction chemotherapy, surgery and radiotherapy for patients with breast carcinoma larger than 3 cm. *Cancer* 1994; **74:** 1283–8.

17. Smith IE, Walsh G, Jones A et al. High complete remission rates with primary neoadjuvant chemotherapy for large early breast cancer. *J Clin Oncol* 1995; **13:** 424–9.

18. Chollet P, Charrier S, Brain E et al. Clinical and pathological response to primary chemotherapy in operable breast cancer. *Eur J Cancer* 1997; **33:** 862–6.

19. Rubens RD, Richards MA, Ramirez AJ et al. Large operable breast cancer: the applicability of primary chemotherapy. *Breast* 1997; **6:** 45–50.

20. Remvikos Y, Beuzeboc P, Zajdela A et al. Correlation of pre-treatment proliferative activity of breast cancer with the response to cytotoxic chemotherapy. *J Natl Cancer Inst* 1989; **81:** 1383–7

21. Spyratos F, Briffod M, Tubiana-Hulin M et al. Sequential cytopunctures during preoperative chemotherapy for primary breast carcinoma. II. DNA flow cytometry changes during chemotherapy, tumor regression, and short-term follow-up. *Cancer* 1992; **69:** 470–5.

22. O'Reilly SM, Camplejohn RS, Rubens RD, Richards MA. DNA flow cytometry and response to preoperative chemotherapy for primary breast cancer. *Eur J Cancer* 1992; **28:** 681–3.

23. Gardin G, Alama A, Rosso R et al. Relationship of variations in tumour cell kinetics induced by primary chemotherapy to tumor progression and prognosis in locally advanced breast cancer. *Breast Cancer Res Treat* 1994; **32:** 311–18.

24. MacGrogan G, Mauriac L, Durand M et al. Primary chemotherapy in breast invasive cancer: predictive value of the immunohistochemical detection of hormonal receptors, p53, c-erbB-2, MiB1, pS2 and GSTπ. *Br J Cancer* 1996; **74:** 1458–65.

25. Scholl SM, Fourquet A, Asselain B et al. Neoadjuvant versus adjuvant chemotherapy in premenopausal patients too large for breast conserving surgery: preliminary results of a randomised trial: S6. *Eur J Cancer* 1994; **30A:** 645–52

26. Mauriac L, Durand M, Avril A, Dilhuydy J-M. Effects of primary chemotherapy in conservative treatment of breast cancer patients with operable tumors larger than 3 cm. *Ann Oncol* 1991; **2:** 347–54.

27. Scholl SM, Asselain B, Palagie T et al. Neoadjuvant chemotherapy in operable breast cancer. *Eur J Cancer* 1991; **27:** 1668–71.

28. Semiglazov VF, Topuzov EE, Bavli JL et al. Primary (neoadjuvant) chemotherapy and

radiotherapy compared with primary radiotherapy alone in stage IIb-IIIa breast cancer. *Ann Oncol* 1994; **5:** 591–5.

29. Powles TJ, Hickish TF, Makris A et al. Randomised trial of chemoendocrine therapy started before or after surgery for treatment of primary breast cancer. *J Clin Oncol* 1995; **13:** 547–52.

30. Mansi JL, Smith IE, Walsh G et al. Primary medical therapy for operable breast cancer. *Eur J Cancer* 1989; **25:** 1623–7.

31. Anderson EDC, Forrest APM, Hawkins RA et al. Primary systemic therapy for operable breast cancer. *Br J Cancer* 1991; **63:** 561–6.

32. Soubeyran I, Quenél N, Coindre J-M et al. PS2 protein: a marker improving prediction of response to neoadjuvant tamoxifen in postmenopausal breast cancer patients. *Br J Cancer* 1996; **74:** 1120–5.

33. Forouhi P, Dixon JM, Leonard RCF, Chetty U. Prospective randomised study of surgical morbidity following primary systemic therapy for breast cancer. *Br J Cancer* 1995; **82:** 79–82.

34. Zurrida S, Greco M, Veronesi U. Surgical pitfalls after preoperative chemotherapy in large size breast cancer. *Eur J Surg Oncol* 1994; **20:** 641–3.

14

Adjuvant therapy

I've got to admit it's getting better
It's a little better all the time.

John Lennon

Adjuvant radiotherapy • Adjuvant chemotherapy • Adjuvant endocrine therapy

Deaths from metastatic breast cancer after apparently successful local treatment underline the need to develop systemic adjuvant therapies that will destroy tumour cells disseminated before or during surgery. Even the most bigoted surgeon cannot ignore the evidence showing reduction in relapse and mortality in patients who have received certain types of adjuvant therapy. But, as in any area of human investigation, arguments still rage as to who should receive adjuvant therapy and what form that treatment should take. Nevertheless some guidelines can, and have been, drawn up. As long as the questions remain there will be a need for further, larger, randomized trials.

For patients with operable disease the major prognostic indicators are the extent of axillary nodal involvement, tumour size, and tumour type and grade. Those fortunate enough to work with pathologists experienced in grading will have come to appreciate how useful grade can be as a prognostic indicator and, indeed, quite often as a substitute for oestrogen receptor (ER) status. Others who are less fortunate may have to rely on substitutes for grade, such as measures of tumour proliferation or differentiation. Indeed a prognostic factor industry has evolved which has tried, unsuccessfully, to replace the grading pathologist with a labora-tory investigation that generates a numerical value.

Who needs adjuvant therapy?

There is almost universal agreement that patients with histologically confirmed axillary nodal metastases will benefit from adjuvant therapy. Yet, within this group there are some cases who will be cured by effective primary treatment. In a cohort of 227 women with operable breast cancer treated at Guy's Hospital before 1961, 51 (22%) were alive without recurrence 20 years later.[1] Of these long-term survivors 35% had pathologically involved axillary nodes and 32% had grade III cancers. Quiet et al examined the long-term outcome in 501 women with axillary nodal involvement treated by mastectomy at the University of Chicago Medical Center.[2] Of those patients who had only one node involved, 61% were alive without relapse 20 years later. However, survival was dependent upon tumour size with 81% survival in those with tumours sized 2 cm or less but only 59% in those with cancers larger than 2 cm. Thus it may be possible to select a group of patients with one, apparently bad, prognostic factor who will actually have a good outlook and therefore not require adjuvant therapy.

In 1988 the National Cancer Institute took a contrary view and issued a Clinical Alert which stated 'chemotherapy can have a meaningful impact on the natural history of node-negative breast cancer patients'.[3] This provocative message was taken by some as *carte blanche* approval of chemotherapy for every woman with breast cancer, and to some extent this has been backed up by subsequent meta-analyses. Luckily the folly of this type of sweeping approach to treatment of a heterogeneous disease such as breast cancer has been appreciated by most clinicians.

Within the group of women with node-negative disease, there is an identifiable subgroup with such a good prognosis that their life expectancy is the same as that of women of the same age without breast cancer. These individuals have single breast cancers sized 1 cm or less, without axillary nodal involvement.[4] A similar group can also be identified using the Nottingham Prognostic Index (NPI).[5] The index is derived from tumour size, tumour grade, and nodal status:

$$NPI = 0.2 \times Size + Stage + Grade.$$

The size of tumour is measured clinically in centimetres, and stage is derived from a triple node biopsy (low axillary, apical axillary and internal mammary). This is a discontinuous variable – 1, 2, 3 – derived from stage A, B and C: stage A is absence of metastases in any node and scores 1; if there is involvement of the low axillary node alone this is stage B, and scores 2; stage C is defined by tumour deposits in either the apical or internal mammary node. Grade is another discontinuous variable 1–3 based on a modification of the Bloom and Richardson system.[6]

From these integers a prognostic index between 2 and 7 is derived. Those patients with an index of less than 3.4 carry a good prognosis and those with NPI over 5.4 fare badly. The index continues to predict for prognosis up to 10 years after treatment, not only in those treated by mastectomy but also in women treated by breast conservation therapy.[7] With

the increasing availability of pathologists who can grade both ductal and lobular cancers, this index may prove useful in defining groups requiring adjuvant therapy and, equally important, others who do not.

Barbareschi et al evaluated a variety of prognostic variables in a group of 178 node-negative patients followed for a median of 5 years.[8] These included expression of gene products of *Bcl-2* and *p53*, together with oestrogen receptor status, tumour size, tumour grade and nodal status. In a multivariate analysis the only independent prognostic variable was the NPI. Thus the Nottingham Prognostic Index is an exportable method of identifying women with a need for adjuvant therapy.

Fisher et al examined 22 pathological features of tumours from 950 node-negative patients who participated in the National Surgical Adjuvant Breast and Bowel Project (NSABP) B06 trial.[9] In a univariate analysis, 10 factors were significant at a 1% level (tumour grade, nuclear grade, tumour type, necrosis, mucin production, DCIS component, mitotic rate, ER/PR and race). However, in a multivariate analysis, only nuclear grade, tumour type and race were independently significant factors.

Another approach to the identification of long-term survivors not needing adjuvant therapy is the microvessel count (MVC). Heimann et al used immunohistochemistry of CD34 antigen on microvessel-associated endothelial cells in archival tumour specimens from 167 patients with node-negative disease.[10] Median follow-up was 15.4 years. A high MVC was defined as 15 or more microvessels per high-power field. The 20-year disease-free survival rate was 93% for those with low MVC compared with 69% in those with high MVC. In a multivariate analysis, which included tumour size, age, grade, oestrogen receptor status and MVC, the only independently significant prognostic variable was microvessel count.

ADJUVANT RADIOTHERAPY

It is important to be clear about what constitutes adjuvant radiotherapy. Women with

Table 14.1 Meta-analysis of 10 year relative risk of survival in irradiated cases		
Trial	Node negative	Node positive
Manchester Q	0.9	1.1
Manchester P	0.9	0.9
Oslo I	1.0	1.2
Oslo II	0.9	1.1
Heidelberg	3.8	1.5
Stockholm	1.3	0.8

Table 14.2 Standardized mortality ratios (SMR) for cardiac disease of patients in radiotherapy trials surviving more than 10 years			
Trial	RT SMR	No RT SMR	RR
Radical ± RT	1.3	0.7	1.8
Total ± RT	0.9	0.6	1.4
Overall	1.1	0.7	1.6
From Cuzick et al.[13]			

operable breast cancers managed by conservation therapy receive radiotherapy as an intrinsic part of primary treatment. Adjuvant radiotherapy is chest wall or gland field irradiation given after mastectomy. Like so many aspects of breast cancer management, its use has been subject to changes in fashion, which until recently were based on improving local control of disease, rather than having any impact on survival.

In the first overview of trials in which patients treated by mastectomy had been randomly allocated to receive adjuvant radiotherapy, Cuzick et al examined the long-term mortality effects.[11] Overall there was no reduction in mortality among the irradiated cases after 10 years of follow-up. However, as Table 14.1 shows, there was a trend towards a lower death rate in node-positive irradiated cases. Compared with the non-irradiated cases (relative risk, RR = 1), there was no consistent effect on mortality in node-negative cases. In contrast, there was small overall increased relative risk of survival for node-positive women who received adjuvant radiotherapy. More recently, the Stockholm study has reported that there was a reduction in local and distant relapses in the node-positive irradiated cases.[12]

However, what the meta-analysis showed was a significantly increased mortality rate after 10 years in the irradiated cases: 12% at 10–15 years and 18% at over 15 years. As many of the patients were treated with kilovoltage rather than megavoltage irradiation, which led to more local morbidity, the late mortality effects might have occurred because of fibrosis of underlying myocardium and lung. To test the hypothesis that left-sided breast or chest wall irradiation would increase the risk of subsequent myocardial infarction, Rutqvist and Johansson examined cause-specific mortality in 55 000 Swedish patients. Those patients with left-sided breast cancers had a significantly higher mortality rate from myocardial infarction than those with right-sided tumours.

In a second meta-analysis Cuzick et al examined cause-specific mortality in 10 randomized trials (Manchester Q, Manchester P, Oslo I, Oslo II, Heidelberg, Stockholm, Manchester Regional I, Cancer Research Campaign, NSABP B04 and Edinburgh).[13] There was still an increased all-cause mortality rate in those who had received adjuvant radiotherapy although this was no longer statistically significant. Table 14.2 shows the standardized mortality ratios for cardiac disease in cases treated by radical mastectomy ± radiotherapy and total mastectomy ± radiotherapy. For both subgroups and overall there was a significantly increased mortality in those who had received adjuvant radiotherapy. Within the irradiated

Table 14.3 Relative risks of events in patients receiving adjuvant radiotherapy compared with untreated controls

Event	Node negative	Node positive	All
Local relapse	0.2	0.3	0.3
Distant relapse	1.1	0.7	0.8
Overall deaths	0.92	0.8	0.9

From Arriagada et al.[14]

group there was a slightly increased risk in those who had left-sided tumours (RR + 1.34). However, the breast cancer deaths in the irradiated group were less than in those who were untreated, particularly in the later trials, with a significant trend towards better survival.

As a result of this suggestion of improved survival after adjuvant radiotherapy, Arriagada et al re-analysed the Stockholm trial using a competing risk approach.[14] There were 960 trial participants, all aged under 71 years and treated by modified radical mastectomy. There was a three-way randomization: preoperative radiotherapy, postoperative radiotherapy and no radiotherapy. Megavoltage radiotherapy was given to the chest wall, axilla, supraclavicular fossa and internal mammary chain.

As Table 14.3 shows, there was a significantly reduced risk of local relapse in those who were irradiated. In addition, overall there were significantly fewer distant relapses in the treated group. This effect was significant only in those who had histologically involved axillae. Using local relapse as a time-dependent co-variate, this was predictive of distant recurrence, and nullified the significance of adjuvant radiotherapy. This implies that adjuvant radiotherapy, by preventing local relapse, has a significant impact on reducing distant metastases.

One particular group of patients at high risk of local relapse are those with extranodal spread from axillary metastases, and usually

these cases are advised to have axillary irradiation.[15] In a series of 110 node-positive patients treated by modified or radical mastectomy, 34 demonstrated extranodal spread.[16] Of these half had extensive extranodal spread (>10 foci per high-power field) and half had focal spread (<10 per high-power field). Adjuvant radiotherapy was given to 47% of those with extensive spread and 59% of those with focal involvement. After a median follow-up of 92 months one of each group relapsed within the axilla, and neither had been irradiated. Irrespective of whether radiotherapy had been given, there was a high relapse rate and the 5-year overall survival rate was 59% for those with focal spread and only 25% in those with extensive extranodular spread. This suggests that these cases need systemic therapy rather than adjuvant local radiotherapy.

In 1995, the Early Breast Cancer Trialists' Collaborative Group reported a meta-analysis of 36 trials comparing surgery plus radiotherapy with radiotherapy alone.[17] Overall there was a significant reduction in local relapse in the irradiated group (7% vs 20%). Furthermore there were significantly fewer relapses (38% vs 46%), but the 10-year survival rates of the two groups were not significantly different (40% vs 41%). There was a significant reduction in risk of death from breast cancer in irradiated women (odds ratio, OR = 0.94), representing up to five fewer deaths per 100 women. However, there were more non-cancer deaths after radiotherapy (OR = 1.24), particularly in those aged over 60 at the time of treatment (< 50: 2.5% and 2%; >60: 15% and 11%). In this analysis there did not appear to be any difference between non-breast cancer mortality in trials using orthovoltage and megavoltage radiation.

The magnitude of benefit of systemic adjuvant therapy

For many years, opponents of systemic adjuvant therapy, particularly chemotherapy, had argued that the treatment might lengthen the time to first relapse, but that there was no effect on overall survival. This position became untenable with

Table 14.4 Reduction in annual odds of death in adjuvant therapy trials		
Comparison	**Aged <50 (%)**	**Aged ≥ 50 (%)**
Tamoxifen versus nil	1	23
Single CT versus nil	11	–4
CMF versus nil	26	8
PolyCT versus single CT	21	17
Prolonged CT versus 6 months CT	–8	–12

CT, chemotherapy.
From EBCTCG.[18]

Table 14.5 Meta-analysis of systemic adjuvant therapies: reduction in annual odds of death		
Type of adjuvant therapy	**Aged <50 (%)**	**Aged ≥ 50 (%)**
Ovarian ablation	30	0
Tamoxifen	6	20
Polychemotherapy	25	13
Immunotherapy	–3	–3

From EBCTCG.[19]

the publication by the Early Breast Cancer Trialists' Collaborative Group (EBCTCG) of the first adjuvant overview in 1988.[18] The meta-analysis pooled data from 28 randomized trials, comprising over 16 000 patients. Results are summarized in Table 14.4, which shows significant mortality reductions in women aged 50 or over given tamoxifen and those under 50 treated with polychemotherapy, predominantly cyclophosphamide, methotrexate and fluorouracil (CMF). There was a significantly better survival in those receiving polychemotherapy as compared with single agent treatment, and no advantage to extending chemotherapy treatment beyond 6 months. Thus, it was concluded that, in certain subgroups with breast cancer, systemic adjuvant therapy could significantly reduce 5-year mortality rates.

The second meta-analysis, published in 1992, was a much more ambitious project which analysed 133 randomized trials of hormonal, cytotoxic and immune adjuvant therapy which included 75 000 women.[19] Survival curves were plotted out to 10 years. Outline results of the meta-analysis are shown in Table 14.5.

The most unexpected finding to emerge was the significantly reduced mortality in pre-menopausal women who had adjuvant ovarian ablation, by surgery or radiotherapy. The annual reduction in odds of death was 30% and the benefit continued for at least 10 years after treatment. Ovarian suppression had no effect in postmenopausal women. For node-positive premenopausal patients, the 15-year effect was a 13% absolute reduction in mortality rate compared with 7% in node-negative cases.

There was a small but non-significant effect of tamoxifen in premenopausal women (probably because of relatively small numbers so treated), but a 20% significant reduction in annual odds of death in postmenopausal cases. This effect was dependent upon length of treatment, less than 2 years giving an 11% reduction in odds of death, 2 years causing an 18% reduction and more than 4 years leading to a 24% reduction. There was a 39% reduction in contralateral breast cancers in those who took tamoxifen. When those with oestrogen receptor (ER)-positive and (ER)-negative tumours were analysed with respect to the effect of tamoxifen on reduced odds of mortality, this was 3% in ER-negative women aged less than 50 and 19% in ER-positive cases. For those aged 50 or over, the reductions were 16% and 36% respectively.

Polychemotherapy reduced the odds of mortality by 25% in those aged under 50 and by 13% in women aged 50 or over. For those who had either polychemotherapy or tamoxifen, the main impact on reducing relapse occurred in the first 4 years, but the effect on mortality was greater at 10 years than at 5 years. There did appear to be a small survival advantage with a combination of endocrine treatment and chemotherapy. In premenopausal women, ovarian ablation gave a 28% reduction in odds which rose to 30–40% with added polychemotherapy. Postmenopausal women receiving tamoxifen and polychemotherapy had a further 10% reduction in odds of death compared with those given tamoxifen alone.

The trials of so-called immune therapy, including bacillus Calmette–Guérin (BCG), levamisole, *Corynebacterium parvum*, and interferon, did not achieve any reduction in mortality. Thus attempts at adjuvant immunotherapy for breast cancer should be confined to clinical trials. The publication of results from the third meta-analysis of the EBCTCG is awaited with great interest.

ADJUVANT CHEMOTHERAPY

It is now clear that the group who benefit most from adjuvant chemotherapy are node positive cases aged less than 50, but that in women aged 50 or more there is a small positive effect. Bonadonna and Valagussa have suggested that the apparent lack of efficacy in older women is because of dosage reduction leading to inadequate treatment.[20] In the Milan adjuvant trials there was evidence of a dose–response effect. Optimal dosage for the first course was calculated from the patient's surface area and thus the optimal dose for the entire course was either six or twelve times that amount, depending on the number of cycles. Actual dosage was given as a percentage of optimal dose, and the patients were divided into three groups: those who received more than 85% of optimal dose, those who were given 65–84% and those who received less than 65%. The last group fared significantly worse and also contained an over-representation of women more than 50 years.

A similar dose–response effect has been found in two different adjuvant trials,[21,22] whereas two others reported no difference in relapse.[23,24] However, after reviewing the literature, Henderson et al concluded that, although there was some evidence of a dose–response effect in rodent models, there was scant evidence that this had relevance in humans.[25] It was pointed out that retrospective analyses can be flawed because patients who relapse while receiving adjuvant therapy will not have the full course and will anyway have a very poor prognosis.

Hryniuk and Levine recalculated dose intensity in a different way.[26] Taking the original dosages in the Cooper regimen,[27] they made an assessment of the percentage given, taking the control untreated group as receiving 0%. So that trials of melphalan could be included, they equated 1 mg melphalan to 40 mg cyclophosphamide. There was a significant correlation between dose intensity and 3-year relapse-free survival. This approach was refuted by Gelman and Henderson who argued that giving equal weighting to each component of a chemotherapy regimen was inconsistent with the experimental evidence.[28] In addition, they asserted that it was illogical to take no treatment as the lowest dosage, and also inappropriate to lump together a variety of cytotoxic regimens.

In a randomized trial of treatment for advanced disease a combination of fluorouracil, doxorubicin (Adriamycin) and cyclophosphamide (FAC) was given either in a standard manner or with escalating dosages of doxorubicin and cyclophosphamide.[29] There was no difference in response rate or duration of remission in the two groups. In an adjuvant trial, the Cancer and Acute Leukemia Group B (CALGB) tested two different dosages of CMF with vincristine and prednisone.[30] After a median follow-up of 45 months there was no difference in either relapse-free or overall survival between the two groups.

Role of anthracyclines in adjuvant therapy

As CMF became recognized as the standard adjuvant regimen, so evidence emerged

Table 14.6 Randomized adjuvant trials comparing CMF with anthracycline-containing regimens

Patients	No.	CMF	Anthracycline	5-year OS (%)	Reference
Node+ve, ER−ve	2194	× 6	AC × 4 or AC × 4–CMF	80 vs 80 vs 80	Fisher et al[31]
Node+ve or ER−ve	228	× 9	MTV × 3–EVM × 3	80 vs 80	Mauriac et al[32]
Node+ve >3	403	× 12	A-CMF or CMF/A	75 vs 62	Bonadonna et al[33]
Node+ve	360	× 6	FEC1	80 vs 72	Coombes et al[34]
	399	× 6	FEC2	78 vs 90	

concerning the value of anthracyclines, particularly doxorubicin, in advanced breast cancer. Consequently trials were set up to compare CMF with regimens containing either doxorubicin or epirubicin.[31–34] With varying indications for entry, different drug dosages and scheduling, the results have, not surprisingly, been diverse as shown in Table 14.6. In NSABP trial B-15, 2194 patients with node-positive and ER-negative disease were randomized to receive either six cycles of standard CMF or four cycles of doxorubicin and cyclophosphamide (AC), or AC followed by CMF.[31] After 3 years, the overall survival of the three groups was the same.

Mauriac et al treated 228 women with either node-positive or ER-negative diseases and compared nine cycles of CMF with three cycles of mitomycin C, thiotepa and vindesine (MTV) followed by three cycles of epirubicin, vincristine and methotrexate (EVM).[32] The overall survival of both groups was the same, but MTV/EVM caused more alopecia and neurotoxicity whereas CMF led to greater haematological toxicity.

Bonadonna et al adopted a different approach and examined different scheduling of anthracyclines.[33] A total of 403 patients with more than three positive nodes were randomized to receive either four courses of doxorubicin followed by eight cycles of CMF (sequential regimen), or two cycles of CMF alternating with one course of doxorubicin for a total of 12 courses (alternating regimen).

Those who received the sequential regimen fared better with a 5-year survival rate of 75% versus 62%. Dose intensity was the same in both randomization arms. However, there were four cases of congestive cardiac failure, two of which were fatal.

The International Collaborative Group ran two parallel trials which compared two CMF dosages and two FEC regimens.[34] CMF1 had a dose intensity of C (350), M (20) and F (300 mg/m^2 per week) as compared with CMF2, C (300), M (20) and F (300 mg/m^2 per week). The dose intensity of FEC1 was F (200), E (17), C (200 mg/m^2 per week) and for FEC2, F (300), E (13), C (300 mg/m^2 per week). Overall, severe nausea and vomiting occurred more frequently in those given FEC (46% vs 22%), as did alopecia (41% vs 9%).

At 5 years there was no difference in overall survival of those given CMF or FEC (80% vs 82%) and those given CMF1 and FEC1 had similar outcome (80% vs 78%). However, there was a survival disadvantage for those given FEC2 compared with CMF2 (87% vs 74%). This difference was present in those with three or fewer nodes or four or more nodes. There is a subgroup of node-positive patients who will benefit from an anthracycline-containing regimen, but this is achieved with increased toxicity and occurs only with appropriate scheduling.

Once a cytotoxic agent has been found to be active in patients with advanced breast cancer, there is usually pressure to test it in an adjuvant role. As paclitaxel (Taxol) and docetaxel (Taxotere) have been responsible for marked remissions in patients with heavily pre-treated disease, these are emerging as costly but important new therapies. It is likely that taxanes will be tested as adjuvant therapy in patients with high-risk disease such as those with four or more nodes involved. Studies are also under way to examine the role of high-dose chemotherapy with bone marrow transplantation in high-risk cases. Cost–benefit analyses are awaited with great interest.

Endocrine effects of adjuvant chemotherapy

As the major effect of adjuvant chemotherapy is seen in premenopausal women, this does suggest that part of the action might be through a hormonal mechanism, possibly as a result of ovarian suppression. This was suggested by the results of the Guy's/Manchester adjuvant trial in which 411 patients were randomized to receive 12 cycles of CMF or serve as untreated controls.[35] The major effect was seen in premenopausal women and the trial was re-analysed to examine the relationship between ER/PR status and the impact of permanent amenorrhoea on outcome.[36] The results are shown in Table 14.7.

In the premenopausal patients, those with PR-positive tumours had a significantly better outcome if treated with CMF. This did not occur in postmenopausal cases. Of the premenopausal patients, 61% of those given CMF developed permanent amenorrhoea. The survival of those cases was significantly better than that of untreated controls, and also of those given CMF who did not stop menstruating.

The Danish Breast Cancer Co-operative Group ran a trial for premenopausal women who were either node positive or had cancers larger than 5 cm.[37] There was a three-way randomization to observation, 12 cycles of CMF or 12 cycles of cyclophosphamide alone (C), 130 mg/m^2 on days 1–14. As Table 14.8 shows, both cyclophosphamide and CMF were equally

Table 14.7 Five-year survival of patients in CMF trial in relation to tumour ER/PR status and development of amenorrhoea

Group	Control	CMF
Overall	75	80
ER +ve	90	90
ER –ve	70	90
PR +ve	70	95
PR –ve	45	65
Amenorrhoea +ve	**75**	**90**
Amenorrhoea –ve	75	75

From Padmanabhan et al.[36]

Table 14.8 Five-year relapse-free survival in relation to treatment, ER status and development of amenorrhoea

Feature	C	CMF
Amenorrhoea +ve	78	70
Amenorrhoea –ve	63	70
ER +ve	**77**	65
ER –ve	**80**	65

From Brincker et al.[37]

effective and reduced recurrence by 17% at 7 years. The improvement in overall survival was 14%. Amenorrhoea developed in 70% of C and 63% of CMF cases.

These results suggested that part of the effect of adjuvant chemotherapy in premenopausal women is the result of ovarian suppression. Partly because of this, the Guy's Breast Unit joined with the Scottish Cancer Trials Breast Group in an adjuvant study which compared ovarian ablation with CMF in premenopausal node-positive cases.[38] The trial was of factorial 2 × 2 design:

Table 14.9 Eight-year survival of patients treated with adjuvant ovarian ablation or CMF

Group	CMF (%)	Ovarian ablation (%)
All	60	60
ER +ve	65	75
ER −ve	72	55

- Ovarian ablation
- Ovarian ablation + prednisolone 7.5 mg daily
- CMF
- CMF + prednisolone 7.5 mg daily.

The 8-year survival rate of those treated by either ovarian ablation or CMF was 60%, and no effect of prednisolone was detectable. However, when cases were subdivided on a basis of ER status of the primary tumour (< 20 fmol/mg protein negative, $> + 20$ fmol/mg protein positive) the results changed, as shown in Table 14.9. Those patients with ER-positive tumours fared significantly better if treated by ovarian ablation whereas ER-negative cases had a better survival after adjuvant CMF.

Thus, in patients with ER-negative tumours, CMF is exerting a direct cytocidal effect but this may be partly combined with an endocrine effect in premenopausal women with ER-positive tumours.

Duration of treatment

In the original studies adjuvant CMF treatment was given for 12 cycles, but a subsequent trial compared six cycles of CMF with 12 cycles.[39] After 5 years the overall survival rate of those given 12 cycles was 73% and that of those who received six cycles was 77%. This suggests that the effect of CMF occurred within the first 6 months, with no additional gain for prolonging

the treatment and with an extra burden of side effects.

Levine et al compared a 12-week regimen of cyclophosphamide, methotrexate, fluorouracil, vincristine, prednisone, doxorubicin and tamoxifen (CMFVP + AT) with a 36-week course of CMFVP.[40] After a median follow-up of 37 months relapse occurred in 57% of those who had the short course but in only 42% of those given 36 weeks of treatment. The 3-year overall survival rates were 78% for the 12-week group and 85% in those who received the 36-week regimen. Thus, short-term intensive adjuvant treatment was less effective than more prolonged therapy.

The Dutch Breast Cancer Working Party and the European Organization for Research and Treatment of Cancer (EORTC) ran a joint trial for node-positive women who were either given no adjuvant therapy or received low-dose CMF for 2 years.[41] This comprised monthly courses of cyclophosphamide 50 mg/m^2 on days 1 and 14, methotrexate 15 mg/m^2 on days 1 and 8, and fluorouracil 359 mg/m^2 on days 1 and 8. There was a significantly better survival in the low-dose CMF arm (59% vs 50%). However, even though the dosage was reduced by 50% there was substantial toxicity, with nausea in 88%, vomiting in 59% and alopecia in 35%. It was concluded that a standard 6-month course of CMF was to be preferred.

The International Breast Cancer Study Group entered 1554 node-positive cases into a 2×2 factorial design randomized trial.[42] The options were as follows:

- CMF$\times$ 6 months
- CMF $\times$ 6 months + CMF on months 9, 12, 15
- CMF $\times$ 3 months
- CMF $\times$ 3 months + CMF on months 6, 9, 12.

Among those given CMF for three cycles, without re-introduction of CMF, the 5-year relapse-free survival was 53%, whereas for each of the other randomized groups it was 58%. Thus, again, 6 months of CMF emerged as the optimum duration of treatment, in terms of both efficacy and minimization of toxicity.

Perioperative chemotherapy

The action of adjuvant systemic therapy may be either to destroy pre-existing micrometastases present at the time of diagnosis, or alternatively to neutralize tumour emboli shed during surgery. Possibly chemotherapy acts by a combination of both. If the reversal of iatrogenic dissemination is important then perioperative chemotherapy would be a useful adjunct. Should this type of treatment be beneficial, how much is gained by how many and at what cost?

Hypothesizing that a short perioperative course of chemotherapy might be beneficial, with fewer side effects than long-term treatment, Nissen-Meyer coordinated the Scandinavian Adjuvant Chemotherapy Study Group Trial.[43] All patients were treated by mastectomy and then were given either a 6-day postoperative course of cyclophosphamide (total dose 30 mg/kg) or no adjuvant therapy. There were 507 treated patients and 519 controls and, after 10 years of follow-up, the relapse-free survival rate was 75% in the treated group and 55% in the controls. Also, overall survival was significantly better for the treated group (71% vs 62%).

A similar pattern of benefit was seen in all the 11 collaborating centres, with one exception. In that hospital the course of chemotherapy was delayed for 3 weeks postoperatively and no effect on relapse-free or overall survival was observed in that group of treated patients. This does suggest that the efficacy of perioperative chemotherapy depends upon scheduling immediately after surgery, either because it acts on relatively unprotected tumour emboli or because tumour removal serves to induce mitosis in metastases which are then more susceptible to cyclophosphamide.

Side effects of treatment included nausea in most, alopecia in a few and, only rarely, cystitis. In terms of postoperative wound healing no significant differences were noted between the treated and control groups.

As a result of the potential importance of this mortality reduction, the Cancer Research Campaign re-examined the effect in a factorial 2 × 2 design trial with the following randomizations:

- No treatment
- Cyclophosphamide (30 mg/g i.v. in 6 days)
- Tamoxifen (10 mg twice daily for 2 years)
- Cyclophosphamide plus tamoxifen.

The trial started in 1980 and in 5 years accrued 1070 participants who received no cyclophosphamide and 1126 cyclophosphamide-treated cases.[44] Patients were treated either by modified radical or total mastectomy, with or without radiotherapy or breast conservation therapy (tumorectomy, axillary sampling and radiotherapy). After a median follow-up of 2.5 years, fewer events had occurred in the cyclophosphamide-treated group (75% vs 70%), but there was no difference in terms of overall survival. Compliance with chemotherapy was 91%. Nausea occurred in 56%, 8% had alopecia sufficient to require a wig, and severe leukopenia was reported in 7%.

A second analysis after 3.3 years of follow-up showed that there was still a better event-free survival in the cyclophosphamide-treated group (73% vs 70%).[45] For tamoxifen-treated cases versus controls the event-free survival rates were 74% and 64% respectively. No effect was seen on overall survival and the only significant prognostic indicator of breast cancer mortality was axillary nodal status. Thus, there were only marginal benefits from a short course of cyclophosphamide given after disparate surgical procedures.

More recent studies have examined the role of perioperative polychemotherapy, in comparison with postoperative standard chemotherapy, or no adjuvant therapy in node-negative cases. The results of these trials are outlined in Table 14.10. The Ludwig Breast Cancer Study Group in Ludwig Trial V randomized 1275 node-negative patients to postoperative chemotherapy (CMF plus leucovorin on days 1 and 8) or no treatment.[46] There was a small but significant improvement in disease-free survival at 4 years and a small insignificant difference in overall survival rate (90% vs 86%). Similar effects were seen in both pre- and postmenopausal cases.

Table 14.10 Trials of adjuvant perioperative chemotherapy versus no treatment for node negative cases

Group	Perioperative chemotherapy (%)	Control (%)	Reference
Premenopausal	76	71	The Ludwig Breast Cancer Study Group[46]
Postmenopausal	78	74	
All	77	73	
Premenopausal	–	–	Sertoli et al[47]
Postmenopausal	–	–	
All	80	75	
Premenopausal	79	75	Clahsen et al[48]
Postmenopausal	79	76	
All	79	76	

The Genoa Institute of Oncology ran a trial in which 167 node-negative cases received perioperative therapy (cyclophosphamide, epirubicin and fluorouracil on day 2 or 3), and 152 had no adjuvant treatment.[47] The 4-year disease-free survival of the group given perioperative chemotherapy was significantly better, but this was only observed among those with ER-negative tumours. There was no significant difference in overall survival.

The EORTC Breast Cancer Co-operative Group conducted EORTC Trial 10854 in which 727 node-negative cases received perioperative treatment (one course of fluorouracil, doxorubicin and cyclophosphamide within 24 hours of surgery), and 716 were untreated controls.[48] The 4-year local relapse-free survival rate was significantly better after perioperative chemotherapy (94% vs 91%). There was also a better disease-free survival but no effect on overall survival.

In the Scandinavian trial only after 5 years was there any effect of perioperative chemotherapy on overall survival and so the lack of any significant mortality reduction in these three trials is not surprising. However, if there is any effect it is likely to be small (<5%) and so more than 95% of node-negative cases given perioperative chemotherapy will not benefit.

This type of therapy is not without toxicity. In the Ludwig study there was a high rate of wound breakdown, possibly because of an interaction between nitrous oxide and methotrexate which inhibited wound healing.[49] In EORTC trial 10854, thromboembolic complications occurred in 2.1% of those given perioperative therapy and in 0.8% of controls. This took the form of phlebitis, venous thrombosis and pulmonary embolus which in three of six cases was fatal.[50] The frequency of complications was significantly higher in postmenopausal women, and after mastectomy rather than tumourectomy. To reduce this risk it was suggested that prophylactic heparin should be given with perioperative chemotherapy.

Canavese et al quantified the surgical complications in 275 patients participating in the Genoa Trial.[51] The median hospital stay was similar in the treated and control groups as was the incidence of wound infections and need for postoperative seroma drainage. Toxicity was as would be expected with nausea and vomiting in 55%, hair loss in 55% (total in only 3%) and stomatitis in 3%. Only 9% of treated cases had grade III/IV toxicity.

If the benefits of perioperative chemotherapy are marginal in node-negative cases, they are undetectable in node-positive cases who receive treatment or are controls when both groups are given subsequent standard chemotherapy. In the Ludwig study, the disease-free survival rate of those node-positive cases who had perioperative chemotherapy was 62% compared with 60% in those who had standard postoperative therapy.[47] In the Genoa trial 82% of treated and untreated node-positive cases were disease free at 5 years.[47] None of these studies show any benefit in terms of relapse-free or overall survival for node-negative cases given perioperative chemotherapy. Overall significant improvement in survival of breast cancer cases is more likely to be achieved by preoperative rather than perioperative systemic therapy.

ADJUVANT ENDOCRINE THERAPY

The endocrine sensitivity of some breast cancers provides an opportunity to use less toxic endocrine therapies for women at risk of recurrence, even among those with only a slight hazard of relapse. At present there is clear evidence of benefit for some premenopausal cases treated by ovarian ablation and for both node-positive and -negative, ER-positive cases given adjuvant tamoxifen. Attention is now focusing on whether survival can be improved further with extra endocrine therapies or a combination treatment of endocrine treatment and chemotherapy.

Ovarian ablation

After the second Oxford Overview had demonstrated the unexpected long-term benefit of ovarian ablation,[19] another meta-analysis was conducted which contained data from 15 years of follow-up of 12 randomized trials.[52] As a result of lack of uniformity in definition of menopausal status, the analyses were based on

Table 14.11 Fifteen-year overall survival in adjuvant trials of ovarian ablation versus no treatment

Age (years)	Ovarian ablation (%)	Control (%)
< 50	52	46
≥ 50	37	35

From EBCTCG.[52]

age less than 50 and 50 or over. Outline results are shown in Table 14.11. For those aged less than 50 there was a significantly better 15-year relapse-free survival rate after ovarian ablation (45% vs 39%) and a better overall survival rate (52% vs 46%), with an approximate 20% reduction in event rate. There was no significantly different relapse-free or overall survival in treated and control cases aged 50 or over.

In the five trials that examined ovarian ablation with or without chemotherapy, there was a 25% improvement in relapse-free survival in those aged less than 50 who had ovarian suppression. However, for those who also received chemotherapy, the improvement in relapse-free survival race was only 10%, suggesting that the combination of endocrine and chemotherapy may be deleterious.

Ovarian ablation improves survival in both node-positive and -negative cases. In the node-negative cases treated by ovarian ablation the 15-year overall survival rate was 77% compared with 71% in controls, representing five to six fewer deaths per 100 patients. For the node-positive cases the respective 15-year survival rates were 42% and 29%, a reduction of 12.5 deaths per 100 women resulting from ovarian suppression. There was no difference in non-breast cancer deaths of the treated and control cases, and surprisingly no significant reduction in contralateral breast cancers.

With such a prolonged and significant reduction in risk of dying from breast cancer, many will wish to offer this less toxic treatment to premenopausal patients. Eligible cases are those with ER-positive node-positive disease and ER-positive node-negative disease in those with tumours larger than 1 cm in diameter. Ovarian ablation can be achieved surgically, using the laparoscope, medically with gonadotrophin-releasing hormone (GnRH) analogues, such as goserelin, and radiotherapeutically with external pelvic irradiation. At Guy's Hospital the preferred method for the past 20 years has been ovarian irradiation delivering 15 Gy in five daily fractions. This gives a rapid ovarian suppression with most of patients developing immediate amenorrhoea. It avoids the discomfort of surgery and is considerably cheaper and easier than depot injections of goserelin.

For node-negative cases it would be worthwhile conducting a trial comparing ovarian suppression with tamoxifen alone, looking not only at relapse and mortality but also at quality of life, bone density, and changes in lipoproteins and cholesterol. Some patients may wish to become pregnant subsequently and this would be possible after tamoxifen but not after ovarian irradiation. In addition, there is a considerable expense involved in 2 years of goserelin treatment.

There is still some doubt in the minds of many clinicians about the interaction of endocrine therapy and chemotherapy. For these individuals the ABC trial is being run by the United Kingdom Co-ordinating Committee on Cancer Research (UK CCCR) to test pragmatically various therapies. For premenopausal patients the randomization options are as follows:

- All have ovarian ablation then chemotherapy versus none
- All have chemotherapy then ovarian ablation versus none
- Chemotherapy versus none and ovarian ablation versus none.

Chemotherapy is not specified but CMF or an anthracycline-containing regimen is advised. All postmenopausal patients receive tamoxifen and are randomized to chemotherapy versus none. The study aims to accrue 4000 patients.

Adjuvant tamoxifen

The overview by the EBCTCG[19] has convinced all oncologists that tamoxifen is beneficial, particularly in postmenopausal ER-positive patients, but paradoxically many are still striving to demonstrate an unacceptable profile of side effects and a future risk of more cancers as a result of genotoxicity.

The overview suggests that a dosage of 20 mg daily should be given for 5 years. There is no value in giving higher dosages as adjuvant treatment and this will lead to more side effects. Also, the pharmacokinetics of tamoxifen are such that a single daily dose can be given, although a few women will suffer fewer side effects if given 10 mg twice daily. There is still an argument about whether tamoxifen treatment should continue beyond 5 years but preliminary results are available from three randomized trials.[53-55] In the NSABP B-14, patients with ER-positive, node-negative disease were randomized to tamoxifen (1404) or placebo (1414).[55] After 5 years disease-free patients who had received tamoxifen were then randomized to a further 5 years of tamoxifen or placebo. In addition, a further 1211 cases similar to the randomized cases were registered and those who remained disease free after 5 years were also randomized to another 5 years of tamoxifen (261) or placebo (249).

Four years after the second randomization 89% of those taking tamoxifen were disease free compared with 94% of the placebo group. The overall survival rates were 96% and 98% respectively. The trial was brought to a close after analyses had indicated almost zero probability that any benefit of prolonged tamoxifen would be demonstrable after longer follow-up.

The Eastern Co-operative Oncology Group examined the value of prolonged tamoxifen in node-positive patients who had received 12 cycles of chemotherapy and tamoxifen, followed by a further 4 years of tamoxifen.[55] After 5 years they were randomized to continue or stop tamoxifen. There were 193 women with a median follow-up of 5.6 years after the 5-year randomization. In those who continued tamoxifen beyond 5 years, the overall survival rate was 86% compared with 89% in those who stopped.

In the Scottish Cancer Trials Breast Group study 169 women were re-randomized to continue tamoxifen after 5 years and 173 to stop the drug.[56] After a median follow-up of 6 years following re-randomization, the relapse-free survival rate of those who continued tamoxifen was 78% and for those who stopped, it was 83% (hazard ratio = 1.27).

Furthermore, there was an increased rate of endometrial carcinoma among the women who took a prolonged course of tamoxifen. With a slightly worse outcome, it was concluded that further gain in disease control from more than 5 years of tamoxifen was unlikely.

Although a small benefit from prolongation of tamoxifen cannot be excluded on a basis of these three trials, it is likely if positive to be extremely small and possibly further prolongation could lead to more toxicity, such as an increased incidence of endometrial cancer. With an increasingly restricted budget for clinical research, investigation of more prolonged courses of tamoxifen would not seem to be a high priority.

Tamoxifen and prednisolone

In patients with advanced breast cancer prednisolone can improve the response to primary endocrine therapy as was shown in a trial conducted at Guy's Hospital.[56] The study included 220 women with advanced disease who were treated by ovarian irradiation, if premenopausal, and tamoxifen if post-menopausal. They were randomized to receive or not receive prednisolone 5 mg twice daily. Those who received prednisolone were more likely to have a complete or partial response (49% vs 30%) and a more prolonged remission (14 vs 9 months).

Evidence of a potential adjuvant role for prednisolone came from the Princess Margaret Hospital Toronto Trial in which 224 premenopausal women received post-mastectomy radiotherapy and were then randomized to observation, ovarian irradiation or ovarian irradiation and prednisolone 7.5 mg daily for 5

years. After 10 years of follow-up, the disease-free and overall survival rate was significantly better in those who received prednisolone.

As a result of this evidence a trial was run at Guy's Hospital, London and the Christie Hospital, Manchester in which 254 post-menopausal women with node-positive and -negative breast cancer were randomized to tamoxifen 20 mg daily for 5 years (128) or tamoxifen plus prednisolone 7.5 mg daily for the same duration (126).[57] After a median follow-up of 4 years there was no significant difference in survival of the two groups.

Survival slightly favoured tamoxifen and, as the confidence intervals of the hazard ratio indicated that a 5% difference in favour of prednisolone was very unlikely, the study indicated the lack of efficacy of prednisolone in this particular adjuvant role. Interestingly, as a parallel study, bone density was measured in both groups to determine whether there was a significant reduction in those taking prednisolone, and no significant difference was found, indicating that tamoxifen may protect against steroid-induced bone loss.[58]

SYNOPSIS

- Most patients benefit from systemic adjuvant therapy other than those with well-differentiated node-negative cancers sized 1 cm or less.
- Adjuvant radiotherapy may reduce local relapse and thereby prevent distant metastases.
- Ovarian ablation can be achieved simply by irradiation at less cost than by surgery or luteinizing hormone-releasing hormone (LHRH) agonists and achieves a 30% reduction in annual odds of death for up to 10 years.
- Six cycles of CMF is the optimum duration and is equivalent to perioperative chemotherapy in node-positive cases.
- Tamoxifen should be given as adjuvant therapy at a dose of 20 mg daily for 5 years and achieves a 20% annual reduction in odds of death.

REFERENCES

1. Fentiman IS, Cuzick J, Millis RR, Hayward JL. Which patients are cured of breast cancer? *Br Med J* 1984; **289:** 1108–11.
2. Quiet CA, Ferguson DJ, Weichelsbaum RR, Hellman S. Natural history of node-positive breast cancer: the curability of small cancers with a limited number of positive nodes. *J Clin Oncol* 1996; **14:** 3105–11.
3. National Cancer Institute. *Clinical Alert*. Bethesda, MD: National Cancer Institute, 1988.
4. O'Reilly SM, Camplejohn RS, Barnes DM et al. Node-negative breast cancer: prognostic subgroups defined by tumour size and flow cytometry. *J Clin Oncol* 1990; **8:** 2040–6.
5. Haybittle JL, Blamey RW, Elston CW et al. A prognostic index in primary breast cancer. *Br J Cancer* 1982; **45:** 361–5.
6. Elston CW, Gresham GA, Rao GS et al. The Cancer Research campaign (King's/Cambridge) Trial for early breast cancer: clinico-pathological aspects. *Br J Cancer* 1982; **45:** 665–9.
7. Todd JH, Dowle C, Williams MR et al. Confirmation of a prognostic index in primary breast cancer. *Br J Cancer* 1987; **56:** 489–92.
8. Barbareschi M, Veronese S, Leek RD et al. Bcl-2 and p53 gene expression in node negative breast cancer. *Hum Pathol* 1996; **27:** 1149–55.
9. Fisher ER, Redmond C, Fisher B et al. Pathologic findings from the National Surgical Adjuvant Breast and Bowel Projects (NSABP). *Cancer* 1990; **65:** 2121–8.
10. Heimann R, Ferguson D, Powers C et al. Angiogenesis as a predictor of long-term survival for patients with node negative breast cancer. *J Natl Cancer Inst* 1996; **88:** 1764–9.
11. Cuzick J, Stewart H, Peto R et al. Overview of randomized trials of postoperative adjuvant radiotherapy in breast cancer. *Cancer Treat Rep* 1987; **71:** 15–29.
12. Rutqvist LE, Cedermark B, Glas U et al. Radiotherapy, chemotherapy, and tamoxifen as adjuncts to surgery in early breast cancer: a summary of three randomized trials. *Int J Radiat Oncol Biol Phys* 1989; **16:** 629–39.
13. Cuzick J, Stewart H, Rutqvist L et al. Cause-specific mortality in long-term survivors of breast cancer who participated in trials of radio-therapy. *J Clin Oncol* 1994; **12:** 447–53.
14. Arriagada R, Rutqvist LE, Mattsson A et al. Adequate locoregional treatment for early breast cancer may prevent secondary dissemination. *J Clin Oncol* 1995; **13:** 2869–78.
15. Fisher ER, Gregorio RM, Redmond C et al. Pathologic findings from the National Surgical Adjuvant Breast Project (protocol No. 4): III. The significance of extranodal extension of axillary metastases. *Am J Clin Pathol* 1976; **65:** 439–44.
16. Leonard C, Corkhill M, Tompkin J et al. Are axillary recurrence and overall survival affected by axillary extranodal tumor extension in breast cancer? Implications for radiation therapy. *J Clin Oncol* 1995; **13:** 47–53.
17. Early Breast Cancer Trialists' Collaborative Group. Effects of radiotherapy and surgery in early breast cancer. *N Engl J Med* 1995; **333:** 1444–55.
18. Early Breast Cancer Trialists' Collaborative Group. Effects of adjuvant tamoxifen and of cytotoxic therapy on mortality in early breast cancer. *N Engl J Med* 1988; **319:** 1681–92.
19. Early Breast Cancer Trialists' Collaborative Group. Systemic treatment of early breast cancer by hormonal, cytotoxic, or immune therapy. *Lancet* 1992; **339:** 1–15. 71–84.
20. Bonadonna G, Valagussa P. Dose response effect of adjuvant chemotherapy in breast cancer. *N Engl J Med* 1981; **304:** 10–15.
21. Hakes T, Geller N, Petroni G et al. Confirmation of dose–survival relationship in breast adjuvant chemotherapy [Abstr]. *Proc Am Soc Clin Oncol* 1984; **3:** 122.
22. Howell A, Rubens RD, Bush H et al. A controlled trial of adjuvant chemotherapy with melphalan versus cyclophosphamide, methotrexate and fluorouracil for breast cancer. In: *Recent Results in Cancer Research. Adjuvant chemotherapy of breast cancer*. Senn HJ, ed. Heidelberg: Springer Verlag, 1984.
23. Mouridsen HT, Rose C, Brincker H et al. Adjuvant systemic therapy in high risk breast cancer: the Danish Breast Cancer Co-operative Group's trials of cyclophosphamide or CMF in premenopausal and tamoxifen in postmenopausal patients. In: *Recent Results in Cancer Research. Adjuvant chemotherapy of breast cancer*. Senn HJ, ed. Heidelberg: Springer Verlag, 1984.
24. Velez-Garcia E, Carpenter JT, Moore M et al. Post-surgical adjuvant chemotherapy with or without radiotherapy in women with breast

cancer and positive axillary nodes. Progress report of a South Eastern Cancer Study Group (SEG) trial. In: *Adjuvant Therapy of Cancer V*. Salmon SE, ed. Philadelphia: Grune & Stratton, 1987.

25. Henderson IC, Hayes DF, Gelman R. Dose–response in the treatment of breast cancer: a critical review. *J Clin Oncol* 1988; **6:** 1501–15.

26. Hryniuk W, Levine MN. Analysis of dose intensity for adjuvant chemotherapy trials in stage II breast cancer. *J Clin Oncol* 1986; **4:** 1162–70.

27. Cooper RG. Combination chemotherapy in hormone resistant breast cancer [Abstr]. *Proc Am Assoc Cancer Res* 1969; **10:** 15.

28. Gelman RS, Henderson IC. A re-analysis of dose intensity for adjuvant chemotherapy trials in stage II breast cancer. *SAKK Bull* 1987; **1:** 10–12.

29. Hortobagyi GN, Bodey SP, Buzdar AV et al. Evaluation of high dose versus standard FAC chemotherapy for advanced breast cancer in protected environment units: a prospective randomized trial. *J Clin Oncol* 1987; **5:** 354–64.

30. Korzun A, Norton L, Perloff M et al. Clinical equivalence despite dosage differences of two schedules of cyclophosphamide, methotrexate 5–fluorouracil, vincristine and prednisone (CMFVP) [Abstr]. *Proc Am Soc Clin Oncol* 1988; **7:** 12.

31. Fisher B, Brown AM, Dimitrov NV et al. Two months of doxorubicin-cyclophosphamide with and without interval reinduction therapy compared with 6 months of cyclophosphamide, methotrexate, and fluorouracil in positive-node breast cancer patients with tamoxifen-nonresponsive tumors: results from the National Surgical Adjuvant Breast and Bowel Project B-15. *J Clin Oncol* 1990; **8:** 1483–96.

32. Mauriac L, Durand M, Chauvergne J et al. Randomized trial of adjuvant chemotherapy for operable breast cancer comparing i.v. CMF to an epirubicin-containing regimen. *Ann Oncol* 1992; **3:** 439–43.

33. Bonadonna G, Zampetti M, Valagussa P. Sequential or alternating doxorubicin and CMF regimens in breast cancer with more than three positive nodes. *JAMA* 1995; **273:** 542–7.

34. Coombes RC, Bliss JM, Wils J et al. Adjuvant cyclophosphamide, methotrexate, and fluorouracil versus fluorouracil, epirubicin, and cyclophosphamide chemotherapy in premenopausal women with axillary node-positive operable breast cancer: results of a randomized trial. *J Clin Oncol* 1996; **14:** 35–45.

35. Howell A, Bush H, George WD et al. Controlled trial of adjuvant chemotherapy with cyclophosphamide, methotrexate and fluorouracil for breast cancer. *Lancet* 1984; **ii:** 307–11.

36. Padmanabhan N, Howell A, Rubens RD. Mechanism of action of adjuvant chemotherapy in early breast cancer. *Lancet* 1986; **ii:** 411–14.

37. Brincker H, Rose C, Rank F et al. Evidence of a castration-mediated effect of adjuvant cytotoxic chemotherapy in premenopausal breast cancer. *J Clin Oncol* 1987; **5:** 1771–8.

38. Scottish Cancer Trials Breast Group and ICRF Breast Unit, Guy's Hospital, London. Adjuvant ovarian ablation versus CMF chemotherapy in premenopausal women with pathological stage II breast carcinoma: the Scottish Trial. *Lancet* 1993; **341:** 1293–8.

39. Tancini G, Bonadonna G, Valagussa P et al. Adjuvant CMF in breast cancer: comparative 5–year results of 12 versus 6 cycles. *J Clin Oncol* 1983; **69:** 2–10.

40. Levine MN, Gent M, Hryniuk WM et al. A randomized trial comparing 12 weeks versus 36 weeks of adjuvant chemotherapy in stage II breast cancer. *J Clin Oncol* 1990; **8:** 1217–25.

41. Clahsen PC, van de Velde CJH, Welvaart K et al. Ten-year results of a randomized trial evaluating prolonged low-dose adjuvant chemotherapy in node-positive breast cancer: a joint European Organization for Research and Treatment of Cancer–Dutch Breast Cancer Working Party Study. *J Clin Oncol* 1995; **13:** 33–41.

42. International Breast Cancer Study Group. Duration and reintroduction of adjuvant chemotherapy for node-positive premenopausal breast cancer patients. *J Clin Oncol* 1996; **14:** 1885–94.

43. Nissen-Meyer R, Kjellgren K, Malmio K et al. Surgical adjuvant chemotherapy. Results of one short course with cyclophosphamide after mastectomy for breast cancer. *Cancer* 1978; **41:** 2988–98.

44. Houghton J, Baum M, Nissen-Meyer R. Is there a role for perioperative adjuvant therapy in the treatment of early breast cancer? *Eur J Surg Oncol* 1988; **14:** 227–33.

45. CRC Adjuvant Breast Working Group. Cyclophosphamide and tamoxifen as adjuvant therapies in the management of breast cancer. *Br J Cancer* 1988; **57:** 604–7.

46. The Ludwig Breast Cancer Study Group. Prolonged disease-free survival after one course of perioperative adjuvant chemotherapy for

node-negative breast cancer. *N Engl J Med* 1989; **320:** 491–6.

47. Sertoli MR, Bruzzi P, Pronzato P et al. Randomized co-operative study of perioperative chemotherapy in breast cancer. *J Clin Oncol* 1995; **13:** 2712–21.

48. Clahsen PC, van de Velde CJH, Julien J-P et al. Improved local control and disease-free survival after perioperative chemotherapy for early-stage breast cancer: a European Organisation for Research and Treatment of Breast Cancer Co-operative Group Study. *J Clin Oncol* 1996; **14:** 745–53.

49. Ludwig Breast Cancer Study Group. Toxic effects of early adjuvant chemotherapy for breast cancer. *Lancet* 1983; **ii:** 542–4.

50. Clahsen PC, van de Velde CJH, Julien J-P et al. Thromboembolic complications after periopera-tive chemotherapy in women with early breast cancer: a European Organisation for Research and Treatment of Breast Cancer Co-operative Group Study. *J Clin Oncol* 1994; **12:** 1266–71.

51. Canavese G, Catturich A, Vecchio C et al. Surgical complications related to perioperative adjuvant chemotherapy in breast cancer. Results of a prospective, controlled, randomized clinical trial. *Eur J Surg Oncol* 1997; **23:** 10–12.

52. Early Breast Cancer Trialists' Collaborative Group. Ovarian ablation in early breast cancer: overview of the randomised trials. *Lancet* 1996; **348:** 1189–96.

53. Fisher B, Dignam J, Bryant J et al. Five versus more than five years of tamoxifen therapy for breast cancer patients with negative lymph nodes and estrogen receptor-positive tumors. *J Natl Cancer Inst* 1996; **88:** 1529–42.

54. Tormey DC, Gray R, Falkson HC. Postchemotherapy adjuvant tamoxifen therapy beyond five years in patients with node-positive breast cancer. *J Natl Cancer Inst* 1996; **88:** 1828–33.

55. Stewart HJ, Forrest AP, Everington D et al. Randomised comparison of 5 years of adjuvant tamoxifen with continuous therapy for operable breast cancer. *Br J Cancer* 1996; **74:** 297–9.

56. Rubens RD, Tinson CL, Coleman RE et al. Prednisolone improves the response to primary endocrine treatment for advanced breast cancer. *Br J Cancer* 1988; **58:** 626–30.

57. Fentiman IS, Howell A, Hamed H et al. A controlled trial of adjuvant tamoxifen, with or without prednisolone, in post-menopausal women with operable breast cancer. *Br J Cancer* 1994; **70:** 729–31.

58. Fentiman IS, Zaad S, Chaudary MA et al. Tamoxifen protects against steroid induced bone loss. *Eur J Cancer* 1992; **28:** 684–5.

15

Pregnancy and exogenous oestrogens

It's as large as life and twice as natural.

Lewis Carroll

**Breast cancer in pregnancy • Pregnancy subsequent to breast cancer • Oral contraception •
Hormone replacement therapy**

As oestrogens play a major role in the promotion of breast cancer, great interest has been taken in those conditions under which the body is exposed to excessive or prolonged levels of these hormones, such as pregnancy, oral contraception (OC) and hormone replacement therapy (HRT). It was assumed, and indeed was standard teaching, that these should all be eschewed by women who had been diagnosed with breast cancer. Furthermore, it was suspected that both OC and HRT might increase the risk of developing the disease. Recent work has both illuminated and complicated the situation. Some of the risks have been quantified so that advice can be based on knowledge rather than bias. Women can now make informed choices about significant aspects of their reproductive life.

BREAST CANCER PREGNANCY

After studying the available evidence it is difficult to escape the conclusion that pregnancy is protective against breast cancer in both the long and short term. However, among those women who develop a cancer during pregnancy the overall prognosis can be worse, particularly as a result of delay in diagnosis. Those breast cancer patients who subsequently become pregnant do not suffer a worsening of their prognosis.

Protective effect of pregnancy

As breast cancer is rare among young women, the expected incidence is low as shown in Table 15.1, which summarizes data on cancers developing during pregnancy reported by the German National Cancer Registry.[1] The most common malignancy was cervical cancer which was detected more frequently than would be expected, possibly because of increased cervical

---

Table 15.1 Standardized incidence rates of cancers in pregnant women

Site	Observed (O)	Expected (E)	O/E	95% CI
Cervix	229	200	1.15	1.01–1.31
Breast	28	78	0.36	0.24–0.52
Ovary	19	36	0.53	0.31–0.82

From Haas.[1]

Table 15.2 Presentation of breast cancer within trimesters of pregnancy

First trimester	Second trimester	Third trimester	Reference
28	16	9	Holleb and Farrow[2]
28	20	26	Bunker and Peters[3]
3	9	13	Clark and Reid[4]
21	20	22	King et al[5]
31	12	27	Ribeiro et al[6]
5	4	11	Tretli et al[7]
116 (38)	**81 (27)**	**108 (35)**	**Total***

* Values in parentheses are percentages.

screening during pregnancy. However, there were significantly fewer cases of breast cancer than were expected, with a two-thirds reduction in incidence.

This substantial reduction may be the result of the process of differentiation and apoptosis of mammary epithelium during pregnancy leading to destruction of premalignant and malignant cells. As there is an almost equal distribution of cancers diagnosed within the trimesters of pregnancy, this inhibitory effect occurs early as shown in Table 15.2.[2–7]

Cancers emerging from this milieu would be unlikely to be hormone dependent and would thus be unaffected by termination of the pregnancy. Several uncontrolled series in which pregnancy was or was not terminated are summarized in Table 15.3.[3–5,8–11] Rather than improving the situation by withdrawal of hormones, 5-year survival of those women who continued with the pregnancy was better (70% vs 44%).

The even more drastic measure of oophorectomy may make matters worse. Deemarsky et al reported that 63% of women who had a termination in the first trimester survived 5 years if the ovaries were conserved compared with only 29% if oophorectomy was

Table 15.3 The effect of termination of pregnancy on 5-year survival of breast cancer patients

Termi-nation (%)	No termi-nation (%)	Reference
0	40	Bunker and Peters[3]
57	100	Holman and Bennett[8]
29	50	Peete et al[9]
75	80	Rissanen[10]
50	63	Clark and Reid[4]
43	88	Deemarsky et al[11]
53	67	King et al[5]
44 (42–46)	**70 (66–74)**	**Total***

* Values in parentheses are 95% confidence interval (95% CI).

performed.[11] When the pregnancy was allowed to go to term, or after early delivery, those treated by oophorectomy had a 5-year survival rate of 86% compared with 100% in those whose ovaries were retained.

That pregnancy has a suppressant effect on mammary carcinogenesis is also suggested by population-based case-control studies from Sweden and Norway, which showed a transient increase in risk of breast cancer after full-term delivery.[12,13] Further evidence of suppression of hormone-dependent tumours and emergence of hormone-resistant cancers is provided by a Japanese case-control study of 192 pregnant or lactating women with breast cancers compared with 191 age-matched non-pregnant controls with breast cancer.[14] Of the pregnant cases, 30% had oestrogen receptor (ER)-positive tumours compared with 61% of the non-pregnant group. Similarly, the rates of progesterone receptor (PR) positivity were 29% and 68% respectively. As another indicator of tumour aggression, vascular invasion was present in 70% of the pregnant cases but in only 45% of non-pregnant controls.

Delay in diagnosis during pregnancy

As a result of the low level of suspicion of breast cancer among midwives and obstetricians, together with the masking effect of breast enlargement during pregnancy, many women have a long duration of symptoms before the diagnosis is made. Results from the case-control study conducted by Ishida et al are shown in Table 15.4.[14] Of the non-pregnant cases 37% had symptoms for more than 3 months compared with 50% of the pregnant patients.

This delay in diagnosis is reflected in the higher stage of pregnancy-associated cancers together with an increased incidence of axillary nodal metastases. Nettleton et al used a mathematical model to determine the risk of axillary metastases with increasing delay in diagnosis.[15] Cases were subdivided on a basis of growth rate of tumour, moderate (doubling time 130 days) and fast (doubling time 65 days). Results are summarized in Table 15.5. For those with moderately proliferating cancers, a 6-month delay was calculated to result in a 5% increased risk of axillary nodal spread compared with 10% in those with fast-growing tumours.

That delay is common during pregnancy is indicated by the reported 75% incidence of

Table 15.4 Delay in diagnosis in pregnant and non-pregnant women with breast cancer

Duration of symptoms (months)	Pregnant cases (%)	Control cases (%)
1	30	43
2–3	20	22
4–6	21	11
7–12	18	16
13+	12	10

From Ishida et al.[14]

Table 15.5 Risk of axillary nodal metastases in pregnant women with increasing delay in diagnosis

	Increased risk (%) of	
Delay (months)	Moderate growth	Rapid growth
1	1	2
3	3	5
6	5	10

From Nettleton et al.[15]

axillary nodal involvement.[2,3,6,11] In a case-control study there was nodal involvement in 58% of pregnant women compared with 46% of non-pregnant controls.[14]

Prognosis of breast cancer in pregnancy

Several studies have shown that, overall, there is a worse prognosis for patients with pregnancy-associated breast cancers.[7,14,16] However, this is

Table 15.6 Five- and ten-year survival by stage in women with pregnancy-associated breast cancer and non-pregnant controls

Stage	Pregnant	Controls	Pregnant	Controls	Reference
I	100	70			Nugent and O'Connell[17]
II	50	48			
I	82	82	77	75	Petrek et al[18]
II	47	59	25	41	
I	90	100	85	93	Ishida et al[14]
II	50	70	37	62	

the result of late diagnosis and hence an over-representation of stage II and more advanced cancers in pregnant cases. When women with cancer in pregnancy are compared stage for stage with non-pregnant age-matched controls their survival is similar, as shown in Table 15.6.[14,17,18] Thus although there are more aggressive cancers diagnosed during pregnancy, if diagnosed early enough these do not appear to lead to any significant worsening of outcome after 10 years of follow-up.

In contrast, Guinee at al reported different results in a multicentre study of prognostic factors for breast cancer in young women aged less than 30 years at the time of diagnosis.[19] Among those who were pregnant at the time of diagnosis there was a threefold increase in risk of dying of breast cancer (relative risk, RR = 3.26) compared with nulliparous women. Even after adjustment for axillary nodal status and tumour size, this relative risk was still significantly increased at 2.83. In this young age

Table 15.7 Comparison of nodal status and 5-year survival of women with pregnancy-associated and lactational breast cancers

Pregnancy associated			Lactational			
No. (%)	Node-positive (%)	5-year survival rate (%)	No. (%)	Node-positive (%)	5-year survival rate (%)	Reference
35 (70)		20	15 (30)	72	33	Tretli et al[7]
154 (62)	72	32	96 (38)	69	39	Clark and Chua[20]
345 (97)	37	70	10 (3)	90	20	Lethaby et al[21]

group of breast cancer patients, the risk of dying from breast cancer decreased by 15% for each year between the previous pregnancy and diagnosis of breast cancer.

Lactational carcinomas

Cancers presenting during the first 12 months after delivery are usually described as lactational tumours. Many authors have not distinguished between cancers diagnosed in the three trimesters and those occurring during lactation, but it is of interest to know whether lactational cancers carry a similar, worse or better prognosis compared with other pregnancy-associated tumours. Results from those recent series that have separately reported details of pregnancy associated and lactational cancers are summarized in Table 15.7.[7,20,21] These suggest a similar rate of nodal involvement and 5-year survival in both groups with the exception of the study from the Auckland Breast Cancer Study Group in which there was only a small proportion of lactational cancers (3%), but these had a poorer prognosis, with none being alive 10 years after diagnosis.[21]

It may be difficult to make a diagnosis of cancer in an engorged lactating breast, either because of deep location or as a result of mistaken diagnosis of a galactocele. This latter may be suspected clinically but can be confirmed only by aspirating milk from the lump with complete resolution. Persistence of the lump is an indication for aspiration cytology. If a lactating woman has an equivocal lump she should be asked to wean rapidly from that side so that the non-engorged breast can be assessed. If there is any doubt the patient should be referred to a breast clinic where fine needle aspiration cytology can be performed.

Treatment

In a pregnant woman with a suspicious breast lesion the simplest method of determining its nature is fine needle aspiration cytology (FNAC). If the result of this is equivocal or inadequate, either a core needle biopsy or an open biopsy should be performed in the first trimester. The procedure should be carried out under local rather than general anaesthesia to minimize risk to the developing fetus. General anaesthesia is suitable for excision or incision biopsy in the second and third trimesters.

Having made the diagnosis of breast cancer, and clinically staged the disease, the situation has to be discussed as a matter of urgency with the patient and her partner. The first question to be addressed is whether the pregnancy should be allowed to continue. As has been described previously, continuation of the pregnancy will not directly affect the patient's prognosis but nevertheless this may have important implications in terms of the future of mother, father and the unborn child.

If the disease is inoperable, stage III or IV, the future outlook is dire and the father needs to be aware that, irrespective of treatment, it is likely that he alone may be looking after the child on its fifth birthday. Expressed in such stark terms some couples will not wish the pregnancy to continue. Treatment is likely to be by a combination of chemotherapy and radiotherapy, and neither of these is compatible with an intrauterine fetus.

Luckily most cancers in pregnancy are operable, albeit sometimes with extensive axillary nodal involvement. The simplest and most rapid method of extirpating the cancer is a modified radical mastectomy, but this may be unacceptable to some women preferring preservation of their breast to continuation of the pregnancy. Under these circumstances either termination or early delivery of a preterm neonate will enable breast conservation therapy to be performed, providing that the tumour is unicentric and no more than 4 cm in diameter.

There should be no compromise on radicality of breast conservation treatment, which should include wide excision, axillary clearance and radiotherapy. After this many women with pregnancy-associated cancers will require adjuvant chemotherapy, because of either nodal involvement or a poorly differentiated (grade III) primary tumour. Those with larger primary tumours (>4 cm in diameter) wanting breast conservation will need first-line chemotherapy and this will also necessitate early delivery or termination.

Advising pregnant women with breast cancer can be particularly harrowing, not least because many will be angry that there has been a delay in diagnosis. In addition, what is considered as a 'happy event' becomes a major threat to the future of a couple and the life of a woman. Confronted for the first time with such a therapeutic dilemma, the surgeon is sensible to seek the advice of a more experienced colleague.

PREGNANCY SUBSEQUENT TO BREAST CANCER

As pregnancy may exert an inhibitory effect on development of breast cancers it might also reduce the risk of recurrence in women who have had breast cancer treated, thereby acting as a form of differentiational adjuvant therapy. Such an idea was for many years regarded as heretical. The increase in plasma oestrogens in pregnancy was seen as a potential stimulant to the growth of dormant micrometastases and so young women were forbidden to become pregnant if they had had a breast cancer, or were treated by oophorectomy so that they were infertile.

For some time there has been evidence available that pregnancy subsequent to breast cancer does not lead to a worse prognosis. Peters examined the 5-year survival of women with breast cancer who became pregnant and compared them with cases who had no further pregnancies.[16] Among those with stage I disease 81% of the pregnant group were alive at 5 years compared with 70% of the non-pregnant cases. Similarly for stage II patients the respective survival rates were 76% and 54%. This does not suggest a worsening of prognosis for those who became pregnant, but the results have to be interpreted with caution because to become pregnant the patient must survive.

Those with a worse prognosis who die rapidly will not become pregnant and therefore diminish the overall survival of the non-

pregnant group. This bias in favour of those who become pregnant has been dubbed the 'healthy mother effect' by Sankila et al.[22] In a study from the Finnish Cancer Registry the relative risk of death from breast cancer was 4.8 in those who never became pregnant after a diagnosis of breast cancer compared with those who subsequently had a full-term delivery.[22]

To carry out an unbiased comparison of the survival rate of breast cancer patients who did or did not become pregnant, it is necessary to take into account the timing of the pregnancies. With this in mind the recurrence rates in 201 Guy's Hospital patients, aged less than 36 at the time of diagnosis, were examined using a time-dependent Cox's regression model.[23] Of this group, 20 patients had subsequently become pregnant. Relative risks of relapse were calculated in the pregnant and non-pregnant cases and adjusted for age, tumour size, stage and tumour type.[24]

The results are shown in Table 15.8. Those who became pregnant within the first year after diagnosis had an increased risk of breast cancer relapse. In contrast, those becoming pregnant in the second year after diagnosis had a reduced risk of relapse and by the third year this was significantly reduced. This implies that those women who have not developed recurrence of breast cancer after 2 years of follow-up can be safely advised to become pregnant. It is possible that this may have a positive impact on their prognosis, but further study is needed.

The Danish Breast Cancer Co-operative Group conducted a follow-up study of 5725 women aged 45 years or younger at the time of diagnosis of breast cancer.[25] Of these, 173 subsequently became pregnant, more than 10 months after diagnosis of breast cancer, of whom 97 had a full-term delivery, 22 miscarried and 92 had induced abortions. The women who had full-term pregnancies had a reduced risk of breast cancer mortality (relative risk, RR = 0.55). There was no reduction in relative risk for those with interrupted pregnancies and the protective effect was not significantly changed after adjustment for age at diagnosis, tumour size, nodal status or premorbid reproductive history.

Table 15.8 Relative risk of relapse, adjusted for age, tumour size and type, in women becoming pregnant after breast cancer

Time of pregnancy	Relative risk for	
	Pregnant group	Non-pregnant group
1st Year 1	1.24	1
2nd Year 2	0.57	1
3rd Year 3	0.13	1

From Stevens et al.[24]

This further evidence supports the hypothesis that pregnancy after breast cancer does not worsen the prognosis and may indeed have a beneficial effect.

ORAL CONTRACEPTION

Problems

Since oral contraceptives were first introduced in 1960 they have been used by an estimated 200 million women.[26] Thus even a very small increase in risk of breast cancer among users could lead to a large number of extra cases, particularly in young women. The issue is made complex by the heterogeneity of use, change in formulation, inaccurate recall of type of oral contraceptive, together with interspersed pregnancies and subsequent use of hormone replacement therapy (HRT). In addition, a prolonged latent interval between tumour stimulation and clinical presentation would need prolonged follow-up to be detectable.

Case-control studies

The earliest case-control studies of oral contraceptives did not indicate any significant increase in risk of breast cancer among users compared with women who had never taken the Pill.[27-29] However, Pike et al reported among Californian women aged less than 32 that there was a doubling in risk after 6 years of oral contraceptive usage before the first-term pregnancy.[30] This was the first suggestion that prolonged usage before pregnancy might lead to an increase in risk. Against this the Cancer and Steroid Hormone (CASH) Study of 2066 women with breast cancer diagnosed before age 45 reported no increase in risk of prior oral contraceptive use compared with 2065 neighbourhood controls.[31]

To try and resolve the paradoxical answers from both case-control and follow-up studies, Romieu et al carried out a meta-analysis of all the published data from 1966 to 1989.[32] In 27 case-control and five cohort follow-up studies there was no increase in relative risk of breast cancer in those who had ever taken oral contraceptives, as shown in Table 15.9. Similarly, even after 10 years of oral contraceptive use, although there was a trend towards increase in relative risk, this was not significant. However, those women who had taken oral contraceptives for more than 4 years before first full-term pregnancy (FFTP) were at significantly increased risk (RR = 1.72). A risk of similar magnitude was also estimated in those who had been diagnosed most recently (since 1980). Among those studies that had considered a potential latent effect there was no increase in risk 10 years after starting oral contraceptives.

Table 15.9 Meta-analysis of case-control and cohort studies of oral contraceptive usage and risk of breast cancer

Type	Relative risk	95% CI	p value
Ever	1.06	0.98–1.14	NS
>10 years	1.14	0.90–1.42	NS
>4 years before FFTP	1.72	1.36–2.19	0.0001

NS, not significant.
From Romieu et al.[32]

Table 15.10 Relative risk of breast cancer in women taking oral contraceptives

Usage of oral contraceptives	Relative risk	p value
Current	1.24	0.00001
1–4 years after	1.16	0.00001
5–9 years after	1.07	0.009
10 years after	1.01	NS

From CGHFBC.[33]

The results were consistent over all types of study design and it was calculated that there was a 46% increase in risk after 10 years of contraceptive use, predominantly among women who used oral contraceptives before first full-term pregnancy.

In 1992 the Collaborative Group on Hormonal Factors in Breast Cancer (CGHFBC) was formed with the intention of collating and re-analysing as many as possible of the available worldwide data. This resulted in a meta-analysis of results from 54 studies which included 53 297 breast cancer cases and 100 239 controls which comprised 90% of the available data.[33] When those who had ever used oral contraceptives were compared with never users they had a small but significant increase in relative risk of 1.24. As those who had ever taken oral contraceptives had taken a variety of formulations for a range of exposures, separate analyses of relative risk were estimated for 400 different variables.

There was no difference in pattern of risk associated with combined or progesterone-only oral contraceptives, nor between parous and nulliparous women. Height, weight, ethnic origin and family history of breast cancer did not alter relative risk. However, overall there was a small but statistically significant increase in risk up to 10 years after cessation of use as shown in Table 15.10.

Thus although there is a small increase in risk lasting for 10 years after taking oral contraceptives, this does not represent an increased lifetime effect. However, it remains to be determined whether use of HRT results in a renaissance and possible enhancement of this risk.

A particularly encouraging result of the overview was that women who had taken combined oral contraceptives were more likely to have cancers localized to the breast, as shown in Table 15.11. The relative risk estimates given are the probability that those with axillary nodal involvement and distant metastases were ever users compared with those with tumours localized to the breast being ever users.

The more favourable breast cancers among those who have taken oral contraceptives might result from earlier diagnosis or because less biologically aggressive cancers are promoted by oral contraceptive use. It is unlikely that women taking oral contraceptives have been under increased surveillance because up to now they have not been regarded as being at significantly increased risk of breast cancer. Thus it is more likely that the hormone-dependent oral contraceptive-promoted tumours are slower growing and more cohesive so that distant spread is not an early event.

The World Health Organization (WHO) Collaborative Study on Neoplasia and Steroid

Table 15.11 Extent of breast cancer in relation to use of oral contraceptives	
Spread of cancer	Relative risk
Breast only	1.00
Axillary nodes	0.89
Distant metastases	0.70
From CGHFBC.[33]	

Table 15.12 Estimated numbers of cancers in two cohorts of 10 000 women using or not using oral contraceptives		
Age (years)	Users	Non-users
16–19	4.5	4
20–24	17.5	16
25–29	49	44
30–34	110	100
35–39	180	160
40–44	260	230
From CGHFBC.[33]		

Hormones had previously examined the risk of breast cancer in women who were taking oral contraceptives around the time of the menopause to determine if they were at increased risk of developing breast cancer.[34] No increase in relative risk was found in older compared with younger premenopausal women, irrespective of whether their menopause was natural or induced. These findings were confirmed in the CGHFBC meta-analysis.[33]

What advice should be given?

It is most important to place the small risks associated with oral contraceptive use in context with the social and medical gains from avoidance of unwanted pregnancy. Calculated numbers of cancers in two cohorts of 10 000 women are given in Table 15.12.[33]

For a particular duration of use, the age at which oral contraceptives are taken does not increase relative risk. Thus, younger women are not putting themselves at increased risk compared with older women and for both groups the risk reverts to that of no-users 10 years after cessation. Excess breast cancers are more likely to be localized to the breast and thus more likely to be cured by effective local treatment. Women with a family history can be reassured that they are not amplifying their risk of breast cancer by taking oral contraceptives. More mature women can take combined oral contraceptives secure in the knowledge that they are not placing themselves at increased risk of dying of breast cancer.

HORMONE REPLACEMENT THERAPY

Until recently the decision to take hormone replacement therapy (HRT) was based largely on anecdotal information from friends, sometimes polarized advice from general practitioners and a public debate dominated by demagogues yielding more heat than light. It is now possible for a woman to make an informed choice, accepting that the formulation of HRT that worked wonderfully for her age and size-matched neighbour may, in her case, produce unacceptable side effects.

Potential benefits of HRT are both immediate and long term. For those women who have been incapacitated by hot flushes and drenching sweats, these are rapidly relieved. Also those who have lost their drive and libido may regain control of their lives, sometimes made worse by the coincident departure of children from the family home. There is a restored sense of well-being and vaginal dryness is usually improved together with quality of skin and hair.

Set against this, there may be nausea, weight gain, fluid retention, breast swelling and tenderness. In addition, some women may not wish to have monthly withdrawal bleeds associated with HRT. Skin patches may produce local irritation and implants may produce a refractory state in which menopausal symptoms recur despite apparently supraphysiological plasma levels of oestrogen. Recent work has also shown that there is a two- to fourfold increase in risk of venous thromboembolism in women taking HRT.[35–37] Thus it should be used with great caution in those with a prior history of deep vein thrombosis.

Benefits

In relation to long-term benefits, the most major effects are on the vascular system, bone and brain. The Nurses Health Study comprised a cohort of 121 700 female nurses, followed for 10 years.[38] The results, which were adjusted for age, smoking and weight, showed that the relative risk of a myocardial infarction was 0.56 in current users of HRT, and the relative risk of fatal cardiovascular disease was 0.72. There was no reduction in risk of stroke.

Nabulsi et al analysed data from 4958 women in the Atherosclerosis in Communities Study.[39] All were postmenopausal and they were divided into four groups: current users of oestrogen, current users of combined HRT, past users and never users. Blood was analysed for a variety of lipid factors and markers of cardiovascular risk. Current users of HRT had lower mean levels of low-density-lipoprotein cholesterol, apolipoprotein B, lipoprotein A, fibrinogen, antithrombin III, and higher levels of high-density-lipoprotein cholesterol, high-density lipoprotein and apolipoprotein A-1. There were higher levels of triglycerides, factor VII and protein C among those taking oestrogen alone. It was calculated that these changes would result in a 42% reduction in risk of coronary heart diseases in HRT users, and an even greater reduction in those taking a combination of oestrogen and progesterone.

Osteoporosis is a major cause of morbidity and premature death in postmenopausal women. The accelerated bone loss after the menopause can be prevented or halted by HRT.[40,41] This results in a substantial reduction of pathological fractures. However, to achieve a significant impact on bone density, HRT has to be taken for a minimum of 2 years.[42] Recent work has suggested that an additional benefit of HRT may be a reduction in risk of Alzheimer's disease. Not only are there fewer cases of Alzheimer's among those taking HRT but also the age of onset of dementia is delayed.[43,44]

HRT and malignancy

For more than two decades there has been evidence from case-control studies that unopposed oestrogen replacement therapy leads to an increased risk of endometrial carcinoma.[45–47] However, because of problems in selection of an appropriate control group and lack of long-term follow-up, Paganini-Hill conducted a cohort study of 5160 women with a high prevalence of prior oestrogen use.[48] They were aged 44–100 and none had had a hysterectomy. There was a tenfold increase in relative risk of endometrial cancer in women who had ever taken oestrogens. For those who took oestrogen for 15 years or more the relative risk rose to 20. Even after stopping oestrogen, there was a persistent elevation of risk which was still present after 15 years.

Whatever else HRT does, it effectively prolongs the length of time that a women spends in a premenopausal state. Epidemiological data have shown consistently that the more periods a woman has in her reproductive lifetime, the greater her risk of breast cancer. Thus both an early menarche and a late menopause increase the chances of developing breast cancer. In terms of age incidence, on a semi-logarithmic scale, there is a gradual increase from age 25 to 50, and at that time an inflexion with a subsequent linear increase of reduced slope.[49] The menopause is causing a reduction in incidence of breast cancer and may prevent some women from developing the

Table 15.13 Meta-analyses of relative risks of breast cancer in women taking HRT

Type of use	Dupont and Page[50]	Steinberg et al[51]	Sillero-Arenas et al[52]
Ever	1.07	1.0	1.06
Dose <0.625 mg	1.08		1.0
Dose >1.25 mg	2.0		1.0
Duration <5 years		1.0	1.0
Duration >5 years		1.3	1.2
Combined	1.08		1.0
Oestrogen alone	1.08		1.08
Benign breast cancer	1.16	1.2	
Family history		2.3	

disease. This would mean that increasing the age at which periods stop would be responsible for more breast cancers being diagnosed.

Hence, a priori, HRT should increase the number of women with breast cancer. Just before the menopause, however, many of the menstrual cycles are irregular and anovular. Without a functioning corpus luteum, there will be oestrogen stimulation of the breast tissue without any opposing progesterone. If a combination of oestrogen and progesterone were given as HRT this might have a beneficial effect with possibly fewer breast cancers than in perimenopausal women undergoing anovular cycles.

HRT and breast cancer risk

Case-control and cohort studies have varied greatly in their ability to detect an effect. This is the result of numbers of women studied and variation in duration of exposure, together with difficulties in ascertainment of histology, formulation of HRT and exclusion or inclusion of premenopausal women. As it is likely that any effect might be small, it has been necessary to combine results in meta-analyses to get answers to some of the important questions. Three overviews have been conducted and,

although these have led generally to similar conclusions (owing to selection and rejection of different studies), some of the individual conclusions have not been in agreement.[50–52] The results are summarized in Table 15.13.

The first meta-analysis was conducted by Dupont and Page, who included 28 studies, selected on a basis of 12 quality control criteria.[50] Overall there was no significant increase in risk for the entire group of women who had ever taken HRT (relative risk, RR = 1.07). Women who took 1.25 mg or more of oestrogen daily had a doubling of relative risk. Those taking 0.625 mg daily had no significant increase in risk. There was a slight increase in risk among women with prior benign breast disease.

Steinberg et al combined data from 16 case-control studies and found that there was no increase in risk among women who had ever taken HRT.[51] Thus the relative risk was 1. Dose–responses were calculated which showed that there was no increase in risk until HRT had been taken for 5 years or more. Thereafter, risk rose progressively so that after 15 years there was a 30% increase (RR =1.3). After a subgroup analysis it emerged that there was a doubling of risk among HRT users with a family history of breast cancer (RR = 2.3). Also there was a slight increase among those with a prior history of benign breast disease (RR = 1.2).

Sillero-Arenas et al carried out the third overview of 23 case-control studies, 13 cohort studies and one clinical trial.[52] The overall risk was slightly but significantly increased (RR = 1.06). There was no significant increase in the case-control studies; this emerged from the cohort follow-up studies. There was no rise in risk with increase in dose, nor did formulation (conjugated vs non-conjugated) affect risk. Risk was affected by duration, with significant increases occurring after 5 years of treatment. Thus, overall, the meta-analyses have shown slight increases in risk after 5 years or more of either oestrogen alone or combined with progestin. Women at slightly increased risk over and above this have a family history of breast cancer, or a previous history of benign breast disease.

Combination HRT, comprising oestrogen and progestin, has only been used relatively recently making long-term follow-up unavailable, but recent reports suggest that the combination may not increase risk and indeed might be protective. Risch and Howe reported a record-linkage cohort study of 33 003 women aged 43–49, living in Saskatchewan.[53] Among these, 742 developed breast cancer. Information on all drugs that had been prescribed to the cohort was available because this was recorded on the Province's Prescription Drug Plan Database. For women who had taken unopposed oestrogens, there was a significantly increased risk of breast cancer (RR = 1.072), amounting to a 7% increase in risk for each year of use. In contrast, there was no increase in risk of breast cancer among those women who received a combination of oestrogens and progestins.

Against this Colditz et al reported from the Nurses Health Study that there were similar increases in relative risk for those taking oestrogen alone (RR = 1.32) or a combination (RR = 1.41).[54] This provided no support for the hypothesis that progestins were protective.

In a study from Washington State, Stanford et al compared 537 breast cancer patients with 492 population controls selected by random digit dialling.[55] Those individuals who had taken combination HRT for more than 8 years were at reduced risk of breast cancer compared with non-takers (RR = 0.4). In a case-control study, La Vecchia et al compared HRT usage in 2569 breast cancer cases and 2588 hospital controls.[56] There was a slight increase in breast cancers among those who had taken HRT (RR = 1.2), which increased with duration, but by 10 years after stopping treatment there was no detectable increase in risk.

Tavani et al combined data from two Italian case-control studies in order to carry out an age-specific analysis of HRT and breast cancer risk.[57] There were 5984 breast cancer cases aged less than 75 and 5504 controls and the odds ratio for those that took HRT was 1.2, with an increasing trend following from more prolonged duration of use. When subdivided by age at diagnosis a difference in risk was seen with the odds ratio for women aged under 55 being 0.9, for those aged 55–64, 1.2, and among those aged 65–74, 1.6. Only in the group aged 65–74 was there a significant increase in risk with duration of use (OR = 1.6 for < 5 years and 2.2 for ≥ 5 years). Thus women who are further away from their natural menopause may be at increased risk of breast cancer after prolonged use of HRT.

HRT and prognosis in breast cancer

It is difficult to escape the conclusion that HRT, if taken for more than 5 years, leads to a small but significant increase in risk of developing breast cancer. This then raises the question as to whether HRT increases the chance of dying of breast cancer. In general the available data are reassuring.

Bergkvist et al studied the survival of a cohort of 6617 breast cancer patients of whom 261 had previously taken HRT.[58] In women over 50 there was a 10% better survival at 8 years for those who had taken HRT, corresponding to a 40% reduction in excess mortality. The favourable prognosis was most evident in those who were the most recent users of HRT

Table 15.14 Grade of screen detected breast cancers in users and non-users of HRT		
Grade	Users (*n* = 108) (%)	Non-users (*n* = 325) (%)
I	45	20
II	44	64
III	10	16

From Harding et al.[61]

Table 15.15 Relative risk of breast cancer death after HRT use	
HRT use	Relative risk of mortality
Never	1.00
Ever	0.84
Years of use	
<1 year	0.85
2–5 years	0.78
6–10	0.78
Age at first use	
<40	0.66
40–49	0.84
50+	0.89

From Willis et al.[63]

before diagnosis of breast cancer. In a smaller study of 82 breast cancer cases who had taken HRT and 174 non-user cases, Strickland et al reported no significant differences in outcome after controlling for stage at diagnosis.[59]

To study this problem indirectly Jones et al examined prognostic indices in 39 HRT users with breast cancer and 258 cases who had not taken HRT.[60] There was no difference in distribution of tumour types and grades but the HRT group had a lower rate of axillary nodal involvement (23% vs 40%). The authors suggested that the higher incidence of cancers confined to the breast was the result of early diagnosis because these women were under surveillance. This may be so, but there is a striking similarity between this finding with HRT and that reported by CGHFBC in women who had taken oral contraceptives.[33] Thus possibly these induced tumours are less aggressive.

Support for this hypothesis comes from a study conducted at a screening unit in south Manchester.[61] Tumour grade was determined in 433 postmenopausal women with screen-detected cancers, of whom 108 were taking HRT. The median duration of use was 24 months. Results are shown in Table 15.14. Significantly larger numbers of the women who were taking HRT had grade I cancers (45% vs 20%).

Further evidence is provided by a study from Uppsala which determined a variety of prognostic factors in 1589 breast cancer cases of whom 121 had taken HRT.[62] Those who had taken HRT were less likely to have cancers bigger than 2 cm (RR=0.7) and also had a reduced risk of axillary nodal involvement (RR=0.7). In addition, there were fewer aneuploid tumours in the group who had taken HRT.

As part of Cancer Prevention Study II, a cohort study of 422 373 postmenopausal women, Willis et al analysed breast cancer deaths in relation to prior use of HRT.[63] After 9 years of follow-up there had been 1469 deaths from breast cancer. The relative risks of dying of breast cancer after various patterns of use are shown in Table 15.15. Overall there was a significant 16% reduction in risk of dying of breast cancer in women who had taken HRT. This was most evident among those who had a natural menopause before age 40. There was no trend with regard to duration of use or in terms of number of years since stopping HRT.

All of these studies suggest strongly that there is no deleterious effect of prior HRT usage on the prognosis of women who develop breast cancer and it is more likely that this may lead to an improvement in outcome.

HRT after diagnosis of breast cancer

About two-thirds of breast cancer patients are chronologically postmenopausal and therefore likely to suffer menopausal symptoms, and these may also be induced in premenopausal patients treated with adjuvant chemotherapy or ovarian ablation. Thus, to some extent most patients who have had breast cancer will be troubled with menopausal symptoms. These may be exacerbated by ubiquitously prescribed tamoxifen. One of the main reasons for the widespread acceptance of tamoxifen has been the low profile of reported side effects. However, a recent survey conducted at the Breast Unit at Guy's Hospital, using the Menopausal Symptoms Check List (MSCL), revealed that two-thirds of women receiving tamoxifen were getting troublesome symptoms, in particular hot flushes and night sweats. Other than HRT, there are no effective treatments for these symptoms.

Palshof et al conducted an adjuvant trial in which postmenopausal breast cancer patients were randomized to receive one of three options: diethyl oestradiol (DES 1 mg three times daily), tamoxifen (10 mg three times daily) or placebo three time daily.[64] After 3 years of follow-up there were 91 relapses comprising 37% of the placebo group, 24% of the tamoxifen group and only 18% of the DES group. Thus, in supraphysiological dosage oestrogens reduced rather than increased the relapse rate.

With regard to physiological levels of oestrogens, Stoll and Parbhoo gave a combination of tamoxifen and HRT (Premarin or Prempak-C) to 35 postmenopausal women who had been treated for breast cancer.[65] In most patients menopausal symptoms were controlled and relapse of breast cancer occurred in only two cases. Wile et al gave HRT to 25 women treated for breast cancer and compared the outcome

Table 15.16 Effect of tibolone on DMBA-induced tumours in rats

Treatment	Tumour load (mm³)
DMBA alone	1050
DMBA + tamoxifen	440
DMBA + tibolone	340
DMBA + tamoxifen + tibolone	240

From Kloosterboer et al.[68]

with five age- and stage-matched controls.[66] There were two deaths from cancer in the control group and one in the HRT-treated group.

In a cohort study, DiSaia et al compared the survival of 41 breast cancer patients given HRT and compared them with 82 breast cancer cases not given HRT.[67] The relapse-free and overall survival of the two groups was similar. If HRT does not compromise survival of breast cancer patients it is unlikely that a combination of HRT and tamoxifen would be harmful, and this is being examined in randomized trials that are now in progress.

In a rodent model system, tamoxifen has been shown to reduce significantly the incidence of rat mammary cancers after administration of the carcinogen dimethylbenzanthracene (DMBA). Similarly, if the synthetic progestin tibolone is administered there is a greater reduction in cancers, and this is reduced still further in animals given a combination of both tamoxifen and tibolone, as shown in Table 15.16.[68]

This shows that tibolone inhibits mammary carcinogenesis in rats. It is therefore likely that it might exert a similar effect in women. Tibolone (Livial) has been widely used as HRT and is particularly useful because it induces endometrial hypoplasia so that breakthrough bleeding is rare. The agent relieves menopausal symptoms and prevents bone demineralization. This would make tibolone a potentially very useful drug for women who have had breast cancer.

Tibolone could not only relieve menopausal symptoms in women taking tamoxifen but it might also inhibit the oestrogen agonist effect on the endometrium which can lead to hyperplasia and sometimes neoplasia. A pilot study is under way at Guy's Hospital to determine whether it conveys short-term benefits. If this can be verified, a case could be made for adding the agent to tamoxifen in an adjuvant role to determine whether it can further reduce the risk of breast cancer relapse.

SYNOPSIS

• During pregnancy women are less likely to develop breast cancer than age-matched non-pregnant women.

• Pregnancy cancers are not necessarily more aggressive but may be more advanced because of delay in diagnosis.

• Breast cancer is not a contraindication to pregnancy provided that 2 disease-free years have elapsed.

• Use of oral contraceptives for more than 4 years before first full-term pregnancy leads to a small but significant increase in risk of beast cancer which persists for 10 years after cessation.

• Hormone replacement therapy taken for more than 5 years leads to a small increase in risk of developing breast cancer but no increase in risk of dying of the disease.

• Some breast cancer patients can safely take hormone replacement therapy and some formulations might reduce the subsequent risk of relapse.

REFERENCES

1. Haas JF. Pregnancy in association with a newly diagnosed cancer: a population-based epidemiologic assessment. *Int J Cancer* 1984; **34:** 229–5.
2. Holleb AI, Farrow JH. The relation of carcinoma of the breast and pregnancy in 283 patients. *Surg Gynecol Obstet* 1962; **115:** 65–71.
3. Bunker ML, Peters MV. Breast cancer associated with pregnancy or lactation. *Am J Obstet Gynecol* 1963; **85:** 312–21.
4. Clark RM, Reid J. Carcinoma of the breast in pregnancy and lactation. *Int J Radiat Oncol Biol Phys* 1978; **4:** 693–8.
5. King RM, Welch JS, Martin JK et al. Carcinoma of the breast associated with pregnancy. *Surg Gynecol Obstet* 1985; **160:** 228–32.
6. Ribeiro G, Jones DA, Jones M. Carcinoma of the breast associated with pregnancy. *Br J Surg* 1986; **73:** 607–9.
7. Tretli S, Kvalheim G, Thoresen S et al. Survival of breast cancer patients diagnosed during pregnancy or lactation. *Br J Cancer* 1988; **58:** 382–4.
8. Holman P, Bennett MB. Breast cancer and pregnancy. *S Afr Med J* 1963; **37:** 1236–9.
9. Peete CH, Hunlycutt HC, Cherry MB. Cancer of the breast and pregnancy. *NC Med J* 1966; **27:** 514–17.
10. Rissanen PH. Pregnancy following treatment for mammary cancer. *Acta Radiol* 1969; **8:** 315–22.
11. Deemarsky LJ, Neishtadt EL, Brea SL. Cancer and pregnancy. *Breast* 1980; **7:** 17–21.
12. Leon DA, Carpenter LM, Broeders MJM et al. Breast cancer in Swedish women before age 50: evidence of a dual effect of completed pregnancy. *Cancer Causes Control* 1995; **6:** 283–91.
13. Albrektsen G, Heuch I, Kvale G. The short-term and long-term effects of a pregnancy on breast cancer risk: a prospective study of 802,457 parous Norwegian women. *Br J Cancer* 1995; **72:** 480–4.
14. Ishida T, Yokoe T, Kasumi F et al. Clinicopathologic characteristics and prognosis of breast cancer patients associated with pregnancy and lactation: analysis of case-control study in Japan. *Jpn J Cancer Res* 1992; **83:** 1143–9.
15. Nettleton J, Long J, Kuban D et al. Breast cancer during pregnancy: quantifying the risk of treatment delay. *Obstet Gynecol* 1996; **87:** 414–18.
16. Peters MV. The effect of pregnancy in breast cancer. In: *Prognostic Factors in Breast Cancer.* Forrest APM, Kunkler PB, eds. Livingstone: Edinburgh, 1968.
17. Nugent P, O'Connell TX. Breast cancer and pregnancy. *Ann Surg* 1985; **120:** 1221–4.

18. Petrek JA, Dukoff R, Rogatko A. Prognosis of pregnancy-associated breast cancer. *Cancer* 1991; **67**: 869–72.

19. Guinee VF, Olsson H, Moller T et al. Effect of pregnancy on prognosis for young women with breast cancer. *Lancet* 1994; **343**: 1587–9.

20. Clark RM, Chua T. Breast cancer and pregnancy: the ultimate challenge. *Clin Oncol* 1989; **1**: 11–18.

21. Lethaby AE, O-Neill MA, Mason BH et al. Overall survival from breast cancer in women pregnant or lactating at or after diagnosis. *Int J Cancer* 1996; **67**: 751–5.

22. Sankila R, Heinavaara S, Hakulinen T. Survival of breast cancer cases after subsequent term pregnancy: 'Healthy mother effect'. *Am J Obstet Gynecol* 1994; **170**: 818–23.

23. Cox DR. Regression models and life tables. *J R Stat Soc* 1972; **34**: 197–220.

24. Stevens A, Richards MA, De Stavola BL et al. Pregnancy after treatment for breast cancer: risk or benefit? Manuscript in preparation.

25. Kroman N, Jensen M-B, Melbye M et al. Should women be advised against pregnancy after breast cancer? *Lancet* 1997; **350**: 319–22.

26. Kleinman, EL, ed. *Hormonal Contraception*. London: IPPF Medical Publications, 1990.

27. Paffenbarger RS, Fasal E, Simmons ME et al. Cancer risk as related to use of oral contraceptives during fertile years. *Cancer* 1977; **39**: 1887–91.

28. Vessey MP, MacPherson K, Doll R. Breast cancer and oral contraceptives. Findings in Oxford Family Planning Association Contraceptive Study. *BMJ* 1981; **282**: 2093–4.

29. Royal College of General Practitioners. Breast cancer and oral contraceptives. findings in Royal College of General Practitioners Study. *BMJ* 1981; **2**: 89–93.

30. Pike MC, Henderson BE, Casagrande JJ et al. Oral contraceptive use and abortion as risk factors for breast cancer in young women. *Br J Cancer* 1981; **43**: 72–6.

31. Stadel BV, Rubin GL, Webster LA. Oral contraceptives and breast cancer in young women. *Lancet* 1985; **ii**: 970–3.

32. Romieu I, Berlin JA, Colditz G. Oral contraceptives and breast cancer. Review and meta-analysis. *Cancer* 1990; **55**: 2253–63.

33. Collaborative Group on Hormonal Factors in Breast Cancer. Breast cancer and hormonal contraceptives: collaborative re-analysis of individual data on 53 297 women with breast cancer and 100 239 women without breast cancer from 54 epidemiological studies. *Lancet* 1996; **347**: 1713–27.

34. Thomas DB, Noonan EA and the WHO Collaborative Study of Neoplasia and Steroid Contraceptives. Risk of breast cancer in relation to use of combined oral contraceptives near the age of the menopause. *Cancer Cases Control* 1991; **2**: 389–94.

35. Daly E, Vessey MP, Hawkins MM et al. Risk of thromboembolism in users of hormone replacement therapy. *Lancet* 1996; **348**: 977–80.

36. Jick H, Derby LE, Wald Myers M et al. Risk of hospital admission for idiopathic venous thromboembolism among users of postmenopausal oestrogens. *Lancet* 1996; **348**: 981–3.

37. Grodstein F, Stampfer MJ, Goldhaber SZ et al. Prospective study of exogenous hormones and risk of pulmonary embolism in women. *Lancet* 1996; **348**: 983–7.

38. Stampfer MJ, Colditz GA, Willatt WC et al. Postmenopausal estrogen therapy and cardiovascular disease. *N Engl J Med* 1991; **325**: 756–62.

39. Nabulsi AA, Folsom AR, White A et al. Association of hormone replacement therapy with various cardiovascular risk factors in postmenopausal women. *N Engl J Med* 1993; **328**: 1069–75.

40. Kiel DP, Felson DT, Anderson JJ et al. Hip fracture and the use of estrogens in postmenopausal women: the Framingham study. *N Engl J Med* 1987; **317**: 1169–74

41. Steiniche T, Hasling C, Charles P et al. A randomised study of the effects of estrogen/gestagen or high dose oral calcium on trabecular bone remodelling in postmenopausal osteoporosis. *Bone* 1989; **10**: 313–20.

42. Fentiman IS, Wang DY, Allen DS et al. Bone density of normal women in relation to endogenous and exogenous oestrogens. *Br J Rheumatol* 1994; **33**: 808–15.

43. Paganini-Hill A, Henderson VW. Estrogen deficiency and risk of Alzheimer's disease in women. *Am J Epidemiol* 1994; **140**: 256–61.

44. Tang M-X, Jacobs D, Stern Y et al. Effect of oestrogen during menopause on risk and age at onset of Alzheimer's disease. *Lancet* 1996; **348**: 429–32.

45. Smith DC, Prentice R, Thomson DJ et al. Association of exogenous estrogen and endometrial cancer. *N Engl J Med* 1975; **293**: 1164–7.

46. Ziel HK, Finkle WD. Increased risk of endometrial carcinoma among users of conjugated estrogens. *N Engl J Med* 1975; **293:** 1167–9.

47. Mack TM, Pike MC, Henderson BE et al. Estrogens and endometrial cancer in a retirement community. *N Engl J Med* 1976; **294:** 1262–5.

48. Paganini-Hill A, Ross RK, Henderson BE. Endometrial cancer and patterns of use of oestrogen replacement therapy: a cohort study. *Br J Cancer* 1989; **59:** 445–7.

49. Henderson BE, Ross RK, Bernstein L. Estrogens as a cause of breast cancer: the Richard and Hinda Rosenthal Foundation Award Lecture. *Cancer Res* 1988; **48:** 246–253.

50. Dupont WD, Page DL. Menopausal estrogen replacement therapy and breast cancer. *Arch Intern Med* 1991; **151:** 67–72.

51. Steinberg KK, Thacker SB, Smith J et al. A meta-analysis of the effect of estrogen replacement therapy on the risk of breast cancer. *JAMA* 1990; **265:** 1985–90.

52. Sillero-Arenas M, Delgado-Rodriguez M, Rodigues-Canteras R et al. Menopausal hormone replacement therapy and breast cancer: a meta-analysis. *Obstet Gynecol* 1992; **79:** 286–94.

53. Risch HA, Howe GR. Menopausal hormone usage and breast cancer in Saskatchewan: a record linkage study. *Am J Epidemiol* 1994; **139:** 670–683.

54. Colditz GA, Hankinson SE, Hunter DJ et al. The use of estrogens and progestins and the risk of breast cancer in postmenopausal women. *N Engl J Med* 1995; **332:** 1589–93.

55. Stanford JL, Weiss NS, Voigt LF et al. Combined estrogen and progestin hormone replacement therapy in relation to risk of breast cancer in middle-aged women. *JAMA* 1995; **274:** 137–42.

56. La Vecchia C, Negri E, Franceschi S et al. Hormone replacement therapy and breast cancer risk: a co-operative Italian study. *Br J Cancer* 1995; **72:** 244–8.

57. Tavani A, Braga C, La Vecchia C et al. Hormone replacement treatment and breast cancer risk: an age-specific analysis. *Cancer Epidemiol Biomark Prev* 1997; **6:** 11–14.

58. Bergkvist L, Adami H-O, Persson I et al. Prognosis after breast cancer diagnosis in women exposed to estrogen and estrogen-progestogen replacement therapy. *Am J Epidemiol* 1989; **130:** 221–8.

59. Strickland DM, Gambrell RD, Butzin CA et al. The relationship between breast cancer survival and prior postmenopausal estrogen use. *Obstet Gynecol* 1992; **80:** 400–4.

60. Jones C, Ingram D, Mattes E et al. The effect of hormone replacement therapy on prognostic indices in women with breast cancer. *Med J Aus* 1994; **161:** 106–10.

61. Harding C, Knox WF, Faragher EB et al. Hormone replacement therapy and tumour grade in breast cancer: prospective study in screening unit. *BMJ* 1996; **312:** 1646–7.

62. Magnusson C, Holmberg L, Norden T et al. Prognostic characteristics in breast cancers after hormone replacement therapy. *Breast Cancer Res Treat* 1996; **38:** 325–34.

63. Willis DB, Calle EE, Miracle-McMahill HL et al. Estrogen replacement therapy and risk of fatal breast cancer in a prospective cohort of postmenopausal women in the United States. *Cancer Causes Control* 1996; **7:** 449–57.

64. Palshof T, Mouridsen HT, Daehnfeldt JL. Adjuvant endocrine therapy of primary operable breast cancer. Report of the Copenhagen breast cancer trials. *Eur J Cancer* 1980; **Suppl 1:** 183–7.

65. Stoll BA, Parbhoo S. Treatment of menopausal symptoms in breast cancer patients. *Lancet* 1988; **i:** 1278–9.

66. Wile AG, Opfell DA, Margileth DA et al. Hormone replacement therapy does not affect breast cancer outcome. *Proc Am Soc Clin Oncol* 1991; **10:** 58

67. DiSaia PJ, Grosen EA, Kurosaki T et al. Hormone replacement therapy in breast cancer survivors: a cohort study. *Am J Obstet Gynecol* 1996; **174:** 1494–8.

68. Kloosterboer HJ, Schoonen WGEJ, Deckers GH, Klijn JGM. Effects of progestagens and Org OD14 in in vitro and in vivo tumor models. *J Steroid Biochem Mol Biol* 1994; **49:** 311–18.

16

Lobular carcinoma in situ

A false friend is more dangerous than an open enemy.

Francis Bacon

Histology • Clinical aspects • LCIS and risk of invasive breast cancer • Endocrine function and LCIS • Prevention of progression

No patient has ever died of non-infiltrating carcinoma, but many may have suffered because of inadequate treatment leading to the development of potentially life-threatening invasive disease. Both lobular carcinoma in situ (LCIS) and ductal carcinoma in situ (DCIS) were rare, forming only 5% of all breast cancers. Now, as a result of increasing availability of mammographic screening, DCIS comprises 15–20% of all screen-detected cancers because of microcalcification on mammograms. As LCIS has no specific radiological signs, this condition is still an incidental histological finding on a surgical biopsy.

It is customary to think of the evolution of cancer as a gradual progression from normal epithelium to hyperplasia, followed by atypia, then non-invasive carcinoma and finally invasive disease. Considered in this way the fossil record is incomplete. Some infiltrating cancers do not appear to have any surrounding non-invasive disease and many cases of DCIS have become diffuse within the breast, without evolving into an invasive lump. Despite the gaps in our knowledge about the classification and behaviour of non-invasive cancers, it is nevertheless of great interest to pick up these lesions and test out interventions in the hope of preventing the subsequent progression to invasive disease. At last there are also trials

under way that may both provide some answers and spawn an even greater number of unanswered questions.

HISTOLOGY

In 1898, Shield wrote *A Clinical Treatise on Disease of the Breast*,[1] and described a morbid proliferation of the acinous epithelium, which was subsequently called lobular carcinoma in situ by Foote and Stewart.[2] This is their definition of the abnormality.

> Microscopically the process shows the following characters: there is a sudden and abrupt alteration in lobular cytology. A group of normal lobules is interrupted by the presence of a lobule or group of lobules in which the cells are large. They are perhaps twice the size of those in normal lobules and their nuclei are in proportion. The nuclei tend to be clear, the cytoplasm is apt to be opaque. The compact orderly arrangement of the epithelium gives place to a decided looseness, a loss of cohesion. Cells are progressively displaced towards the lumina in a disorderly fashion eventually obliterating the space. Mitoses are rare. The cells lose polarity, varying in shape, while maintaining surprisingly uniform size.

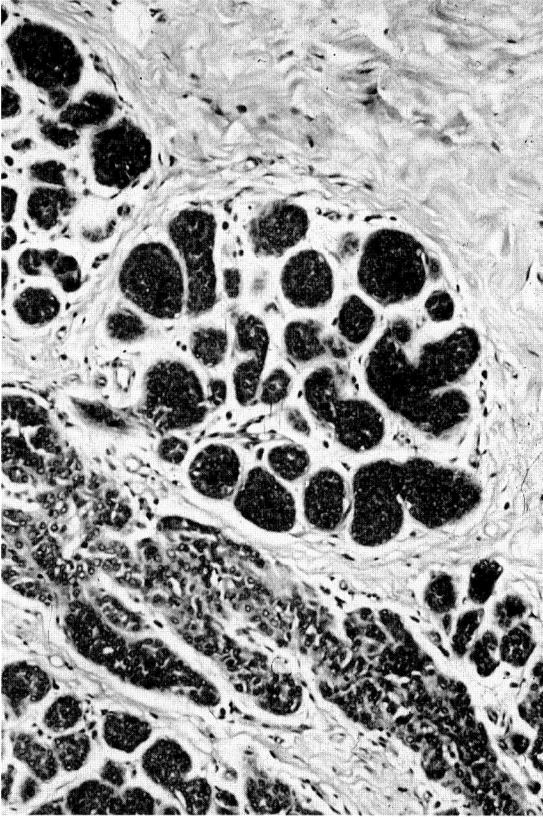

Fig. 16.1 Lobular carcinoma in situ (LCIS).

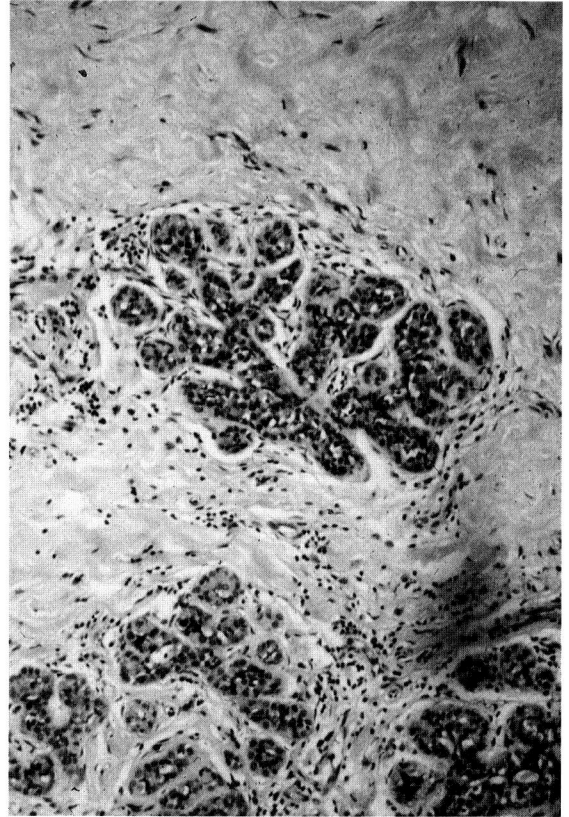

Fig. 16.2 Atypical lobular hyperplasia (ALH).

An example of LCIS is shown in Fig. 16.1, and this illustrates the excellent description given by Foote and Stewart. They also stated that cells could spread into the terminal lobular duct which they dubbed 'pagetoid spread'. Unless the process was present in at least three lobules they would not make a diagnosis of LCIS.

This quantitative aspect of the diagnosis was challenged by Wheeler and Enterline because no relationship had been demonstrated between outcome and number of lobules involved.[3] However, when there is limited involvement of the terminal ducts and lobules by LCIS it may be difficult distinguishing this from atypical lobular hyperplasia (ALH) which is shown in Fig. 16.2.

Haagensen et al have argued that LCIS should be re-named lobular neoplasia, so that the surgeon is not moved to consider radical surgery, and the patient not unnecessarily worried by an unexpected diagnosis.[4] Whatever the histological finding is called, however, what is most important is that both surgeon and patient understand the implications of the diagnosis as a marker of risk rather than a direct precursor of invasive cancer.

CLINICAL ASPECTS

The proliferating monomorphic cells within the lobules do not form tumours, nor do they elicit an inflammatory reaction, so that the lesions are not palpable. In addition, LCIS does not lead to a nipple discharge and only rarely to necrosis which calcifies and so is undetectable mammographically. For all these reasons the diagnosis

Table 16.1 Histological findings after mastectomy for LCIS

Cases	Contralateral biopsy	Contralateral LCIS	Residual LCIS	Invasion	Axillary metastases	Reference
26	18	6	27	0	0	Newman[7]
13	5	2	13	0	0	Benfield et al[8]
28	15	6	21	0	?	Lewison and Finney[9]
118	?	?	79	0	0	Farrow[10]
24	?	1	14	0	0	Dall'Olmo et al[11]
49	44	27	31	3	1	Carter and Smith[12]
258	**82 (71)**	**42 (30)**	**185 (72)**	**3 (1)**	**1 (0.4)**	**Total***

* Values in parentheses are percentages.

is histological rather than clinical or radiological, but there may be dispute among pathologists about the diagnosis and difficulty of distinguishing between LCIS and ALH.

The National Surgical Adjuvant Breast Project (NSABP) registered cases of LCIS in protocol B-17, and of 218 cases diagnosed by hospital pathologists only 182 (83%) were deemed to be true LCIS on review.[5] Of the cases 50% were aged less than 49, whereas among patients with invasive cancer approximately one-third will be aged less than 49. In a comparative review from the Alberta Cancer Registry the mean age at diagnosis of women with LCIS was 50, compared with 55 for those with DCIS.[6] Hence individuals with LCIS are from a younger age group than those with either DCIS or invasive disease.

Although there is still confusion among surgeons about the nature of the condition, this is as nothing compared to the mayhem in the past when luckless women diagnosed with LCIS suffered indiscriminate, sometimes bilateral, mastectomies. This unnecessary surgery has at least enabled pathologists to describe the histological characteristics and distribution of LCIS within the breasts.

Table 16.1 gives the histological findings from various series of mastectomy specimens after a biopsy had shown the presence of LCIS.[7–12] In almost three-quarters of cases a mirror image or random contralateral biopsy was taken and this revealed contralateral LCIS in 30%. Further LCIS was present in 72% of resected breasts. However, with the exception of one series,[12] coexistent ipsilateral invasion and axillary nodal metastases were not found. This indicates that mastectomy represents overtreatment in terms of the contralateral breast for most patients with LCIS.

To determine the incidence of undetected LCIS in the general population, histological studies have been carried out on breasts removed at postmortem from women dying of other diseases.[13–15] In 185 random postmortem autopsies Alpers and Wellings found no evidence of LCIS in any.[13] However, in 63 cancer-containing breasts, six showed evidence of LCIS, four within the group aged 39–49 and two in women aged 50–59. In 44 breasts contralateral to those containing cancer, LCIS was found in eight of whom two were aged 39–49, four 50–59, one 60–69 and one 70–79. They suggested that a premenopausal endocrine environment might be necessary for the continued existence of LCIS.

Nielsen et al studied specimens from medicolegal postmortem examinations of 110

Table 16.2 Long-term risk of ipsilateral invasive breast after biopsy showing LCIS

Cases	Follow-up (years)	5 years (%)	10 years (%)	15 years (%)	20 year (%)	Reference
50	19.5	8	15	27	35	McDivitt et al[18]
25	17.5	–	–	4	4	Newman[7]
47	15	9	11	13	17	Andersen[19]
211	14	3	7	10	18	Haagensen et al[4]
99	24	–	–	–	19	Rosen et al[20]
39	19	–	–	11	13	Page et al[21]
Total		**5**	**8**	**13**	**18**	

women aged 20–54, using extensive histological examination and correlative specimen radiology.[14] Breast malignancy was found in 22 (20%) and only one case was known to have breast cancer. In a mere four cases (4%) was LCIS alone present and in one other a combination of LCIS and DCIS was seen. In a previous study of 83 hospital-derived postmortem examinations LCIS was found in 10% and DCIS and LCIS in 4%.[15] The authors calculated that, if all invasive breast cancers evolved from in situ lesions, without complete spontaneous regression, about one-third of LCIS cases would proceed to invasive disease.

These studies suggest that LCIS is a rare asymptomatic finding in ostensibly normal individuals and is not a direct precursor of invasive disease but rather an indicator of increased risk. Extensive local surgical approaches are an inappropriate and inadequate response to this condition.

LCIS AND RISK OF INVASIVE BREAST CANCER

As surgeons began to understand that mastectomy represented overtreatment for LCIS, so a more conservative approach of long-term observation was adopted which has provided information on the natural history of the condition. As the finding of LCIS is to some extent an indicator of the assiduousness of the pathologist and the number of slides cut and examined, review of apparently benign specimens shows the presence of undetected LCIS in about 3%.[16,17] These previously undiagnosed cases gave another opportunity to quantify the risk of invasive disease.

Long-term follow-up series are summarized in Table 16.2.[4,7,18–21] In general the cumulative risk of ipsilateral invasive cancer is similar in most of the series, occurring in 5% of cases at 5 years, rising to 8% at 10 years, 13% at 15 and 18% after 20 years. However, the ipsilateral breast is not the only tissue at risk of invasive disease and Table 16.3 gives the cumulative risk for development of contralateral disease in the same series.

This shows that there is a significant risk on the opposite side, albeit slightly less than that in the ipsilateral breast. After 20 years of follow-up, 14% of cases developed contralateral invasive cancer. In toto 32% of women with LCIS had developed invasive disease after 20 years of follow-up; of these 56% were ipsilateral and 44% contralateral. Taking the mean age at diagnosis as 45, and with an average life expectancy of another 35 years, this would

Table 16.3 Risk of contralateral invasive cancer after biopsy showing LCIS

Cases	Follow-up (years)	5 years (%)	10 years (%)	15 years (%)	20 years (%)	Reference
50	19.5	4	11	16	25	McDivitt et al[18]
25	17.5	0	7	12	12	Newman[7]
47	15	0	4	6	9	Andersen[19]
211	14	6	7	9	15	Haagensen[4]
99	24	–	–	–	16	Rosen et al[20]
39	19	–	–	6	7	Page et al[21]
Total		**3**	**7**	**9**	**14**	

place the lifetime risk for an affected individual as being greater than 50%. Thus LCIS is a very major risk factor and those diagnosed with this condition need, at very least, close surveillance and would be appropriate candidates for intervention trials.

Page et al found that family history of breast cancer and postmenopausal use of oestrogens did not increase the risk of invasive disease.[21] During the first 15 years of follow-up, women with LCIS had a tenfold increase in risk of breast cancer compared with age-matched women with biopsied benign breast disease who had no histological evidence of epithelial proliferation.

As stated above, LCIS is a marker of risk for invasive breast cancer rather than being an obligate precursor of invasive lobular carcinoma. Table 16.4 shows the types of invasive cancers that developed after 24 years of follow-up of a cohort of 99 women with LCIS.[20] Of the 35 invasive cancers, 20 (57%) were invasive ductal and 13 (37%) were invasive lobular lesions. This is a higher proportion of invasive lobular cancers than among the distribution in breast cancer cases of which invasive lobular lesions comprise about 10–15%. Nevertheless, most subsequent invasive lesions, both ipsilateral and contralateral, were of invasive ductal type.

Table 16.4 Subsequent invasive cancers after follow-up of LCIS

Tumour type	Ipsilateral No.	(%)	Contralateral No.	(%)
Infiltrating ductal	11	(58)	9	(56)
Infiltrating lobular	8	(42)	5	(31)
Mucoid	0		1	(6.5)
Tubular	0		1	(6.5)

From Rosen et al.[20]

ENDOCRINE FUNCTION AND LCIS

More than half the cases of LCIS are aged less than 50 at the time of diagnosis,[5] and most of these are premenopausal. This propensity for younger women suggests that in some cases there is spontaneous regression as a result of the reduction of steroid hormones at the time of the menopause. Possibly the nature of LCIS may change after the menopause, with cells being capable of autocrine stimulation or alternatively the proliferation may be maintained by elevated levels of endogenous or exogenous steroids in some individuals.

Nevertheless, the study of Page et al did not find any relationship between risk of invasive breast cancer and use of hormone replacement therapy in women with LCIS.[21] In addition, in a study comparing 59 women with LCIS and 190 with ductal carcinoma, Rosen et al found no evidence linking HRT use and incidence of LCIS in postmenopausal women.[22] In view of the bilateral nature of the risk of malignancy a systemic rather than a local intervention would seem most logical and some form of endocrine modulation would appear to offer the most appealing form of experimental therapy.

PREVENTION OF PROGRESSION

At present the International Breast Cancer Intervention Study (IBIS) is under way, and one of the entry criteria is a histological diagnosis of lobular carcinoma in situ. The intention is to recruit 15 000 women into the trial, all of whom have at least a two- to threefold increase in risk of breast cancer compared with the general population. Volunteers will be given either tamoxifen 20 mg once daily or placebo, for 5 years. The main study group will be women with a family history of breast cancer but also those aged 35–65 who have had a histological diagnosis of LCIS, without evidence of invasion, will be eligible for the trial. The main endpoint will be incidence of invasive cancer in the treated and control groups.

The most important matter, however, is to determine whether tamoxifen can lead to a reduction in mortality from breast cancer in the treated group. Even with 15 000 volunteers, the trial is unlikely to answer this question but it should be possible to carry out a meta-analysis of the results of this study, and a parallel one being run in the USA, to find out whether 5 years of tamoxifen reduces mortality in those at risk, including women with LCIS.

SYNOPSIS

- Lobular carcinoma in situ is a marker of increased risk of invasive cancer in either breast and cases should be carefully monitored or entered into prevention trials.
- Extensive surgery is an inappropriate first response to a histological diagnosis of LCIS.

REFERENCES

1. Shield AM. *A Clinical Treatise on Disease of the Breast.* London: Macmillan, 1898.
2. Foote FW, Stewart FW. Lobular carcinoma in situ. A rare form of mammary cancer. *Am J Pathol* 1941; **17**: 491–6.
3. Wheeler JE, Enterline HT. Lobular carcinoma of the breast in situ and infiltrating. *Pathol Annu* 1976; **11**: 161–8.
4. Haagensen CD, Lane N, Lattes R et al. Lobular neoplasia (so-called lobular carcinoma in situ) of the breast. *Cancer* 1978; **42**: 737–69.
5. Fisher ER, Costantino J, Fisher B et al. Pathologic findings from the National Surgical Adjuvant Breast Project (NSABP) Protocol B-17. Five year observations concerning lobular carcinoma in situ. *Cancer* 1996; **78**: 1403–16.
6. Temple WJ, Jenkins M, Alexander F et al. Natural history of in situ breast cancer in a defined population. *Ann Surg* 1989; **210**: 653–7.
7. Newman W. In situ lobular carcinoma of the breast: report of 26 women with 32 cancers. *Ann Surg* 1963; **157**: 591–9.
8. Benfield JR, Jacobson M, Warner NE. Lobular carcinoma in situ of the breast. *Arch Surg* 1965; **91**: 130–5.
9. Lewison EF, Finney GC. Lobular carcinoma in situ of the breast. *Surg Gynecol Obstet* 1968; **126**: 1280–6.
10. Farrow JH. Clinical considerations and treatment of in situ lobular carcinoma breast cancer. *AJR* 1968; **102**: 652–6.
11. Dall'Olmo CA, Ponka JL, Horn RC et al. Lobular carcinoma of the breast in situ, Are we too radical in its treatment? *Arch Surg* 1975; **110**: 537–42.

12. Carter D, Smith RRL. Carcinoma in situ of the breast. *Cancer* 1977; **40**: 1189–93.
13. Alpers CE, Wellings SR. The prevalence of carcinoma in situ in normal and cancer-associated breasts. *Hum Pathol* 1985; **16**: 786–807.
14. Nielsen M, Thomsen JL, Primdahl S et al. Breast cancer and atypia among young and middle-aged women: a study of 110 medicolegal autopsies. *Br J Cancer* 1978; **56**: 814–19.
15. Nielsen M, Jensen J, Andersen J. Precancerous and cancerous breast lesions during lifetime and at autopsy. *Cancer* 1984; **54**: 612–15.
16. Gaton E, Czernobilsky B. Lobular carcinoma in situ of the breast. *Isr J Med Sci* 1978; **71**: 106–11.
17. Harvey DG, Fechner RE. Atypical lobular and papillary lesions of the breast: a follow-up study of 30 cases. *South Med J* 1978; **71**: 361–4.
18. McDivitt RW, Hutter RVP, Foote FW et al. In situ lobular carcinoma. A prospective follow-up study indicating cumulative patient risks. *JAMA* 1967; **201**: 82–6.
19. Andersen JA. Lobular carcinoma in situ: a long-term follow-up in 52 cases. *Acta Pathol Microbiol Scand* 1974; **82**: 519–33.
20. Rosen PP, Kosloff C, Lieberman PH et al. Lobular carcinoma in situ of the breast. *Am J Surg Pathol* 1978; **2**: 225–51.
21. Page DL, Kidd TE, Dupont WD et al. Lobular neoplasia of the breast: Higher risk for subsequent invasive cancer predicted by more extensive disease. *Hum Pathol* 1991; **22**: 1232–9.
22. Rosen PP, Senie RT, Farr GH et al. Epidemiology of breast carcinoma: age, menstrual status, and exogenous hormone usage in patients with lobular carcinoma in situ. *Surgery* 1979; **85**: 219–24.

17

Ductal carcinoma in situ

In nature's infinite book of secrecy
A little I can read

William Shakespeare

**Risk factors • Histology • Biological features • Steroid receptors • Expression of oncogene *c-erbB-2*
• Tumour suppressor gene *p53* • Clinical features • Mastectomy findings • Bilaterality of DCIS •
Follow-up of biopsied DCIS • Radiosensitivity of DCIS • Clinical trials • The future**

Whereas a defined place cannot be assigned to lobular carcinoma in situ (LCIS) in the genesis of invasive cancer, there is a close relationship between ductal carcinoma in situ (DCIS) and invasive ductal carcinoma. There are other differences. DCIS may be symptomatic, producing a discrete lump or area of nodularity or Paget's disease of the nipple, and may give rise to a haemoglobin-containing nipple discharge. Most importantly, as a result of cell necrosis and subsequent calcification, DCIS is being detected with increasing frequency because of more widespread use of mammography in symptomatic cases and in screening programmes.

The pick-up rate for LCIS is not significantly increasing whereas DCIS now forms 15–20% of cancers detected by screening. As most surgeons have treated cases of DCIS, many will hold strong views about optimum treatment, whether by mastectomy or breast conservation, with or without the use of radiotherapy. However, some of these views have been uninfluenced by the available evidence. Some guidelines are possible but, as with all areas subjected to research, the emerging answers raise a new series of questions and indicate the complexity of the lesions which have been collectively termed DCIS.

RISK FACTORS

As a result of its prior rarity, the epidemiology of DCIS had not been studied until recently. In a case-control study of women from Los Angeles County, 233 patients with DCIS and 2057 with invasive breast cancer (IBC) were compared with 2203 age- and neighbourhood-matched controls.[1] Although there were many similarities between risk factors for invasive and non-invasive disease, such as parity and age at first full-term pregnancy, the magnitude differed for benign breast disease which almost doubled the risk of DCIS compared with IBC. In premenopausal women there was an inverse association between obesity as measured by Quetelet's index (kg/m^2) and risk of DCIS, but no effect on invasive disease. Late age at menarche (>14 years) gave greater protection against DCIS than IBC. As shown in Table 17.1, family history disproportionately increased the risk of DCIS rather than invasive cancer in both pre- and postmenopausal women.

Table 17.1 Comparison of risk factors for DCIS and invasive breast cancer

Factor	Premenopausal		Postmenopausal	
	DCIS	Invasive	DCIS	Invasive
Age (per 10 years)	2.3*	6.1	1.2	1.5
Family history	2.7†	2.1	2.1	1.9
	2.4*	1.7	2.2	1.5
Menarche >14	0.4†	0.6	1.1	0.9
	0.7*	0.8	1.1	0.5
Benign breast disease	2.4†	1.3	1.5	1.4
	1.0*	1.4	0.9	1.1
BMI > 27 kg/m^2	0.4†	1.1	1.4	2.0
	0.4*	0.6	1.1	0.9

* From Kerlikowske et al.[2]
† From Longnecker et al.[1]

Kerlikowske et al conducted a cross-sectional study of 39 542 women who had screening mammography in San Francisco between 1985 and 1995.[2] Their findings were broadly similar to those of Longnecker et al,[1] as outlined in Table 17.1. In terms of age incidence, in the premenopausal woman each decade led to a doubling of risk of DCIS and a sixfold increase for IBC. This gap narrowed in the postmenopausal woman but there was still a greater risk of IBC. There was a disproportional increase in risk of DCIS associated with a family history. Late age at menarche was again shown to have a greater effect on DCIS than IBC for premenopausal cases, but no impact in the postmenopausal cases.

Contrary to the findings of Longnecker et al, prior breast surgery (a surrogate for benign breast disease) did not affect risk. The protective effect of being overweight in terms of development of premenopausal DCIS was again seen.

HISTOLOGY

A major obstruction to the understanding of DCIS was the lack of a good histological classification. Pathologists tended to subdivide lesions into six types, based on architecture: solid, cribriform, comedo, clinging, papillary and low papillary. Sometimes the presence or absence of necrosis was mentioned, but many lesions were mixed and in at least 10% of cases no pathological consensus could be achieved.

A group of pathologists associated with the EORTC Breast Cancer Co-operative Group have tackled this problem and proposed a new classification.[3] They recognized the heterogeneity of DCIS in terms of pattern of mammographic microcalcification, differences in distribution of lesions within the mammary tree, and different relapse rates of DCIS after breast-conserving treatment. Also, in patients with invasive cancer and associated DCIS, there

Table 17.2 Proposed histological classification of DCIS

Feature	Well differentiated	Intermediately differentiated	Poorly differentiated
Primary			
Nuclei	Monomorphic	Pleomorphic +	Pleomorphic +++
Chromatin	Uniform fine	Fine to coarse	Coarse clumped
Nucleoli	Insignificant	Evident	Prominent
Mitoses	Rare	Present	Often present
Secondary			
Architectural differentiaton	Marked	Present	Absent or minimal

From Holland et al.[3]

was an association between grade of invasive component and grade of DCIS.[4]

The proposed classification both introduced a new terminology based on cytonuclear differentiation and architectural pattern, and derived three grades from these features; these were well differentiated (WD), intermediately differentiated (ID) and poorly differentiated (PD). The components of the classification are shown in Table 17.2. Primary features are the morphology of nuclei, chromatin, nucleoli and mitoses. The secondary feature is cell polarization (architectural differentiation).

One reason for using the classification is that there may be great variation within an individual lesion in terms of architecture and necrosis whereas cytonuclear features are much more consistent. Furthermore, as the components of the classification are well characterized this should reduce the interobserver variation.

It remains to be confirmed whether the classification does define groups of lesions with different biological behaviour. There are indicators that this may be so because there is close correlation between the appearance of microcalcifications on mammograms and presence of poorly differentiated DCIS. In addition, three-

Table 17.3 Van Nuys' classification of DCIS and local relapse

	Non-high grade without necrosis	Non-high grade with necrosis	High grade
No.	80	90	68
Local relapse after 6.5 years (%)	4	11	27

From Silverstein et al.[7]

dimensional studies indicate that poorly differentiated lesions are continuous, whereas well-differentiated DCIS may be discontinuous within a breast segment. In terms of biological features, poorly differentiated DCIS is more likely to be *c-erbB-2* and *p53* positive and oestrogen and progesterone receptor negative.[5]

Table 17.4 DNA ploidy and S-phase fraction in DCIS

Number	Variant	Aneuploidy (%)	S-phase fraction	Reference
12		30	–	Carpenter et al[9]
74	Cribriform	13	3.5	Locker et al[10]
	Solid	57	6.5	
	Comedo	61	9.5	
	Micropapillary	75	6.5	
	Mixed	43	6.8	
	Overall	46		
74	Comedo	55	–	Aasmundstad and Haugen[11]
	Non-comedo	27		
	Overall	38		
56	WD	17	–	Killeen and Namiki[12]
	ID	39		
	PD	65		
	Overall	39		
46	DCIS	63	–	Pallis et al[13]
	LCIS	17		

WD, well-differentiated; ID, intermediately differentiated; PD, poorly differentiated.

A different classification of DCIS using grade based on nuclear features and necrosis was described by Lagios et al.[6] This divides the lesions into three groups: high, intermediate and low grade. After wide excision, none of those with low-grade DCIS relapsed, as compared with one with an intermediate grade and 12 with high-grade lesions.

Another prognostic system has been proposed by Silverstein et al.[7] The Van Nuys' prognostic index uses a combination of nuclear grade and comedo-type necrosis, defining three groups: non-high grade without necrosis, non-high grade with necrosis and high grade.

As is shown in Table 17.3, there were significantly different local relapse rates after breast conservation treatment, after a median follow-up of 6.5 years. It remains to be determined how universally applicable the Van Nuys' classification will be. Douglas-Jones et al applied six different classifications to the DCIS component associated with invasive cancers and found close correlation of the differentiation of DCIS to the grade of the invasive component.[8] When interobserver variation was assessed independently, the Van Nuys' classification emerged as the best. It will be important in the analysis of clinical trials of treatment of DCIS that pathological review takes into account the different proposed classifications so that, eventually, an acceptable worldwide system can be adopted which will be of value in determining treatment and prognosis.

BIOLOGICAL FEATURES

As changes in nuclear morphology are a major component of the histological diagnosis and classification, this would probably be associated with changes in DNA ploidy and cell proliferation. Several studies have shown that DNA aneuploidy is common in DCIS and these are summarized in Table 17.4.[9–13] Overall, aneuploidy was found in 30–60% of DCIS specimens.

Carpenter et al reported that cribriform lesions were least likely to be aneuploid (13%), and had the lowest S-phase fraction, so they hypothesized that this might be the least biologically aggressive of the DCIS variants.[9] Others reported that comedo types were the most aneuploid or that well-differentiated DCIS was the most likely to be diploid.[10] With a different method of measuring cell proliferation, thymidine labelling index (TLI), Meyer found a significantly reduced TLI in non-comedo variants compared with comedo DCIS (1–2% vs 5.2%).[14]

Nielsen et al carried out a cytogenetic analysis of eight DCIS lesions and found that all contained abnormal metaphases, with involvement of several chromosomes of which chromosome 1 was the most common.[15] Using fluorescence in situ hybridization (FISH) to study 30 archival DCIS specimens, Murphy et al observed extensive genetic alterations, particularly in chromosomes 1, 3, 10, 16, 17 and 18.[16] Stratton et al used polymorphic short tandem repeats and the polymerase chain reaction (PCR) to look for loss of heterozygosity (LOH) at loci of reported allele loss in invasive cancers using a series of 46 DCIS cases and 86 invasive cancers with associated DCIS.[17] Of the pure DCIS lesions there was LOH on chromosome 17 in 29% compared with 52% of the DCIS cases associated with invasive disease. Similarly, on chromosome 17, LOH was seen in 28% and 55% respectively. In some cases LOH was found in the invasive but not in the non-invasive component, suggesting that abnormalities at more than one genetic locus are responsible for, or associated with, the progression of DCIS to invasive disease.

After carrying out a microdissection of ducts followed by DNA extraction, Munn et al found allelic imbalance (AI) on chromosome 17q in the region of the *BRCA-1* gene in 74% of DCIS lesions.[18] In two cases AI was found distal to *BRCA-1*, suggesting a possible second tumour suppressor gene on the chromosome. To examine the role of loss of heterozygosity on 11q13, Chuaqui et al carried out microdissection of normal, hyperplastic, and tumour cells from 24 paraffin-fixed DCIS specimens and 12 cases of atypical ductal hyperplasia (ADH), and then extracted DNA for PCR testing.[19] There was LOH in one of 11 (9%) ADH cases and in six of 22 (27%) of those with DCIS. Of the low-grade cases of DCIS none displayed LOH, whereas this was observed in 35% of those with high-grade DCIS. This may be another site of a tumour suppressor gene which is mutated in the evolution of high-grade DCIS.

STEROID RECEPTORS

In a comparison of invasive cancers and DCIS, Hawkins et al measured oestrogen receptors (ER) using the dextran charcoal method and found that, at a cut-off of 5 fmol/mg protein,

Table 17.5 Oestrogen and progesterone receptor status in relation to new DCIS classification

Well-differentiated (%)		Intermediately differentiated (%)		Poorly differentiated (%)		Reference
ER +ve	PR +ve	ER +ve	PR +ve	ER +ve	PR +ve	
83	75	90	65	74	74	Zafraniet et al[24]
75	64	88	80	44	56	Leal et al[25]

Table 17.6 Histological classification of DCIS and percentage of lesions expressing *p53* mutation

Well differentiated (%)	Intermediately differentiated (%)	Poorly differentiated (%)	Reference
0	4	60	Lagios[6]
5	35	61	Poller et al[23]

77% of the invasive cancers were ER-positive compared with only 44% of the DCIS cases.[20] Other immunohistochemical studies compared ER status of non-comedo and comedo DCIS and reported ER-positive rates of 39–90% and 16–57% respectively.[21–23]

Since the proposed histological grading system for DCIS,[3] other groups have examined both ER and progesterone receptor (PR) status in relation to the new classification.[24,25] These results are shown in Table 17.5. The lowest percentage ER and PR positivity is seen in those with poorly differentiated lesions, but the highest among those with intermediately differentiated DCIS.

EXPRESSION OF ONCOGENE *c-erbB-2*

A series of 189 invasive cancers and 45 DCIS cases were examined for amplification of *c-erb-2* (*neu*) expression by van de Vijver et al.[26] Of the invasive cancers there was overexpression of c-erbB-2 protein in 14%, compared with 42% of DCIS cases. All non-invasive lesions showing amplification were of comedo type. Similar results were reported by Alfred et al who suggested that *c-erbB-2* might be involved in initiation rather than progression of DCIS.[27]

Evans et al compared the mammographic appearance of DCIS and attempted to relate this to expression of *c-erbB-2*.[28] They found that *c-erbB-2*-positive tumours were more likely than negative cases to show calcification (92% vs 72%), which was ductal (78% vs 57%), granular (97% vs 86%) and rod-shaped (82% vs 54%). Tumours that were *c-erbB-2* negative were more

likely not to show any calcification (28% vs 8%). As *c-erbB-2* positivity was usually associated with a large cell comedo variant which was a more rapidly proliferating variant, Barnes et al examined the relationship between the oncoprotein expression and thymidine-labelling index (TLI) in 70 cases of DCIS.[29] Of the 37 with a low TLI (2), 14% were *c-erbB-2* positive, whereas among those with a high TLI (>2) 43% overexpressed the protein. Of the comedo carcinomas 75% were *c-erbB-2* positive and 85% had a high TLI.

TUMOUR SUPPRESSOR GENE *p53*

The tumour suppressor gene *p53* has been found in invasive tumours, but its role in mammary carcinogenesis has not been defined. Two large immunohistochemical studies have examined both *p53* mutations and histological classification of DCIS and are summarized in Table 17.6. This indicates the close association between *p53* expression and lack of differentiation in DCIS with a negligible incidence of mutation in well-differentiated lesions, rising to 60% in poorly differentiated cases.

CLINICAL FEATURES

For patients with DCIS the average age at the time of diagnosis is 52 years, which is approximately 7 years later than that of women with LCIS. The presenting features of cases in four large series are given in Table 17.7.[30–33] Despite increasing use of mammography the most common symptom was a breast lump. A nipple discharge, usually

Table 17.7 Presenting features of patients with DCIS

No.	Mean age (years)	Lump	Discharge	Paget's disease	X-ray mammography	Reference
101	52	54	15	11	21	Fentiman et al[30]
100	52	40	0	1	59	Silverstein et al[31]
112	48	33	17	0	62	Ottesen et al[32]
183	54	125	28	0	30	Cataliotti et al[33]
Total*	52	252 (51)	60 (12)	12 (2)	172 (35)	

* Values in parentheses are percentages.

containing haemoglobin, was the presenting feature in 12% of cases. Just over one-third of cases were mammographically detected, without any clinical signs being present.

However, not all patients with breast symptoms and DCIS will have a lump or a discharge as a direct result of the disease. Symptoms may arise from coexisting duct ectasia or a duct papilloma, with DCIS being a coincidental finding. There is no evidence to suggest that mammographically detected DCIS has a different behaviour from that which presents with clinical symptoms.

MASTECTOMY FINDINGS

Only in recent years has breast conservation become more widely used in patients with DCIS. Most cases have been treated by either total or modified radical mastectomy, and this has provided an opportunity to examine the extent and distribution of DCIS within the breast, together with the likelihood of coexistent invasive disease and axillary nodal involvement. Several series are summarized in Table 17.8.[8,31,34–39]

The original biopsy had completely cleared the DCIS in 35% of cases, whereas in 40% there

Table 17.8 Histological findings after mastectomy for DCIS

No.	No residual DCIS	Residual DCIS	Multifocal DCIS	Invasion	Axillary meta-stases	Reference
38	5	25	–	7	4	Faverley et al[39]
50	16	20	10	3	0	Rosen et al[34]
53	25	–	17	11	1	Lagios et al[35]
47	23	–	18	6	0	Von Rueden and Wilson[36]
82	30	20	19	13	0	Douglas-Jones et al[8]
45	15	28	–	2	1	Petersee et al[37]
49	11	28	27	–	0	Silverstein et al[31]
61	27	10	24	3	1	Gump et al[38]
Mean (%)	35	40	34	12	2	

Table 17.9 Histological classification of DCIS and growth pattern

DCIS type	Number (%)	Continuous No. (%)	Multifocal No. (%)
Number	60	30 (50)	30 (50)
WD	27 (45)	8 (30)	19 (70)
ID	9 (15)	4 (44)	5 (56)
PD	19 (32)	17 (90)	2 (10)
Mixed	5 (8)	1 (20)	4 (80)

WD, well differentiated; ID, intermediately differentiated; PD, poorly differentiated
From Faverley et al.[39]

was residual DCIS. An associated invasive carcinoma was present in 12% and this was more likely if there was multifocal DCIS,[29] present overall in 34%. Axillary nodal metastases were found in 2%, usually when an invasive cancer had been identified, but occurring sometimes in individuals with extensive DCIS in whom it was not possible for the pathologist to take enough levels of the area so that microinvasion was missed.

In a meticulous study carried out in Nijmegen, a series of 60 mastectomy specimens were subjected to serial subgross sectioning with correlative specimen radiography.[39] As well as taking tissue slices for paraffin section, identified blocks were de-waxed before examination by stereomicroscopy. The aim was to determine the detailed three-dimensional distribution, site and extent of DCIS within the mammary tree. Multicentricity was defined as DCIS in two different areas of the breast separated by at least 4 cm of ostensibly normal tissue. If there was a discontinuous pattern of growth separated by uninvolved duct of less than 4 cm, this was called multifocal disease.

The distribution of DCIS, continuous or multifocal in relation to histological classification, is shown in Table 17.9. There was an equal distribution of continuous and multifocal patterns of DCIS. However, what clearly emerges is that well-differentiated DCIS is most likely to be multifocal (70%), whereas poorly differentiated DCIS is usually continuous (90%). Although DCIS was rarely multicentric, it was frequently extensive, and usually multifocal in well-differentiated cases. In terms of the length of uninvolved duct in multifocal cases, this was less than 5 mm in 63%, 5–10 mm in 20% and more than 10 mm in 17%. Thus, if there is 10 mm of uninvolved breast tissue around an area of excised DCIS, complete excision is likely to be achieved in 83% of cases.

It is often assumed that a total mastectomy provides a cure for DCIS, with a zero risk of local recurrence. Unfortunately this is not true. Residual breast tissue may be left behind, particularly in the axillary tail and in the most inferior part of the breast. Recurrence may be invasive rather than non-invasive and lead to premature death of the patient from metastatic disease.[5,40] Thus it is important that patients and surgeons realize that even a total mastectomy is not a guarantee of local cure, although it is likely that close attention to surgical technique should minimize the risk of relapse in residual breast tissue.

Table 17.10 Development of contralateral invasive and non-invasive cancer after DCIS

Number	Follow-up (year)	Women-years	DCIS	Invasive	Reference
101	5	505	2	0	Nielsen et al[15]
70	8	560	1	2	Murphy et al[16]
116	9	1044	0	0	Webber et al[42]
183	10	1830	1	5	Aasmundstad and Haugen[11]
80	17.5	1400	0	1	Eusebi et al[43]
1929	4.5	8681	21	53	Habel et al[44]

BILATERALITY OF DCIS

When considering the optimal management of DCIS, the risk of contralateral disease has to be quantified. In a study of 79 patients with non-comedo DCIS, contralateral mastectomy was performed in 25, of whom 3 (12%) were found to have DCIS.[41] However, this would appear to be an overestimate of risk of contralateral disease. Studies with long-term follow-up are summarized in Table 17.10.[11,15,16,42–44]

After a total of 14 020 women-years of follow-up, 86 contralateral cancers had been diagnosed, of which 25 (29%) were DCIS and 61 (71%) invasive. This represents an annual contralateral cancer rate of 0.02% for women with DCIS, compared with 0.6% for patients with invasive cancer. This is a not a high risk and therefore routine contralateral breast biopsy or mastectomy cannot be justified.

FOLLOW-UP OF BIOPSIED DCIS

For various reasons some patients with DCIS have been biopsied with no further treatment. These would have comprised a mixture of cases

Table 17.11 Development of ipsilateral invasive cancer and recurrence of DCIS after a biopsy for DCIS

Number	Follow-up (years)	DCIS	Invasive carcinoma	Reference
11	10	0	2	Carter et al[45]
10	10	1	6	Betsill et al[46]
15	18	0	10	Rosen et al[47]
25	15	0	7	Page et al[48]
35	9	10	12	Price et al[49]
68	4.5	12	1	Silverstein et al[7]
164		**23 (14)**	**38 (23)**	**Total**

Table 17.12 Development of ipsilateral DCIS and invasive cancer after wide excision for DCIS

Number	Follow-up (years)	DCIS	Invasive carcinoma	Reference
11	10	0	2	Millis and Thynne[50]
20	4	2	1	Aasmundstad and Haugen[11]
22	3	3	2	Page et al[48]
44	5	11	2	Fisher et al[51]
38	5	2	3	Arnesson et al[52]
102	4.5	14	10	Schreer[53]
237		**32 (14)**	**20 (8)**	**Total**

with involved and uninvolved biopsy margins. The main reasons for biopsy alone have been refusal by the patient to undergo further surgery, or a missed pathological diagnosis of DCIS which was picked up at a subsequent histological review. Table 17.11 shows the results of follow-up of such cases.[7,45–49] Overall, 23% of these cases developed an invasive cancer in the same breast, and a further 14% developed further DCIS. Thus more than one-third relapsed after an excision biopsy.

Under circumstances when a wide local excision had been carried out, with a greater likelihood of uninvolved margins, it would be expected that there would be a reduced risk of progression to invasive disease and local relapse of DCIS. Larger series of wide excision for DCIS are shown in Table 17.12.[11,48,50–53]

This suggests that a wide excision does reduce both the incidence of recurrent DCIS (to 14%) and progression to invasive disease (8% vs 23% after excision biopsy). As more is being understood about the extent and distribution of the disease, so it has become even more important for there to be close cooperation between surgeon, radiologist and pathologist. This will maximize the chance of a complete local excision, with 1 cm margins of normal tissue in as many cases as possible at the time of first surgery for suspected DCIS.

RADIOSENSITIVITY OF DCIS

Until recently, no clinical trials had specifically addressed the treatment of DCIS. However, there were two randomized trials in which patients were treated by either breast conservation or mastectomy, and on subsequent histological review it was found that some cases of DCIS had been included and treated by irradiation. In the Guy's Wide Excision Trial six patients with DCIS were treated by wide excision and external radiotherapy (38 Gy).[54] None has developed recurrence but it is impossible to determine whether this success was the result of the surgery or radiotherapy.

The NSABP Trial B-06 compared total mastectomy and axillary clearance with wide excision, with or without breast irradiation (50 Gy).[51] Of the 2072 cases entered, 78 (3.8%) had DCIS without invasion. There were 51 cases treated by wide excision and relapse occurred in five of 22 (23%) of the non-irradiated group and two of 29 (7%) of those who had breast irradiation. This did suggest that there might be some benefit from radiotherapy.

There had been several non-randomized studies in which patients with DCIS were treated by wide excision followed by radiotherapy, and these are outlined in Table 17.13.[55–63] A variety of radiation treatments was used, the

Table 17.13 Results of non-randomized studies treating DCIS by wide excision and post-operative radiotherapy

Number	Radiotherapy	Follow-up (months)	DCIS	Invasive	Reference
44	45–55 Gy+B	92	0	4	Stotter et al[55]
51	45–50 Gy+B	68	3	2	Solin et al[56]
67	58 Gy+B	104	2	5	Fourquet et al[57]
259	50 Gy+B	78	14	14	Solin et al[58]
104	50 Gy+B	51	5	3	Silverstein et al[59]
38	46 Gy+B	81	3	5	Bornstein et al[60]
56	50 Gy+B	61	4	1	Ray et al[61]
70	50 Gy +B	48	0	3	Kuske et al[62]
52	50 Gy+B	68	2	1	White et al[63]
741			**33 (4)**	**38 (5)**	**Total**

B, boost.

most common dose being 50 Gy, with or without a boost to the excision site. The largest study was derived from nine centres in the USA and Europe, and this showed that 11% of cases developed a local relapse after a median follow-up of 6.5 years.[58] Of those who relapsed, half had DCIS and half had an invasive recurrence. Overall the relapse rate in these series was 9% of which invasive disease was slightly more frequent (5% vs 4%).

Thus the non-randomized studies indicate a 22% relapse rate after wide excision alone and a 9% local recurrence rate in those treated by wide excision and radiotherapy.

CLINICAL TRIALS

In the mid-1980s the EORTC Breast Cancer Co-operative Group decided to conduct a trial for patients with DCIS. No previous prospective randomized clinical trials had examined treatment options for DCIS because of the rarity of the condition. As a result of changing attitudes of patients and doctors towards informed consent, it would have been impossible to conduct a study randomizing between mastectomy and breast conservation. At the time of study design the published results were consistent with there being some benefit but none had enough cases or sufficiently long follow-up for definite conclusions to be drawn. Thus it seemed ethical to conduct a trial randomizing to radiotherapy or no radiotherapy after complete local excision of DCIS.

While the trial was underway, results were reported by the NSABP of trial B-12.[64] The trial comprised 818 women with DCIS which had been completely excised and they were randomized to observation (405) or whole breast irradiation (413). After a median follow-up of 43 months ipsilateral breast cancer developed in 64 of the non-irradiated group (32 DCIS, 32 invasive), and in 28 of those irradiated (20 DCIS, 8 invasive). The 5-year cumulative breast relapse rate was reduced from 10% to 7.5% for DCIS, and from 10.5% to 3% for invasive cancers. These represent preliminary results and thus need to be interpreted with caution. They should not be taken as unequivocal proof of the value of radiotherapy after wide excision of DCIS, particularly as different subtypes may have different biological behaviour.

As complete clearance was to be a prerequisite for entry to the EORTC trial, this would mean that a certain proportion of cases would be ineligible because a mastectomy would be necessary to achieve clearance. One object of the study would be to determine the percentage of patients with DCIS detected clinically or by mammography, who would be suitable for wide local excision. In terms of axillary surgery, previous studies had shown that about 2% of patients with DCIS had nodal involvement.[5,6,30-34] and so it was agreed that axillary sampling or clearance should be avoided, unless a clinically suspicious node was present.

It was recognized that pathological quality assurance would need to form an intrinsic part of any trial in which confirmation of complete local excision was essential. Thus specimen handling would need to be performed in a structured way, with marking of margins and appropriate sampling of the specimen. Classification of DCIS was in a process of flux and in many cases a mixture of types was seen. There was a suspicion that the comedo variant was the most likely to evolve into an invasive tumour, but it was not felt that any subtype should be excluded from entry, provided that it had been completely excised. Indeed, one aim of the study was to determine whether certain types of DCIS should be treated by local surgery, mastectomy or possibly radiotherapy.

Study design of EORTC 10853

Eligible cases for the EORTC Trial 10853 had DCIS, without invasion, completely excised, who were then randomized to either no further treatment or breast irradiation (50 Gy) in 5 weeks, with no axillary treatment and without a boost to the excision site. If the first biopsy showed involved margins a wider excision would be performed. Should this also fail to achieve clearance, either a quadrantectomy or a total mastectomy would be carried out depend-

ing on how keen the patient was on breast conservation and that she understood that this would be possible only if the quadrantectomy succeeded in clearing the DCIS.

Excluded from the trial were those with DCIS larger than 5 cm, Paget's disease of the nipple and pregnant women. Also ineligible were those with prior malignancy, other than adequately treated basal cell carcinoma of the skin or cone-biopsied carcinoma in situ of the cervix. Others exclusions were age of 70 years or more, those with mental conditions or social circumstances precluding long-term follow-up and also those with a WHO performance status of 2 or more.

Pre-study investigations were defined in the protocol. All study parameters, including surgical and radiotherapeutic features of each case, were to be recorded on EORTC trial sheets. Each patient had a full clinical history taken and physical examination performed. The WHO performance status was recorded and mammograms of both breasts were taken together with a chest radiograph, full blood count and biochemical screen. Patients were entered up to a maximum of 12 weeks after histological confirmation of complete excision.

The first diagnostic biopsy had samples taken from the whole macroscopic lesion or at least eight blocks, to exclude invasion. A radiograph of the specimen was taken and all macroscopic or radiological lesions sampled. This included the area of suspicion and the breast tissue closest to the nipple, marked by a suture at the time of excision. Details of the histopathology procedure to be adopted were given in an appendix to the protocol, together with illustrations of appropriate handling of specimens. All cases were to be reviewed subsequently by Dr JL Peterse of the Netherlands Cancer Institute, to confirm eligibility.

Those patients randomized to radiotherapy started treatment not later than 12 weeks after wide excision. It was recommended that patients were treated with cobalt-80 apparatus or a 4 MeV linear accelerator. When photons were used with an energy greater than 4 MeV, bolus over the whole breast should be used

Table 17.14 Reasons for non-entry of DCIS cases to EORTC Trial 10853

Protocol exclusions		Extensive DCIS	
Prior breast cancer	25	Margins involved	48
Patient refusal	6	Microcalcification >3 cm	16
Delay in histology	9	Lump >3 cm	6
Borderline lesion	3	Multifocal DCIS	3
Protocol violation	4	Uncertain margins	2
Suspected invasion carcinoma	3		
Previous other carcinoma	3		
>70 years	2		
Contralateral DCIS	2		
Doctor omission	2		
Unfit	2		

during one week out of five. The radiation dose was to be 50 Gy in 25 fractions (2 Gy/fraction) over 5 weeks, irradiating the patient five times a week. The dose was specified at the intersection of the central axis of the beams or, if outside the target volume because of divergency correction, the dose was to be specified in the centre of the target volume. Being the first joint trial of the EORTC Breast Cancer Co-operative Group and the EORTC Radiotherapy Group, it was deemed necessary to include quality assurance as an intrinsic part using site visits as necessary to confirm that the specified dosages had been delivered.

Follow-up visits were at the discretion of the participating centres but follow-up forms were completed annually. All cases had a clinical examination at each follow-up visit and annual bilateral single-view mammograms. Suspected recurrences found clinically or radiologically were confirmed histologically. After completely excised relapse in a non-irradiated breast, radiation could be given or the patient treated by mastectomy. Relapse within an irradiated breast was treated by mastectomy with an axillary clearance if the recurrence was invasive.

The trial has now closed, having accrued 1010 cases from 46 centres in 13 countries, between 1986 and 1996.[65] After a slow start there was a progressive annual increase which improved greatly after 1990, particularly as a result of participation of large French centres. One of the aims of the trial was to register non-eligible cases, together with the reasons for non-entry, in order to determine the proportion of patients with DCIS to whom the eventual trial results would be applicable. When the trial had been in progress for 4 years an analysis was conducted of all the cases of DCIS diagnosed during this time in six of the main collaborating centres.[66]

The six centres were: Centre Henri Becquerel, Rouen; Antoni van Leeuwenhoekhuis, Amsterdam; Daniel den Hoed Hospital, Rotterdam; Longmore Hospital, Edinburgh; Guy's Hospital, London; and Centre Jules Bordet, Brussels. At that time these hospitals had entered into the trial 30, 14, 13, 7, 7 and 6 cases respectively. However, these 77 cases comprised only 36% of the total 216 patients diagnosed with DCIS.

The reasons for non-entry are outlined in Table 17.14. Of the cases 46% were excluded because they did not fulfil non-pathological criteria, such as having had a prior invasive or non-invasive breast cancer (27 or 19%), being too old or frail (4 or 3%), or because of their refusal or the doctor's omission (8 or 6%). Most cases who were not entered had DCIS that was too extensive: 75 (54%). Most of these patients were treated by total mastectomy.

With stringent selection criteria, most symptomatic DCIS cases are unsuitable for breast conservation. At the time of that analysis the entry criteria excluded those with palpable lumps or microcalcification larger than 3 cm (21 or 15%). To try and improve accrual, this was relaxed and cases with lumps or microcalcification up to 5 cm became eligible, provided that complete excision had been achieved.

The major question that was asked in the study was the effect of radiotherapy on this condition. Although the trial has taken 10 years to accrue, most of the cases have been relatively recent and so a longer follow-up will be necessary before a definitive answer can be obtained. It is too early to give a breakdown of results by randomization arm. With a median follow-up of 50 months, there had been 83 ipsilateral relapses in the study, of which 46 (55%) were DCIS and 37 (45%) were invasive. Of the cases with invasive disease who underwent an axillary clearance as part of mastectomy there was histological evidence of nodal involvement in 30%.

UK DCIS trial

When national mammographic screening was introduced in the UK in 1988, it was apparent that this would give rise to the diagnosis of up to 900 cases of DCIS every year, and this would provide an opportunity to investigate different treatment options. The proposed trial, for patients with completely excised DCIS, was of factorial 2 × 2 design.[67] The four treatment arms were: complete local excision (CLE) alone, CLE plus radiotherapy (RT), CLE plus tamoxifen (Tam), and CLE plus RT plus Tam. To increase accrual, individual surgeons could select one half of the trial, CLE versus CLE + RT, or CLE versus CLE + Tam. By Spring 1997, 1254 women had entered the trial, of whom 674 (54%) were in the 2 × 2 randomization, and 580 (46%) in the two-way randomization.

THE FUTURE

The main aim of the NSABP, EORTC and UK DCIS trials was to determine the effectiveness of breast-conserving treatment in women with completely excised disease. Pathological review of the EORTC 10853 trial is starting to suggest that the most important determinant of local control is completeness of excision; this may override any effect of radiotherapy. The studies have underlined the need for good histological control of surgical endeavour, and the very complexity of the histopathological handling of these specimens, with inking of specimen, margins, radiology of specimen slices and meticulous examination of multiple sections may make this unsuitable for overburdened routine laboratories.

What is most worrying is the incidence of nodal involvement in women relapsing with invasive disease. This suggests that it is difficult to detect early changes of invasive disease clinically and, radiologically, possibly made worse by fibrosis after radiotherapy. Worse than this, however, this is an indicator that a proportion of these women will die of metastatic breast cancer, which might have been prevented if they had been treated by mastectomy originally.

This is the continuing paradox. Many women with DCIS may need to be treated by mastectomy in order to prevent subsequent invasive disease. Of the totality of cases of DCIS, the proportion that can be treated safely by breast conservation may be small. Some may need radiotherapy, others may be safely treated by complete local excision alone. It is to be hoped that a detailed analysis of the trials will enable the identification of these lucky individuals.

SYNOPSIS

- Ductal carcinoma in situ is a forerunner of ipsilateral invasive breast cancer which is now classified on a basis of grade and presence or absence of necrosis.

- Ductal carcinoma in situ is often extensive but rarely multicentric with a substantially reduced risk of contralateral disease compared with invasive breast cancer.
- Complete excision with a margin of 1 cm

of normal tissue minimizes the risk of relapse and progression to invasive breast cancer.

- Postoperative radiotherapy may reduce the risk of subsequent invasive carcinoma but the costs and benefits of this are still being studied in clinical trials.

REFERENCES

1. Longnecker MP, Bernstein L, Paganini-Hill A et al. Risk factors for in situ breast cancer. *Cancer Epidemiol Biomark Control* 1996; **5:** 961–5.
2. Kerlikowske K, Barclay J, Grady D et al. Comparison of risk factors for ductal carcinoma in situ and invasive breast cancer. *J Natl Cancer Inst* 1997; **89:** 77–82.
3. Holland R, Peterse JL, Millis RR et al. Ductal carcinoma in situ: a proposal for a new classification. *Semin Diagn Pathol* 1994; **11:** 167–80.
4. Lampejo OT, Barnes DM, Smith P et al. Evaluation of infiltrating ductal carcinomas with a DCIS component: correlation of the histologic type of the in situ component with grade of the infiltrating component. *Semin Diagn Pathol* 1994; **11:** 215–22.
5. Bobrow LG, Happerfield LC, Gregory WM et al. The classification of ductal carcinoma in situ and its association with biological markers. *Semin Diagn Pathol* 1994; **11:** 199–207.
6. Lagios M. Heterogeneity of ductal in situ carcinoma of the breast. *J Cell Biochem* 1993; **17G:** 49–52.
7. Silverstein MJ, Poller DN, Waisman JR et al. Prognostic significance of breast ductal carcinoma in situ. *Lancet* 1995; **345:** 1154–7.
8. Douglas-Jones AG, Gupta SK, Attanoos RL et al. A critical appraisal of six moderm classifications of ductal carcinoma in situ of the breast (DCIS): correlation of associated invasive carcinoma. *Histopathology* 1996; **29:** 397–409.
9. Carpenter R, Gibbs N, Matthews J, Cooke T. Importance of cellular DNA content in pre-invasive carcinoma of the female breast. *Br J Surg* 1987; **74:** 905–6
10. Locker AP, Horrocks C, Gilmour AS et al. Flow cytometric and histological analysis of ductal carcinoma in situ of the breast. *Br J Surg* 1990; **77:** 564–7.
11. Aasmundstad TA, Haugen OA. DNA ploidy in intraductal breast carcinomas. *Eur J Cancer* 1990; **26:** 956–9.
12. Killeen JL, Namiki H. DNA analysis of ductal carcinoma in situ of the breast. *Cancer* 1991; **68:** 2602–7.
13. Pallis L, Skoog L, Falkmer U et al. The DNA profile of breast cancer in situ. *Eur J Surg Oncol* 1992; **18:** 108–11.
14. Meyer JS. Cell kinetics of histologic variants of in situ breast carcinoma. *Breast Cancer Res Treat* 1986; **7:** 171–80.
15. Nielsen KV, Andersen JA, Blichert-Toft M. Chromosome changes of in situ carcinomas in the female breast. *Eur J Surg Oncol* 1987; **13:** 225–9.
16. Murphy DS, Hoare SF, Going JJ et al. Characterisation of extensive genetic alterations in ductal carcinoma in situ by fluorescence in situ hybridisation and molecular analysis. *J Natl Cancer Inst* 1995; **87:** 1694–704.
17. Stratton MR, Collins N, Lakhani SR, Sloane JP. Loss of heterozygosity in ductal carcinoma in situ of the breast. *J Pathol* 1995; **175:** 195–201.
18. Munn KE, Walker RA, Menasce L, Varley JM. Allelic imbalance in the region of the BRCA-1 gene in ductal carcinoma in situ of the breast. *Br J Cancer* 1996; **73:** 636–9.
19. Chuaqui RF, Zhuang Z, Emmert-Buck MR et al. Analysis of loss of heterozygosity on chromosome 11q13 in atypical ductal hyperplasia and in situ carcinoma of the breast. *Am J Pathol* 1997; **150:** 297–303.
20. Hawkins RA, Teasdale A, Ferguson WA, Going JJ. Oestrogen receptor activity in intraduct and invasive breast carcinomas. *Breast Cancer Res Treat* 1987; **9:** 129–33.
21. Bur ME, Zimarowski MJ, Schnitt SJ et al. Estrogen receptor immunohistochemistry in carcinoma in situ of the breast. *Cancer* 1992; **69:** 1174–81.

22. Pallis L, Wilking N, Cedermark B et al. Receptors for estrogen and progesterone in breast carcinoma in situ. *Anticancer Res* 1992; **12:** 2113–15.

23. Poller DN, Snead DRJ, Roberts EC et al. Oestrogen receptor expression in ductal carcinoma in situ of the breast: relationship to flow cytometric analysis of DNA and expression of c-erbB-2 oncoprotein. *Br J Cancer* 1993; **68:** 156–61.

24. Zafrani B, Leroyer A, Fourquet A et al. Mammographically-detected ductal in situ carcinoma of the breast analysed with a new classification. A study of 127 cases: correlation with estrogen and progeaterone receptors, p53 and c-erbB-2 proteins, and proliferative activity. *Semin Diagn Pathol* 1994; **11:** 208–14.

25. Leal CB, Schmitt FC, Bento MJ et al. Ductal carcinoma in situ of the breast. *Cancer* 1995; **75:** 2213–31.

26. van de Vijver MJ, Petersee JL, Mooi WJ et al. Neu-protein overexpression in breast cancer. *N Engl J Med* 1988; **319:** 1239–45.

27. Alfred DC, Clark GM, Molina R et al. Overexpression of HER-2/neu and its relationship with other prognostic factors change during the progression of in situ to invasive breast cancer. *Hum Pathol* 1992; **23:** 974–9

28. Evans AJ, Pinder SE, Ellis IO et al. Correlations between the mammographic features of ductal carcinoma in situ (DCIS) and c-erbB-2 expression. *Clin Radiol* 1994; **49:** 559–62.

29. Barnes DM, Meyer JS, Gonzalez JG et al. Relationship between c-erbB-2 immunoreactivity and thymidine labelling index. *Breast Cancer Res Treat* 1991; **18:** 11–17.

30. Fentiman IS, Fagg N, Millis RR et al. In situ ductal carcinoma of the breast: implications of disease pattern and treatment. *Eur J Surg Oncol* 1986; **12:** 261–6.

31. Silverstein MJ, Rosser RJ, Giersan ED et al. Axillary lymph node dissection for intraductal breast carcinoma – is it indicated? *Cancer* 1987; **59:** 1819–24.

32. Ottesen GL, Graversen HP, Blichert-Toft M et al. Ductal carcinoma in situ of the female breast. Short-term results of a prospective nationwide study. *Am J Surg Pathol* 1992; **16:** 1183–96.

33. Cataliotti L, Distante V, Ciatto S et al. Intraductal breast cancer: review of 183 consecutive cases. *Eur J Cancer* 1992; **28A:** 917–20.

34. Rosen PP, Senie R, Schottenfeld D et al. Noninvasive breast carcinoma. Frequency of unsuspected invasion and implications for treatment. *Ann Surg* 1979; **18:** 377–82.

35. Lagios MD, Westdahl PR, Margolin FR et al. Duct carcinoma in situ. Relationship of extent of noninvasive disease to the frequency of occult invasion, multicentricity, lymph node metastasis and short-term treatment failures. *Cancer* 1982; **50:** 1309–14.

36. Von Rueden DG, Wilson RE. Intraductal carcinoma of the breast. *Surg Gynecol Obstet* 1984; **158:** 105–11.

37. Petersee JL, Gelderman WH, van Dongen JA et al. Ductal carcinoma in situ of the breast: a clinicopathological analysis of 70 cases. *Ned Tijdschr Geneeskd* 1986; **130:** 308–10.

38. Gump FE, Jicha DL, Ozzello L. Ductal carcinoma in situ (DCIS): a revised concept. *Surgery* 1987; **102:** 790–5.

39. Faverley DRG, Burgers L, Bult P, Holland R. Three dimensional imaging of mammary ductal carcinoma in situ: clinical implications. *Semin Diagn Pathol* 1994; **11:** 193–8.

40. de Jong E, Peterse JL, van Dongen JA. Recurrence after breast ablation for ductal carcinoma in situ. *Eur J Surg Oncol* 1992; **18:** 64–6.

41. Griffin A, Frazee RC. Treatment of intraductal breast cancer – noncomedo type. *Am Surg* 1993; **59:** 106–9.

42. Webber BL, Heise H, Neifeld JP, Costa J. Risk of subsequent contralateral breast carcinoma in a population of patients with in situ breast carcinoma. *Cancer* 1981; **47:** 2928–32.

43. Eusebi V, Feudale E, Foschini MP et al. Long-term follow-up of in situ carcinoma of the breast. *Semin Diagn Pathol* 1994; **11:** 223–35.

44. Habel LA, Moe RE, Daling JR et al. Risk of contralateral breast cancer among women with carcinoma in situ of the breast. *Ann Surg* 1997; **225:** 69–75.

45. Carter D, Orr SL, Merino MJ. Intracystic papillary carcinoma of the breast. After mastectomy, radiotherapy or excisional biopsy alone. *Cancer* 1983; **52:** 14–19.

46. Betsill WL, Rosen PP, Lieberman PH et al. Intraductal carcinoma. Long-term follow-up after treatment by biopsy alone. *JAMA* 1978; **239:** 1863–6.

47. Rosen PP, Braun DW, Kinne DF. The clinical significance of pre-invasive breast carcinoma. *Cancer* 1980; **46:** 919–25.

48. Page DL, Dupont AD, Roger LW et al. Intraductal carcinoma of the breast: follow-up after biopsy alone. *Cancer* 1982; **49:** 751–8.

49. Price P, Sinnett HD, Gusterson B et al. Duct carcinoma in situ: predictors of local recurrence and progression in patients treated by surgery alone. *Br J Cancer* 1990; **61:** 869–72.

50. Millis RR, Thynne GSJ. In situ intraduct carcinoma of the breast: a long-term follow-up study. *Br J Surg* 1975; **62:** 957–62.

51. Fisher ER, Sass R, Fisher B et al. Pathologic findings from the National Surgical Adjuvant Breast Project (Protocol 6). 1. Intraductal carcinoma (DCIS). *Cancer* 1986; **57:** 197–208.

52. Arnesson L-G, Smeds S, Fagerberg G, Grontoft O. Follow-up of two treatment modalities for ductal carcinoma in situ of the breast. *Br J Surg* 1989; **76:** 672–5.

53. Schreer I. Conservative therapy of DCIS without irradiation. *Breast Dis* 1996; **9:** 27–36.

54. Atkins HJB, Hayward JL, Klugman DJ et al. Treatment of early breast cancer: report after ten years of a clinical trial. *BMJ* 1972; **2:** 423–9.

55. Stotter AT, McNeese M, Oswald MJ et al. The role of limited surgery with irradiation in primary treatment of ductal in situ breast cancer. *Int J Radiat Oncol Biol Phys* 1990; **18**: 283–7.

56. Solin LJ, Fowble BL, Schultz DJ et al. Definitive irradiation for intraductal carcinoma of the breast. *Int J Radiat Oncol Biol Phys* 1990; **19:** 843–50.

57. Fourquet A, Zafrani B, Campana F et al. Breast-conserving treatment of ductal carcinoma in situ. *Semin Radiat Oncol* 1992; **2:** 116–24.

58. Solin LJ, Recht A, Fourquet A et al. Ten-year results of breast-conserving surgery and definitive irradiation for intraductal carcinoma (ductal carcinoma in situ) of the breast. *Cancer* 1991; **68:** 2337–44.

59. Silverstein MJ, Waisman JR, Gierson ED et al. Radiation therapy for intraductal carcinoma. Is it an equal alternative? *Arch Surg* 1991; **126:** 424–8

60. Bornstein BA, Recht A, Connolly JL et al. Results of treating ductal carcinoma in situ of the breast with conservative surgery and radiation therapy. *Cancer* 1991; **67:** 7–13.

61. Ray GR, Adelson J, Hayhurst E et al. Ductal carcinoma in situ of the breast: results of definitive treatment by conservative surgery and definitive irradiation. *Int J Radiat Oncol Biol Phys* 1993; **28:** 105–11.

62. Kuske RR, Bean JM, Garcia DM et al. Breast conservation therapy for intraductal carcinoma of the breast. *Int J Radiat Oncol Biol Phys* 1993; **26:** 391–6.

63. White J, Levine A, Gustafson G et al. Outcome and prognostic factors for local recurrence in mammographically detected ductal carcinoma in situ of the breast treated with conservative surgery and radiation therapy. *Int J Radiat Oncol Biol Phys* 1995; **31:** 791–7.

64. Fisher B, Costantino J, Redmond C et al. Lumpectomy compared with lumpectomy and radiation therapy for treatment of intraductal breast cancer. *N Engl J Med* 1993; **328:** 1581–6.

65. Fentiman IS. EORTC Trial 10853: Treatment options for DCIS of the breast. In: *Ductal Carcinoma in situ of the Breast*. Silverstein, MJ ed. Baltimore: Williams & Wilkins, 1997.

66. Fentiman IS, Julien J-P, van Dongen JA et al. Reasons for non-entry of patients with DCIS of the breast into a randomised trial (EORTC 10853). *Eur J Cancer* 1991; **27**: 450–2.

67. Fentiman IS. Treatment of screen detected ductal carcinoma in situ: a silver lining within a grey cloud? *Br J Cancer* 1990; **61:** 795–6.

18

Breast cancer in young and elderly women

Dangerous at both ends and uncomfortable in the middle.

Ian Fleming

Breast cancer in young women • Breast cancer in elderly women

BREAST CANCER IN YOUNG WOMEN

Breast cancer is rare in women aged less than 35 years and the unexpectedness of its diagnosis can both cause delays in identification and exert a profound psychological impact on the patient. Neither of these effects is helpful in achieving a cure. As much of the litigation on delay in breast cancer diagnosis relates to younger women, a disproportionately large number are seen in breast clinics. Although a small mobile breast lump in a young woman is likely to be a fibroadenoma, this diagnosis must be regarded as provisional unless there is unequivocal cytological or histological confirmation. There are still too many young women who are falsely assured about an apparently benign lump which subsequently proves to be malignant.

There is in addition a subset of women with early-onset disease who have aggressive cancers not susceptible to conservation treatment with radiotherapy. Consequently, in the age group that might most wish to avoid mastectomy this may sometimes be the best option for local control. Although evidence is mounting that some young women do have particularly aggressive disease, it is important that such individuals are identified effectively

to avoid giving others, who have a good prognosis, an overly pessimistic forecast and subjecting them to unnecessarily radical systemic therapy.

Comparative histopathology

It has been suggested that breast cancer is a disease of good prognosis among the elderly, but has a relatively unfavourable prognosis in young women.[1-4] Alternatively, age may not influence the behaviour of the disease.[5] Relatively few comparative studies of histological features of breast cancer in the young and old have been conducted. Rosen reported that there was a significantly lower mean age for patients with medullary carcinoma, whereas lobular and mucoid carcinomas were relatively more frequent in elderly people.[1] Intracystic papillary carcinoma was also found more frequently in older women.[5] Furthermore, it has been found that younger women have more aggressive high-grade tumours than elderly women.[2]

In view of the uncertainty, histological reports of 1869 consecutive women with breast cancer treated at Guy's Hospital were reviewed. This was to determine the variety of histopathological findings in relation to age and ascertain

Table 18.1 Histopathology in relation to age

Histology	≤ 39 years No. (%)	40–49 years No. (%)	50–69 years No. (%)	≥ 70 years No. (%)
Number	148	355	984	382
Inv. ductal	130 (88)	281 (79)	748 (76)	279 (73)
Grade I	6 (5)	34 (12)	97 (13)	32 (11)
Grade II	39 (30)	128 (46)	368 (49)	142 (51)
Grade III	85 (65)	119 (42)	283 (38)	105 (38)
Inv. Lobular	10 (7)	44 (12)	131 (13)	64 (17)
Mucoid	1	4	12	12
Medullary	0	5	18	3
Tubular	1	5	18	3
Mixed/rare	6	10	67	21

whether there were any indications of less or more aggressive features in different age groups.[6] The patients, treated between 1983 and 1992, were divided into four groups, based on age. There were 148 aged 39 and younger, 355 aged 40–49, 984 aged 50–69 and 382 aged 70 years or more.

The results are shown in Table 18.1. Infiltrating ductal carcinoma, not otherwise specified (NOS), accounted for 77% of all invasive tumours. Only these tumours were graded. The most interesting finding was the increase in incidence of grade III infiltrating ductal carcinoma in those aged 39 years and younger ($p < 0.0001$). As others have also found, certain tumour types, namely lobular, mucoid and intracystic papillary carcinomas, were more frequent in the oldest group.[5]

Examining the histology of 117 948 cases in the Surveillance, Epidemiology and End Results (SEER) programme of the National Cancer Institute, Stalsberg and Thomas found more mucoid and papillary lesions in elderly women, but fewer lobular carcinomas.[7] This latter finding may, however, have been the result of under-reporting by peripheral pathologists' reports because a standardized central review was not conducted.

In addition, there was a significant reduction of axillary lymph node metastases with increasing age, a finding that was independent of tumour grade. In those aged under 39, axillary metastases were found in 60%, compared with only 42% of those aged over 70. There was also a reduction in both vascular invasion and lymphoplasmacytic stromal reaction with increasing age, although these two findings were not independent of tumour grade.

It does appear, therefore, that specific tumour types and patterns of metastasis associated with a more favourable prognosis are found more frequently among elderly women. Nevertheless, it must be remembered that, overall, 27% of the cancers in the over-70 age group were infiltrating ductal carcinoma grade III, a tumour type not necessarily associated with a good prognosis. Treatment should therefore depend not upon the patient's age, but upon the general condition and tumour type.

Diagnosis

There is evidence of delay in many young women with breast cancer. In a series of 36 breast cancer cases aged 30–40 treated at Guy's Hospital in 1985–6, the mean duration of

Table 18.2 Sensitivity of assessment techniques in young women with breast cancer

Clinical (%)	Mammography (%)	Ultrasonography (%)	Cytology (%)	Reference
37	55	58	78	Ashley et al[11]
58	61	–	80	Yelland et al[12]
71	76	–	–	Bennett et al[8]
35	–	–	–	Menon et al[10]
–	70	–	–	Gilles et al[9]

symptoms was 6 months[8] and similar delays have been reported in France[9] and Singapore.[10] As well as delay caused by the patient, once seen in the clinic the diagnosis of malignancy may not be immediate. This is the result of relatively low sensitivity of the components of triple diagnosis; results from recent series are summarized in Table 18.2.[8–12] Clinical evaluation can be inaccurate with a range of sensitivities from 35% to 71%, and the usual reason is a clinical diagnosis of fibroadenoma in a smooth mobile but malignant lump.

Mammography has a sensitivity between 55% and 76%, and in large part this is determined by the density of the breast tissue. Gilles et al classified mammograms as showing a dense breast (type I), mixed dense and fatty (type II) and fatty (type III).[9] Of the cancer patients with dense breasts, the mammograms were normal in 27%, compared with 7% of those with mixed density and none of those with fatty breasts.

Ultrasonography had a sensitivity of 58% which, although better than clinical evaluation, suggested that this was not a good diagnostic test for malignancy. Even cytology, with a false-negative rate of 20%, cannot be relied upon to exclude malignancy in a young woman with a breast lump. The gold standard is an excision biopsy, preferably in the luteal phase of the cycle (see Chapter 7). If a conservative approach to a breast lump is being considered, there has to be unequivocal clinical, ultrasonic and cytological proof of its benign nature.

Prognosis

In a study of 1703 premenopausal breast cancer cases treated at Institut Curie, Paris, De la Rochefordière et al examined the influence of age on prognosis.[3] There was a significantly worse outcome in younger patients and a linear relationship between age and relapse-free survival corresponding to a 4% decrease in risk of relapse for every year of age. In a multivariate analysis of factors predicting for both relapse and survival, the effect of young age was found to be independent of tumour size, grade, oestrogen receptor (ER) status, locoregional treatment and adjuvant therapy.

These conclusions were questioned after undertaking a similar analysis of 557 premenopausal patients treated at Guy's Hospital, of whom 40 were 33 years and younger, 98 aged 34–40 and 419 over 40 years.[13] A significantly worse 10-year overall survival rate was found in those aged 33 and less (50% vs 72%). When the histopathological features of the patients in the two studies were compared, however, there were significantly more grade III cancers in the Guy's series (47% vs 18%). In the multivariate analysis, the independent prognostic variables for relapse were pathological nodal status, histological grade and tumour size, and after taking these into account age was no longer a significant independent variable. We suggested that, because of the subjective nature of tumour grading, there might be an under-representation of grade III cancers in the Curie series.

Table 18.3 Immunohistochemical features of breast cancers in different age groups

Feature	25–29 years (%)	30–34 years (%)	35–39 years (%)	40–44 years (%)	50–67 years (%)
Number	18	30	40	75	70
Grade III	67	70	44	58	37
ER negative	56	43	30	51	33
PR negative	67	63	40	56	51
c-erbB-2 positive	22	20	23	17	17
p53 positive	67	53	45	40	37
Ki67	72	67	40	50	40

From Walker et al.[16]

In a comparative study from Nottingham, of those aged less than 35 years, 76% had grade III cancers, as against 47% of those aged 35–50, and 41% of those aged 51–70.[14] As a result of the high proportion of grade III tumours in younger women, the overall outcome was worse. When the patients were divided into three categories with poor, moderate and good outcome, using the Nottingham Prognostic Index, there was no difference in actuarial survival in terms of age.

Using data from the Hospital Association of Rhode Island Tumour Registry, Chung et al calculated 5-year disease-free survival for 10-year age groups, 40 and younger, 41–50, 51–60, 61–70 and 71–80.[15] Overall those aged 40 or less had the worst prognosis, and this was also true of those with stage II and stage III disease. For those aged 40 or less with stage I breast cancer the 5-year disease-free survival rate was 83%, similar to that of other cases aged 41–70. Thus, some of the effect of young age on worse prognosis resulted from either more aggressive disease leading to higher stage at diagnosis or a similar effect because of delay.

In an immunohistochemical study of breast cancers, Walker et al concluded that tumours in young women were different.[16] Several features,

including tumour grade, ER/PR status, c-erbB-2 and p53 staining, together with proliferation as measured by Ki67, were examined in specimens from women aged 25–44 and compared with findings from women aged 50–67, as shown in Table 18.3. Those aged under 35 years were more likely to have aggressive cancers in terms of all features other than c-erbB-2 staining. It was particularly interesting that 67% of those aged 25–29, and 53% of those aged 30–34, had mutant p53 staining suggesting a genetic instability as a possible aetiological factor in younger women. Although none of those aged under 35 had grade I cancers, 31% had grade II lesions, and 40% were node negative, so that there was a subset with a potentially good prognosis.

Breast conservation therapy

Much of the pioneering work on breast conservation was carried out in France, at the Institute Curie, and in 1981 a review was published on outcome of 314 women with operable breast cancer who were treated by tumourectomy and radiotherapy at that hospital and in the Albert Einstein College of Medicine, New York.[17] Of those who were aged 21–30, breast relapse

Table 18.4 Breast relapse after radiotherapy in relation to age

Age (years)	Percentage breast relapse	Reference
< 40	14	Vilcoq et al[17]
≥ 40	3	
< 40	20	Delouche et al[18]
≥ 40	20	
< 35	38	Recht et al[19]
≥ 35	23	
< 35	11	Matthews et al[20]
≥ 35	7	
< 36	15	Haffty et al[21]
≥ 36	11	
≤ 35	19	Fowble et al[22]
> 35	18	
≤ 35	13	Guenther et al[23]
≥ 35	5	

occurred in 35%, compared with 7% of those aged 31–40, 7% in those aged 41–50 and no recurrences in women aged over 51 years. The results are outlined in Table 18.4, together with comparable data from other studies.[17–23] All show a significantly elevated risk of breast relapse after radiotherapy in younger women, with the exception of the results of Fowble et al who compared outcome of 64 women aged 35 and younger and 916 patients aged over 35 years.[22] Overall there was a similar breast relapse rate in the two groups but in women aged 35 and younger there was a breast relapse in 32% of those who were node negative but in none of the node-positive cases. Not only were there more breast relapses but also the relapse-free and overall survival were significantly worse in younger node-negative cases. Almost all node-positive patients had received adjuvant chemotherapy and this might have had some impact on better local control.

Recht et al examined the influence of extensive intraductal component (EIC) on breast relapse in younger and older women and found that when this was present, local relapse occurred in 38% of those aged 35 or younger and 23% of those over 35 years.[19] Of the cases aged over 35 without EIC, breast relapse occurred in only 3% but in 22% of those aged 35 or younger.

Taken together these results emphasize the need for caution in recommending breast conservation treatment for women aged 35 or younger, particularly in the presence of extensive intraductal component or poorly differentiated cancers, and especially if adjuvant chemotherapy is not going to be advised. Young age is not an absolute contraindication to breast conservation, however, particularly in those with well-differentiated cancers without axillary nodal involvement.

BREAST CANCER IN ELDERLY WOMEN

The most important risk factor for developing breast cancer is age. In western Europe about 50% of cases are aged 65 or older, but these comprise 60% of the deaths, indicating that older women are paying a penalty. The presentation and diagnosis of the disease are beset with misconceptions on the part of the patient and her doctors. There are still too many elderly women who do not consider themselves to be at risk of breast cancer and therefore either disregard symptoms or do not take up the offer of mammographic screening.

Should they decide to consult their general practitioner with a breast lump they may not be referred to hospital as a result of either worries that they will be overtreated with chemotherapy or radiotherapy or a mistaken view that breast cancer in older women is a more indolent disease. Their doctors assume that they will die of other pathology before the malignancy becomes problematic. Should a surgical consultation be arranged, they may receive what is now known to be suboptimal treatment and it is very unlikely that they will be seen by a radiation or medical oncologist.

Table 18.5 TNM stage at presentation of elderly patients

Age (years)	I	II	III	IV	Reference
> 80	23 (31)	15 (20)	18 (24)	19 (25)	Chryssos and Bondi[24]
> 80	73 (52)	24 (18)	8 (6)	35 (24)	Robins and Lee[25]
> 80	39 (25)	77 (49)	24 (15)	16 (10)	Davis et al[26]
> 75	2907 (53)	1221 (22)	686 (12)	698 (13)	Host[27]
> 70	89 (41)	71 (33)	43 (20)	13 (6)	Repetto et al[28]
Overall (%)	51	23	13	13	

Values in parentheses are percentages.

All these aspects conspire to delay diagnosis and deny effective treatment. Ignorance among the general public has to be attacked by good communication of information regarding cancer in elderly people. It is to be hoped that the results of clinical trials will bring about a positive change in the attitude of the medical profession towards breast cancer. Even the politicians, forever demanding financial savings in health care, may realize that effective early treatment will reduce the need for subsequent, more expensive salvage therapy. The great hope for the future is national screening because the awareness of breast problems and understanding of the value of early diagnosis will lead to more older women attending for screening.

Stage at presentation

Although one potential explanation for the worse prognosis in older women is late stage at presentation as a result of delay, the series that examined the TNM stage at presentation are summarized in Table 18.5 and this shows that, overall, three-quarters of older patients had stage I/II disease.[24–28] In the largest series from the Cancer Registry of Norway, which comprised 31 594 patients of all ages, of those aged less than 75 years, 49% were stage I, 37% stage II, 5% stage III and 11% stage IV.[27] Thus

Table 18.6 Age and delay of over 6 months before diagnosis

< 70 years (%)	70+ years (%)	Reference
28	42	Berg and Robbins[29]
28	35	Devitt[30]
22	29	Schottenfeld and Robbins[31]

there were only slight differences between the younger and older group in terms of stage at presentation, although more of the latter group were stage II/IV.

Despite this, there is evidence of increased delay in presentation in older patients as measured by duration of symptoms.[29–31] Table 18.6 shows that more older women delay for more than 6 months before diagnosis. There are many reasons for this delay but only rarely is it because the patient is demented or severely depressed. More usually individuals will have exhibited denial, either because they are caring for a sick husband and cannot take time off or because they are fearful of both a diagnosis of cancer and the possible anger of the medical profession at their not presenting earlier.

These delay statistics are an indictment of our inability to give a clear message to patients in relation to risk and age. In 1995, the British charity Age Concern commissioned a survey of over 1000 women aged over 65 in which a series of questions was asked about breast cancer.[32] One question was:

Given your age, how much risk, if at all, do you think you are at of getting breast cancer?

Of those questioned, 4% said they were very much at risk, 19% somewhat, 36% not very much and 28% regarded themselves as being at no risk at all. Thus almost two-thirds did not consider themselves as being at any great risk of breast cancer, as a result of their age, no family history, a normal mammogram or breast examination, or because they were in good health. Concise clear information about breast cancer should be disseminated as part of the breast cancer screening programmes so that women who are now aged 50–60 will be better informed. If this can be achieved, in 10 years time the problems of delay in those over 70 will have diminished or almost disappeared.

Co-morbidity

One of the main arguments used to justify undertreatment of cancer in elderly people is that they will have concomitant cardiovascular, respiratory and degenerative diseases (co-morbidity) which will lead to their death before cancer becomes problematic. This is not supported by the available evidence. Nicolucci et al examined diagnostic and therapeutic procedures in 1724 women with breast cancer treated in 63 general hospitals in Italy.[33] They assessed co-morbidity using the Comorbidity Index (CI) which comprises two components: Individual Disease Value (IDV) and Functional Status (FS).[34] IDV summates the severity and presence of specific complications for each disease suffered on a scale 0–3, ranging from full recovery (0) to life-threatening disease (3).

Table 18.7 Appropriateness of diagnosis and treatment in relation to co-morbidity and age

	Diagnosis inadequate (%)	Treatment inappropriate (%)
Age (years)		
< 50	20	33
50–70	24	36
> 70	32	46
Co-morbidity index		
0–1	26	38
2–3	18	42
Early disease	25	34
Advanced disease	25	59

From Nicolucci et al.[33]

Functional status is derived from signs and symptoms of 12 system categories and evaluates the impact of all conditions, whether diagnosed or not, on the patient's health status. Both diagnosis and treatment were assessed as being appropriate or inappropriate. The findings are summarized in Table 18.7.

This shows that a substantial proportion of older patients had both inadequate diagnostic work-up and inappropriate treatment, either excessively radical for small tumours or limited surgery, and that this was related mostly to the patient's age and not to co-morbidity.

In another study, from the Virginia Cancer Registry, the records of 2252 female breast cancer patients with non-metastatic disease were examined to assess the effects of age and co-morbidity on treatment.[35] For women aged over 85, the odds of being treated surgically were less than a third of those for women aged 66–74. The odds of receiving breast conservation treatment including radiotherapy were 0.55

Table 18.8 Percentage use of radiotherapy as part of conservation treatment by age and co-morbidity

Co-morbidity	65–69 years (%)	70–74 years (%)	75–79 years (%)	80+ years (%)
0	78	70	65	28
1	65	54	46	20
≥ 2	50	50	44	15

for the older age group. When adjusted for aggregate co-morbidity the odds ratios were virtually unchanged. Thus co-morbidity appeared to exert a minimal effect on treatment decisions for this cohort of patients.

Using data collected as part of the SEER project, Ballard-Barbash et al examined the relationship between use of breast-conserving treatment, including radiotherapy, and both age and co-morbidity.[36] The cohort comprised 18 704 women aged 65 years or more diagnosed between 1985 and 1989. In terms of co-morbidity 84% scored 0, 12% 1 and 4% were 2 or more. Thus only a very small proportion had severe co-morbidity which might have mandated minimal treatment because of limited life expectancy. However, as may be seen in Table 18.8, there was a strong negative association between use of radiotherapy as part of conservation treatment and increasing age, little affected by co-morbidity.

The inescapable conclusion is that co-morbidity is not a significant consideration for most older patients with breast cancer and that treatment decisions are determined by age rather than concomitant pathology. One explanation might be a mistaken belief that older patients might have more toxicity from treatment and therefore fare worse. Crowe et al examined the outcome by age of 1353 patients participating in two multicentre trials.[37] The age range was from 22–75, with a median of 56, and all were treated by modified radical mastectomy, with 35% being node positive who received chemoendocrine therapy.

For the entire cohort, age did not predict for either disease-free or overall survival. When subdivided into three groups – 45 and less, 46–65 and over 65 – the hazard ratios for death from breast cancer were similar in all the age groups. This suggests that, when appropriate local treatment is given, older patients will have as good a prognosis as younger women.

Screening

At present in the UK, mammographic screening is offered to women between the ages of 50 and 64, with recall every 3 years. Women over the age of 65 are eligible for screening, but are not part of the call/recall system. In the Age Concern survey of women over 65, when asked about screening, only 19% had asked for and been offered mammography.[32] Two per cent had asked for and been refused mammography, while 76% had not requested screening.

Women over 65 are being invited in a few areas, and results of screening them in the 12 months ending 31/3/95 were included in the Report of the NHS Screening Programme as shown in Table 18.9.[38] This indicates that there is a gradual decrease in compliance with age, falling from 77% in those aged 50–54 down to 58% in women over 65. It should be appreciated that this is not a static situation. As the 50–64 year olds age so the compliance will rise, provided that they feel that they have been dealt with compassionately and efficiently by the screening system. This is an objective worth aiming for because the pick-up rate of cancers

Table 18.9 Results of NHS screening for 12 months up to 31/3/95

Age (years)	Compliance (%)	Cancers per 1000
50–54	77	4.7
55–59	76	7.2
60–64	66	9.5
65+	58	13.1

Table 18.10 Attendance at seventh screening round in Nijmegen project

Age at invitation (years)	Attendance (%)	Attendants from sixth round (%)
40–49	70	87
50–64	66	90
65–69	54	85
70–74	43	78
75–79	24	68
80+	7	52

From van Dijck et al.[39]

in those over 65 is more than double that in women aged 50–54.

Probably the best evidence of a temporal improvement in compliance has been provided by the Nijmegen Screening Programme. Attendance rates showed a decrease with increasing age by the seventh round of screening.[39] However, the attendance rates in the group who had attended the previous sixth screening round were much higher, as shown in Table 18.10. The range of percentage attendance for those who had participated in the sixth round was from 52% to 90%, with over 70% re-attending from the age group 70–79. Hence, once a commitment to attend mammography can be established, the problem of non-compliance in older women should diminish substantially.

To achieve better results and reduce further the mortality from breast cancer, improving compliance with the offer of screening is essential. One of the most powerful methods of increasing uptake of screening is through general practitioners. Fox et al conducted a telephone survey of 972 women aged over 50 of whom 724 were over 65.[40] In a multivariate analysis of factors predicting for women attending screening, the significant variables were: having a regular doctor, having mammography insurance, doctors talking about mammography during consultations, patient request for referral and doctor's enthusiasm for mammography. However, a study of 129 general practitioners in

Los Angeles showed that, although 73% agreed with annual screening of women aged 65–74, only 21% actually recommended mammography to patients of that age group.[41]

As a different approach, Herman et al conducted a prospective randomized trial to assess methods of increasing the rate of breast examination by doctors and improving compliance with mammography.[42] They used as subjects women aged over 65 attending outpatient medical clinics of three different firms at MetroHealth Medical Center, Cleveland, Ohio. All the internal medicine house staff were asked to complete a questionnaire about their attitudes to prevention in elderly people, doctors and nurses were supplied with a monograph of background articles and invited to a lecture on prevention (attended by about 30%).

In the control firm no further specific interventions were offered. In the second, the patient education firm, nurses provided educational leaflets to patients when they attended the clinic. The third, the prevention firm, provided patients with an opportunity to undergo mammography easily with nurses completing the request form for radiographs. In addition, a

Table 18.11 Results of randomized trial of interventions to increase incidence of breast examination and mammography compliance

Randomization	Breast examination (%)	Mammo- graphy (%)
Control (n = 192)	18	18
Education (n = 183)	22	31
Prevention (n = 165)	32	36

From Herman et al.[42]

health maintenance flow sheet was attached to the patients' charts and updated at each clinic visit.

The results of the study are summarized in Table 18.11, which shows that the highest rate of both breast examination and mammography was achieved by the prevention team. There was a significantly higher rate of breast examination among patients attending the prevention team, compared with the other two groups. However, there was a similar rate of mammography compliance in both the education group and the prevention team. Interestingly, there was a disparity between the attitudes and the actions of doctors. Of the second year residents, 94% believed that they offered mammography to their patients whereas this happened in only 45% of cases. Third year residents also offered mammography to 45%, whereas 72% believed that they suggested this to their patients. The study does add support to the notion that encouragement of older women by motivated doctors and nurses will improve compliance.

Further evidence supporting the value of patient education in improving compliance was given by the National Cancer Institute's Breast Cancer Screening Consortium.[43] They surveyed women in five control communities who were not being offered routine mammography. The

individuals were white non-Hispanic women aged 65 to 74 and two surveys of this age group were carried out in 1987–8 and 1991. Of those eligible for the study in 1987–8, between 65% and 77% were interviewed compared with 76% in the 1991 survey.

In the earlier study, mammography had been carried out in the previous year in 19–33% of those from the five communities, whereas in the later survey this had risen to 35–59%. However, the rates of clinical examination of the breasts fell significantly with time: 47–73% in the first survey and 51–65% in the second. This was probably because women who had undergone mammography did not feel that it was necessary to have a breast examination as well. Rates of breast self-examination did not change significantly with time.

Mortality reduction

Sceptics may question whether it is worthwhile screening an older age group because there may be no impact on mortality, or too high a cost per life saved. This can now be rebutted as more evidence has accumulated showing the benefit of screening older women. Theoretical work using mathematical modelling has suggested a benefit from screening women up to the age of 85, and this is now supported by mortality data from screening studies.

Mandelblatt et al used a decision analysis model, with assumptions of 75% sensitivity and 90% specificity for screening with mammography and clinical examination, and taking incidence data from the SEER programme with interval cancer rates derived from the Breast Cancer Demonstration Detection Project (BCDDP).[44] Calculations of mortality reduction were made for five age bands: 65–69, 70–74, 75–79, 80–84 and 85+. For each age group, saving in life expectancy was computed for those with average health, those with mild hypertension and women with congestive cardiac failure. For those aged 65–84 with average health or with minor or severe co-morbidity there was a significant life saving, although the magnitude of the benefit was less in those with concomitant medical problems. The cost-effectiveness of screening women aged 65–69 was $23 212 per year of life saved. This rose to $27 983 in women 70–74 and $73 000 in those aged over 85.

Brown attempted to make a cost-effectiveness calculation based on a computerized simulation model.[45] This assumed that the US programme initiated in 1990 continues through to 2010, in order to take into account delayed benefits of screening, and used mortality reductions based on the Swedish two-county screening trial.[46] The cost per life year saved was calculated for both annual and biennial results and on whether the 50–65 age group alone was screened, or if older age groups – 65–70, 70–75, 75–80 and 80–85 – were also included.

Table 18.12 shows that biennial mammography is more cost-effective than annual radiographs. Furthermore, screening women aged 50–70 is more cost-effective than restricting screening to those aged 50–65. Although screening women aged 71–75 has little impact on cost-effectiveness of biennial mammography, costs start to rise when 76 to 80 year olds are screened and the inclusion of 81–85 year olds causes a large increase in cost per life year saved.

Using the long-term follow-up data from the Swedish two-county trial, Chen et al examined the effect of mammographic screening on breast cancer mortality rates in women aged 65–74.[47] In the trial, 77 080 women were randomized to undergo screening every 33 months and 55 985 others were in an unscreened control group. Of the screened group, 21 925 were aged 65–74, and there were 15 344 of the same age in the control group. The cumulative mortality in the two groups was analysed after 13 years of follow-up. The relative breast cancer mortality in the screened group was 0.68. This means that an approximately one-third reduction in mortality from breast cancer can be ascribed to screening women aged 65–74.

The Nijmegen screening group also examined breast cancer mortality in women aged 65 or more, but because the programme was not a randomized trial, they carried out a case-control study comparing women who attended for screening with those who were invited but did not attend.[48] Among those who were aged 65–74 and underwent regular screening, the relative breast cancer mortality rate was 0.45 compared with unscreened women. Considered in this way, women who attend screening regularly have less than half the risk of women who do not attend. This may be an apparent exaggeration of benefit, however, because those not attending will include those exhibiting denial who may therefore present with more advanced cancers and thus bias the mortality results further in favour of the screened group.

Taking the economic forecasts and the results from both Sweden and the Netherlands, it is difficult to escape the conclusion that, if it is worthwhile to screen women between ages 50 and 64, it makes more economic and humanitarian sense also to screen those aged 65 and over. At present in Britain, about 7000 women aged over 65 die every year from breast cancer. Reducing this by one-third would save over 2000 lives annually.

Surgery

When an operable breast cancer has been diagnosed in an older woman, a variety of surgical options is possible but it is important

Table 18.12 Cost in $1000 per life year saved of annual and biennial mammography including older age groups

Age group (years)	Annual mammography ($1000)	Biennial mammography ($1000)
50–65	32	27
50–70	28	25
50–75	32	26
50–80	35	30
50–85	47	38

From Brown et al.[46]

Table 18.13 Outline of prospective randomized trials of tamoxifen in operable breast cancer

Trial	Surgery arm	Tamoxifen arm
St George's	Wide excision/simple mastectomy	Tamoxifen 20 mg daily
Nottingham	Wedge mastectomy	Tamoxifen 40 mg daily
CRC	Optimal surgery and tamoxifen 20 mg daily	Tamoxifen 20 mg daily
EORTC 10850	Modified radical mastectomy	Tumour excision and tamoxifen 20 mg daily
EORTC 10851	Modified radical mastectomy	Tamoxifen 20 mg daily

that the patient's wishes are considered in the eventual treatment plan. Ideally, a treatment would be sufficiently effective that the patient did not have to make multiple return visits for follow-up. In general it is agreed by most surgeons that patients with single tumours up to 4 cm diameter can be safely treated by breast conservation, because that is what the NSABP B06 and EORTC 10801 trials have shown.[49,50] Both trials, however, involved tumour excision, axillary clearance and radiotherapy, and also excluded women aged over 70. Biologically there is no reason why these results should not be extrapolated to women aged 70 or more, but there is a reluctance by many radiotherapists to irradiate older patients. This is the result of logistic reasons of daily travel possibly necessitating admission to a precious radiotherapy inpatient bed. Provided that the patient is fit enough and amenable to having daily radiotherapy fractions or three times weekly treatment, this should not be a bar to her receiving proven effective local treatment.

Some surgeons used to generalize that older women were not bothered by the loss of a breast and mastectomy was thus a straightforward option involving a spell in hospital but no need for subsequent radiotherapy. On the contrary, experience with older breast cancer patients has indicated that many older women are concerned about their body image and are very reluctant to undergo mastectomy.

Nevertheless there is a group of patients with larger tumours, or others with smaller lumps, who choose mastectomy. These individuals and their relatives can be reassured that the operation is safe and carries a low operative mortality rate of less than 1%.[51] As 42% of breast cancer patients aged over 70 have axillary nodal metastases, a modified radical rather than a simple mastectomy should be performed to maximize local control.

In an attempt to simplify treatment for older women, many surgeons in the past performed limited surgery (tumour excision) and then gave tamoxifen. Others used tamoxifen alone to try and avoid surgery. These experimental approaches looked promising but needed testing in prospective randomized trials. These studies have now been conducted and enable better informed treatment decisions to be made.

Randomized trials of tamoxifen in elderly women

Four trials have been run that examined the role of tamoxifen in the management of operable breast cancer: three were British and the fourth, a European trial, had a British co-ordinator.[52–55] The outline of the trials is shown in Table 18.13.

The St George's Hospital trial was first published when 116 patients had been entered with a median follow-up of 3 years.[52] At that time the relapse rate and overall survival in the surgery group were similar to that in the tamoxifen-treated group. The study was criticized because the surgery was not standardized, in that, for patients with smaller cancers, total mastectomy was performed in 18% and wide excision in 82%. Among those with larger tumours, total mastectomy was carried out in 67% and wide excision in 33%. Of the patients treated surgically by wide excision, breast relapse occurred in 35%. It was therefore argued that the study had shown that tamoxifen was the equal of inadequate surgery.[56]

A more recent update has changed the picture.[57] After a median follow-up of 6 years the trial had accrued 200 patients, with 100 treated by tamoxifen and 100 by surgery. Local relapse or progression occurred in 56% of the tamoxifen group and 44% of the surgery group. At recurrence or progression, when possible, patients in the tamoxifen group were treated by surgery and vice versa. In the tamoxifen group there were 33 deaths, 17 attributable to breast cancer, and in the surgery group there were 28 deaths of which 15 were the result of breast cancer. Thus the study demonstrated that, if tamoxifen alone is used, there will be progression or relapse in more than half the patients so treated.

The second randomized trial was run at City Hospital, Nottingham and, as shown in Table 18.13, patients were treated by either tamoxifen (40 mg daily) or by wedge mastectomy.[53] This latter procedure was designed to be quick to perform and involved lifting the breast from the chest wall and incising the base, with primary skin closure. Thus it comprised a subtotal mastectomy, without axillary dissection. The trial included 135 patients, 68 treated with tamoxifen and 67 by wedge mastectomy. After a median follow-up of 24 months, 47% of the tamoxifen group were alive without recurrence compared with 70% of the wedge mastectomy group. Mortality rates for the two groups were similar: 11% versus 15%.

A subsequent review was conducted after a mean follow-up of 65 months.[58] By this time there was a significantly increased failure rate for local control in the tamoxifen arm, with 59% developing local relapse or progression, compared with 30% of the wedge mastectomy group. Mortality rates for the two groups were similar: 41% versus 42%. Also the proportion dying of, or with, recurrent disease were similar in both randomization options.

The Cancer Research Campaign (CRC) trial was unlike any other study because both arms received tamoxifen; it was first reported in 1991 when there were 381 participants with a median follow-up of 34 months.[54] At that time, the overall survival of the tamoxifen only and the surgery plus tamoxifen groups was similar, as was quality of life as measured by a sociodemographic questionnaire and the General Health Questionnaire (GHQ). A change of management as a result of recurrence was necessary in 21% of the surgery and tamoxifen group but by 35% of the tamoxifen-alone group.

At subsequent review, when there were 446 participants, significantly more of the tamoxifen group needed a change of treatment (46% vs 21%).[59] Furthermore, 28% of the tamoxifen group had died compared with 21% of the surgery and tamoxifen group, and this difference just reached statistical significance ($p = 0.048$). The largest clinical trial had thus shown that tamoxifen led to an increased mortality from breast cancer. This was a strong argument against the use of tamoxifen for older women with breast cancer who were fit enough to have a predicted survival of more than 12 months.

The EORTC trials 10850 and 10851 are still under review, but a preliminary analysis suggested that, in 10851, there were significantly more recurrences and deaths in the tamoxifen-alone group.[55] Recently, the Guy's Hospital patients who participated in 10850 and others who were in a pilot trial were reviewed. The results are shown in Table 18.14. There were 158 patients in the study, with an average age of 74.5 years on entry and a median follow-up of 9 years. Although there were significantly more breast recurrences in the tumourectomy and tamoxifen

Table 18.14 Ten-year results in Guy's Hospital patients treated by tumourectomy and tamoxifen versus modified radical mastectomy

Survival	Tumourectomy and tamoxifen ($n = 80$) (%)	Modified radical mastectomy ($n = 78$) (%)
Locoregional	55	82
Relapse-free	53	63
Distant	72	72
Overall	43	42

group, the distant relapse and overall survival rates were the same. Relapse within the breast, usually treated by salvage mastectomy, did not lead to any worsening of overall survival and it meant that more than half of the patients treated by tumourectomy and tamoxifen were spared a mastectomy. Of the patients in the mastectomy group, 37 had died, 56% from breast cancer, whereas of the tamoxifen group there were 39 deaths of which 54% were attributed to breast cancer. After 9 years of follow-up more than 50% of the patients were still alive, indicating the relative longevity of this age group.

The trials indicate that there is a subgroup of patients who can be treated by tumourectomy and tamoxifen, or even tamoxifen alone, with long-term effective local control. This subgroup needs to be identified so that they can be given more simplified treatment. As might be expected, considering the site of action of tamoxifen, oestrogen receptor status of the tumour is a major indicator of the likelihood of a response.

The Nottingham group carried out oestrogen receptor immunohistochemical analysis (ER-ICA) of fine needle aspirates from tumours, from 116 patients aged 70 years or more; these 98 (84%) had ER-ICA scores of 100 or more.[60] These were entered into a trial comparing tamoxifen with mastectomy in which 54 received tamoxifen alone. Of the 50 assessable cases at 3 months, only one patient had progressive disease: 28% had complete response, 44% partial and 26% static disease.

Gaskell et al also carried out ER-ICA assays on fine needle aspiration cytology specimens and dichotomized their cases into those with less than 20% cells staining positive and those with 20% or more.[61] At 2 years, 90% of those with less than 20% positive cells had relapsed or progressed, compared with only 20% of the group with a greater proportion of ER-ICA positive cells.

Other approaches to identifying non-responders to tamoxifen have included measurement of epidermal growth factor receptor,[62] and transforming factor β_1,[63] but neither is available

Table 18.15 Meta-analysis of the reduction in odds of relapse and death in postmenopausal women treated with tamoxifen and polychemotherapy

Age (years)	Tamoxifen		Polychemotherapy	
	Relapse	Death	Relapse	Death
50–59	28	19	29	13
60–69	29	17	20	10
70+	28	21	?	?

Table 18.16 Benefit and cost-effectiveness of adjuvant chemotherapy in elderly women

Age (years)	Baseline analysis		Adjusted for life expectancy	
	Months gained	Cost/QALY ($)	Months gained	Cost/QALY ($)
60	2.8	28 200	?	?
65	2.8	31 300	1.3	59 300
70	2.2	36 300	1.0	75 000
75	1.8	44 400	0.7	96 000
80	1.4	57 100	0.4	212 500

From Desch et al.[68]

on a routine basis in most histopathological laboratories. If those individuals who can be safely treated with long-term tamoxifen can be identified, the management of these cases may be greatly simplified, without need for axillary surgery or breast irradiation. This remains as an achievable research endeavour.

Adjuvant therapy

At the time that the EORTC trials were being set up the only available controlled trials had not shown any survival benefit for older women,[64–66] which is why the mastectomy group was not given adjuvant tamoxifen. However, since that time the second meta-analysis of the Early Breast Cancer Trialists' Collaborative Group (EBCTCG) has been conducted and published and this has to alter our attitude towards adjuvant therapy in older women.[67] The overview shows clearly that the magnitude of the effect of tamoxifen is equally large in postmenopausal women of all age groups, and indeed that there may be a slightly larger mortality reduction in women aged over 70, as summarized in Table 18.15.

Although the meta-analysis shows that there is a significant but smaller effect in women aged 50–69, it is not possible to give an accurate estimate of the effect in those aged over 70 because of the small numbers of this age group

in randomized trials of chemotherapy. Despite this, the more hawkish medical oncologists would argue that older women should be allowed the chance of benefiting from adjuvant chemotherapy, particularly those with oestrogen receptor-negative cancers.

To address this problem, Desch et al created a Markov model to assess the survival benefit and cost-effectiveness of adjuvant chemotherapy in older women with node-negative breast cancer.[68] Recurrence rates were calculated from the EBCTCG meta-analysis, together with likelihood of recurrence in node-negative cases from the NSABP B13 study. It was assumed that chemotherapy would comprise cyclophosphamide, methotrexate and fluorouracil (CMF), which would affect only the risk of first relapse and that patients did not have severe co-morbidity. After carrying out a baseline analysis this was then adjusted for active life expectancy, as shown in Table 18.16.

In the baseline analysis there is some small gain in life expectancy in those aged over 70, but this is at great cost per quality of life year (QALY). This gain is almost obliterated when adjusting for life expectancy together with a significant amplification of cost/QALY. When compared with other procedures with known cost/QALY, this was equal to that of liver transplantation and 12 times the cost/QALY of adjuvant tamoxifen or coronary artery bypass.

Table 18.17 Options for treatment of operable breast cancer in elderly patients

Category	Option 1	Option 2	Option 3
≤ 4 cm tumour ER +ve	Standard breast conservation	Modified radical mastectomy	Tumourectomy and tamoxifen
≤ 4 cm tumour ER –ve	Standard breast conservation	Modified radical mastectomy	Tumourectomy and radiotherapy
> 4 cm tumour ER +ve	Modified radical mastectomy	Tamoxifen and then breast conservation	
> 4cm tumour ER –ve	Modified radical mastectomy	Wide excision and radiotherapy	
Severe co-morbidity	Tumourectomy and tamoxifen	Tamoxifen alone	

These data suggest that adjuvant chemotherapy should be used with great caution, and probably not outside randomized clinical trials in patients aged over 70.

Management

Although the definitive treatments for older women with breast cancer are not yet known, various principles can be stated. First, patients should not be undertreated because of their age. Second, both they and their families need to be as involved as they wish in determining optimal treatment. In addition, whenever possible, a core needle biopsy should be performed to confirm the diagnosis of invasive cancer (before discussing treatment) and to ascertain the oestrogen receptor status of the tumour, while as part of the diagnostic work-up of the patient co-morbidity should be determined. Once these aspects have been considered the most appropriate therapy can be instigated, options are outlined in Table 18.17.

The most important principle is to treat the patient's breast cancer at the time of first diagnosis in the most effective way. This is important in order to minimize the probability of subsequent relapse at a time when the patient is less fit and may have to suffer the problems of uncontrolled local disease or unnecessary distant metastases. This should be the overriding basis for the management of all women with operable breast cancer and, if this is neglected in elderly people, it may lead to great personal distress together with the need for costly salvage treatment; with forethought these may be avoided.

SYNOPSIS

- Young women are more likely to have poorly differentiated breast cancers than older women and their prognosis may be worsened by delay in diagnosis.
- There is an increased risk of breast relapse after radiotherapy in younger women, partly because of more extensive cancers and high histological grade.
- Women aged over 70 years are less likely to receive effective treatment for breast cancer.
- In the absence of severe co-morbidity, tamoxifen alone constitutes inadequate treatment for breast cancer.
- Older women should be encouraged to participate in breast screening because increasing age is the major risk factor for malignancy.

REFERENCES

1. Rosen PP, Lesser ML, Kinne DW. Breast carcinoma in the extremes of age: a comparison of patients younger than 35 years and older than 75 years. *J Surg Oncol* 1985; **28:** 90–6.

2. Jacquemier J, Seradour B, Hassoun J et al. Special morphologic features of invasive mammary carcinomas in women under 40 years of age. *Breast Dis* 1985; **1:** 119–22.

3. De la Rochefordière A, Asselain B, Campana F. Age as prognostic factor in premenopausal breast carcinoma. *Lancet* 1993; **341:** 1039–43.

4. Schaefer G, Rosen PP, Lesser ML et al. Breast carcinoma in elderly women: pathology, prognosis and survival. *Pathol Annu* 1984; **19:** 195–219.

5. Carter D, Orr SL, Merino ML. Intracystic papillary carcinoma of the breast. *Cancer* 1983; **52:** 14–19.

6. Fisher CJ, Egan MK, Smith P et al. Histopathology in relation to age. *Br J Cancer* 1997; **75:** 593–6.

7. Stalsberg H, Thomas DB. Age distribution of histologic types of breast carcinoma. *Int J Cancer* 1993; **54:** 1–7.

8. Bennett IC, Freitas R, Fentiman IS. Diagnosis of breast cancer in young women. *Aust N Z J Surg* 1991; **61:** 284–9.

9. Gilles R, Gallay X, Tardivon A et al. Breast cancer in women 35 years old or younger: clinical and mammographic features. *Eur J Radiol* 1995; **5:** 630–2.

10. Menon M, The CH, Chua CL. Clinical and social problems in young women with breast carcinoma. *Aust N Z J Surg* 1992; **62:** 364–7.

11. Ashley S, Royle GT, Corder A et al. Clinical, radiological and cytological diagnosis of breast cancer in young women. *Br J Surg* 1989; **76:** 835–7.

12. Yelland A, Graham MD, Trott PA et al. Diagnosing breast carcinoma in young women. *BMJ* 1991; **302:** 618–20.

13. Richards MA, Gregory WM, Smith P et al. Age as a prognostic factor in premenopausal breast cancer. *Lancet* 1993; **341:** 1484–5.

14. Kollias J, Elston CW, Ellis IO et al. Early-onset breast cancer – histopathological and prognostic considerations. *Br J Cancer* 1997; **75:** 1318–23.

15. Chung M, Chang HR, Bland KI, Wanebo HJ. Younger women with breast carcinoma have a poorer prognosis than older women. *Cancer* 1996; **77:** 97–103.

16. Walker RA, Lees E, Webb MB, Dearing SJ. Breast carcinomas occurring in young women (<35 years) are different. *Br J Cancer* 1996; **74:** 1796–1800.

17. Vilcoq JR, Calle R, Stacey P, Ghossein NA. The outcome of treatment by tumorectomy and radiotherapy of patients with operable breast cancer. *Int J Radiat Oncol Biol Phys* 1981; **7:** 1327–32.

18. Delouche G, Bachelot F, Premont M, Kurtz JM. Conservation treatment of early breast cancer: long term results and complications. *Int J Radiat Oncol Biol Phys* 1987; **13:** 29–34.

19. Recht A, Connolly JL, Schnitt SJ et al. The effect of young age on tumor recurrence in the treated breast after conservative surgery and radiotherapy. *Int J Radiat Oncol Biol Phys* 1988; **14:** 3–10.

20. Matthews RH, McNeese MD, Montague ED, Oswald MJ. Prognostic implications of age in breast cancer patients treated with tumorectomy and irradiation or with mastectomy. *Int J Radiat Oncol Biol Phys* 1988; **14:** 659–63.

21. Haffty BG, Fischer D, Rose M et al. Prognostic factors for local recurrence in the conservatively treated breast cancer patient: a cautious interpretation of the data. *J Clin Oncol* 1991; **9:** 997–1003.

22. Fowble BL, Schultz DJ, Overmoyer B et al. The influence of young age in early stage breast cancer. *Int J Radiat Oncol Biol Phys* 1994; **30:** 23–33.

23. Guenther JM, Kirgan DM, Giuliano AE. Feasibility of breast-conserving therapy for younger women with breast cancer. *Arch Surg* 1996; **131:** 632–6.

24. Chryssos AE, Bondi RP. Breast cancer in women over the age of 80. *Breast* 1984; **10:** 13–15.

25. Robins RE, Lee D. Carcinoma of the breast in women 80 years of age and older: still a lethal disease. *Am J Surg* 1985; **140:** 606–9.

26. Davis SJ, Karrer FW, Moor BJ et al. Characteristics of breast cancer in women over 80 years of age. *Am J Surg* 1985; **150:** 655–8.

27. Host H. Age as a prognostic factor in breast cancer. *Cancer* 1986; **57:** 2217–21.

28. Repetto L, Miglietta L, Costantino M et al. Breast cancer in the elderly: detection and treatment modalities in 341 women. *Int J Oncol* 1994; **5:** 1399–1403.

29. Berg JW, Robbins GF. Modified mastectomy for older, poor risk patients. *Surg Gynecol Obstet* 1961; **113**: 631–4.

30. Devitt JE. The influence of age on the behaviour of carcinoma of the breast. *Can Med Assoc J* 1970; **103**: 923–6.

31. Schottenfeld D, Robbins GF. Breast cancer in elderly women. *Geriatrics* 1971; **26**: 121–32.

32. Age Concern. *Not at my Age: Why the Present Breast Screening System is Failing Women Aged 65 or Over*. London: Age Concern, 1996.

33. Nicolucci A, Mainini F, Penna A et al. The influence of patient characteristics on the appropriateness of surgical treatment for breast cancer patients. *Ann Oncol* 1993; **4**: 133–40.

34. Greenfield S, Blanco DM, Elashoff RM et al. Patterns of care related to age of breast cancer patients. *JAMA* 1987; **257**: 2766–70.

35. Newschaffer CJ, Penberthy L, Desch CE et al. The effect of age and comorbidity in the treatment of elderly women with non-metastatic breast cancer. *Arch Intern Med* 1996; **156**: 85–90.

36. Ballard-Barbash R, Potosky A, Harlan LC et al. Factors associated with surgical and radiation therapy for early stage breast cancer in older women. *J Natl Cancer Inst* 1996; **88**: 716–26.

37. Crowe JP, Gordon NH, Shenk RR et al. Age does not predict breast cancer outcome. *Arch Surg* 1994; **129**: 483–8.

38. NHS Breast Screening Programme. *NHS Breast Screening Review 1995*.

39. van Dijck JAAM, Holland R, Verbeek ALM et al. Efficacy of mammographic screening of the elderly: the Nijmegen Program in the Netherlands. *J Natl Cancer Inst* 1994; **86**: 934–8.

40. Fox SA, Siu AL, Stein JA. The importance of physician communication on breast cancer screening of older women. *Arch Intern Med* 1994; **154**: 2058–68.

41. Roetzheim RG, Fox SA, Leake B. Physician-reported determinants of screening mammography in older women: the impact of physician and practice characteristics. *J Am Geriatr Soc* 1995; **43**: 1398–402.

42. Herman CJ, Speroff T, Cebul RD. Improving compliance with breast cancer screening in older women. *Arch Intern Med* 1995; **155**: 717–22.

43. Coleman EA, Feuer EJ and the NCI Breast Screening Consortium. Breast Cancer Screening among women from 65 to 74 years of age in 1987–88 and 1991. *Ann Intern Med* 1992; **117**: 961–6.

44. Mandelblatt JS, Wheat ME, Monane M et al. Breast cancer screening for elderly women with and without comorbid conditions. *Ann Intern Med* 1992; **116**: 722–30.

45. Brown ML. Economic considerations in breast cancer screening of older women. *J Gerontol* 1992; **47**: 51–8.

46. Tabar L, Fagerberg G, Day NE, Holmberg L. What is the optimum interval between mammographic screening? – an analysis based on the latest results of the Swedish two-county breast cancer screening trial. *Br J Cancer* 1987; **55**: 547–51.

47. Chen H-H, Tabar L, Faggerberg G, Duffy SW. Effect of breast screening after age 65. *J Medical Screen* 1995; **2**: 10–14.

48. van Dijck JAAM, Verbeek ALM, Beex LVAM et al. Mammographic screening after the age of 65 years: evidence for a reduction in breast cancer mortality. *Int J Cancer* 1996; **66**: 727–31.

49. Fisher B, Redmond C, Poisson R et al. Eight-year results of a randomised trial comparing total mastectomy and lumpectomy with or without irradiation in the treatment of breast cancer. *N Engl J Med* 1989; **320**: 822–8.

50. Van Dongen JA, Bartelink H, Fentiman IS et al. Factors influencing local relapse and survival and results of salvage treatment after breast conservation therapy in operable breast cancer: EORTC 10801 trial comparing breast conservation with mastectomy in TNM stage I and II breast cancer. *Eur J Cancer* 1992; **28**: 801–4.

51. Fentiman IS. *Detection and Treatment of Early Breast Cancer*. London: Martin Dunitz, 1990: 197–8.

52. Gazet J-C, Markopoulos C, Ford HT et al. Prospective randomised trial of tamoxifen versus surgery in elderly patients with breast cancer. *Lancet* 1988; **i**: 679–81.

53. Robertson JFR, Todd JH, Ellis IO et al. Comparison of mastectomy with tamoxifen for treating elderly patients with operable breast cancer. *BMJ* 1988; **297**: 311–4.

54. Bates T, Riley DL, Houghton J et al. Breast cancer in elderly women: a Cancer Research Campaign trial comparing treatment with tamoxifen and optimal surgery with tamoxifen alone. *Br J Surg* 1991; **78**: 591–4.

55. Fentiman IS. Treatment of cancer in the elderly – a European view. *Cancer Bull* 1995; **47**: 255–8.

56. Fentiman IS. Breast cancer, tamoxifen and surgery. *Lancet* 1988; **i**: 1044.

57. Gazet J-C, Ford HT, Coombes RC et al. Prospective randomised trial of tamoxifen

versus surgery in elderly patients with breast cancer. *Eur J Surg Oncol* 1994; **20**: 207–14.

58. Robertson JFR, Ellis IO, Elston CW, Blamey RW. Mastectomy or tamoxifen as initial therapy for operable breast cancer in elderly patients: 5 year follow-up. *Eur J Cancer* 1992; **28A**: 908–10.

59. Bates T, Riley DL, Houghton, Baum M. Is tamoxifen adequate treatment for breast cancer in elderly patients: is there still an issue? *Proc SRS* 1992.

60. Low SC, Dixon AR, Bell J et al. Tumour oestrogen receptor content allows selection of elderly patients with breast cancer for conservative treatment. *Br J Surg* 1992; **79**: 1314–16.

61. Gaskell DJ, Hawkins RA, de Carteret S et al. Indications for primary tamoxifen therapy in elderly women with breast cancer. *Br J Surg* 1992; **79**: 1317–20.

62. Nicholson S, Haltren P, Sainsbury JRC et al. Epidermal growth factor status associated with failure of primary endocrine therapy in elderly post-menopausal patients with breast cancer. *Br J Cancer* 1988; **58**: 810–14.

63. Thompson AM, Kerr DJ, Steel CM. Transforming factor β1 is implicated in the failure of tamoxifen therapy in human breast cancer. *Br J Cancer* 1991; **64**: 609–14.

64. Cummings FJ, Gray R, Davis TE et al. Tamoxifen versus placebo: double blind adjuvant trial in elderly women with stage II breast cancer. *NCI Monografh* 1986; **1**: 119–23.

65. Castiglione M, Geller R, Goldhirsch A. Adjuvant systemic therapy for breast cancer in the elderly: competing causes of mortality. *J Clin Oncol* 1990; **8**: 519–26.

66. Mouridsen HT, Andersen AP, Brincker H et al. Adjuvant tamoxifen in post-menopausal high-risk breast cancer patients: present status of Danish Breast Cancer Cooperative Group Trials. *NCI Monograph* 1986; **1**: 115–18.

67. Early Breast Cancer Trialists' Collaborative Group. Systemic treatment of early breast cancer by hormonal, cytotoxic or immune therapy. *Lancet* 1992; **339**: 1–15.

68. Desch CE, Hillner BE, Smith TJ, Retchin SM. Should the elderly receive chemotherapy for node-negative breast cancer? A cost-effectiveness analysis examining total and active life-expectancy outcomes. *J Clin Oncol* 1993; **11**: 777–82.

19

Male breast cancer

A man cannot be too careful in his choice of enemies

Oscar Wilde

Epidemiology • Gynaecomastia • Occupation • Endocrinology

The Imperial Cancer Research Fund produced an information leaflet on male breast cancer in 1993. This aroused major public interest, reflecting the widespread ignorance of this disease. As a result of its rarity and the secrecy surrounding the diagnosis, most men are unaware that breast lumps and nipple changes may be evidence of a potentially fatal disease. This is nothing new. In 1889 Williams reported a series of 100 cases[1] and wrote:

> That fuller information about cancer of the male breast is desirable, both on its own account and because of the value of such knowledge as a factor in the solution of many problems relating to cancerous disease in general, I have not the slightest doubt.

Both public and medical information might lead to earlier diagnosis of male breast cancer and hence an improved prognosis. Evidence that this is being achieved is lacking at present. The larger clinical series, comprising more than 100 cases, are summarized in Table 19.1.[2–11]

These data show that, until recently, the duration of symptoms did not change significantly with time. Specifically, in a series from the Mayo Clinic, for the 42 patients presenting between 1933 and 1958 the median duration of symptoms was 19.5 months, whereas among the 82 treated between 1959 and 1983 the delay was 22 months.[9] However, the two most recent series showed a reduction in duration of symptoms, with a correlation between tumour size and median delay: for T1 tumours, 2 months; for T3, 3 months; and for T4, 10 months.[10,11]

Although male breast cancer differs from the female disease in that the mean age at onset is 60 years, compared with 53 for women, it is similar in terms of laterality of disease (R:L = 1:1.1). The explanation for this phenomenon is not immediately evident. In females the left-sided predominance has been variously attributed to handedness of partners or preference for left-sided breast-feeding. The similar male:female left:right ratios rule out these hypotheses. One possibility is a slightly larger target group of breast epithelial cells on the left side as a result of preferential vascular supply during intrauterine cardiac development.

Table 19.1 Summary data from large series of male breast cancer cases

Number of cases	Symptoms	R:L ratio	Age (years)	Reference
342	29	1:1.13	53	Wainwright[2]
205	23	1:1.13	57	Sachs[3]
146	9	1:1.31	52	Treves and Holleb[4]
237	21	1:1.10	65	Scheike[5]
138	18	1:1	61	Carlsson et al[6]
135	9	1:1	69	Borgen et al[7]
104	18		61	Ramantanis et al[8]
124	21		63	Gough et al[9]
397	6		64	Cutuli et al[10]
169	3	1:1.2	63	Sasco et al[11]

EPIDEMIOLOGY

The rarity of male breast cancer has meant that large case-control studies have been as rare as forthright politicians. However, a recent attempt has been made to conduct a meta-analysis of published case-control studies and determine the underlying epidemiological risk factors.[12] The odds ratio was elevated for unmarried men (1.6), men from Jewish ethnic background (2.1), previous benign breast disease (2.7), gynaecomastia (6.2), testicular pathology (2.2), liver disease (1.6) and family history of breast cancer (2.5). It was found that the two sexes were concordant for risk factors such as age, family history, Jewish ethnic background, benign breast disease, marital status and chest wall irradiation. However, there was discordance in that male breast cancer was more common in black men and gonadal ablation was protective in women, but increased the risk in men.

International variations

In Europe about 1% of breast cancer patients are male, with an annual incidence of one in 100 000, but in Africa the disease is considerably more common in males. An Egyptian study reported a series of 218 breast cancers of which 14 (6%) were male.[13] Of the eight traceable cases, seven were known to have had bilharziasis and it was suggested that hyperoestrogenization resulting from hepatic damage might be the explanation. In Uganda, males comprise 4.8% of cases, with an average age of 60, compared with 35 for females,[14] whereas in Zambia males comprise 15% of cases, the highest rate in the world.[15] It is likely that the sub-Saharan high incidence results from a variety of endemic diseases giving rise to liver damage and consequent hyperoestrogenism.

Among Japanese men there is a reduced incidence of the disease which is between 0.1 and 0.6 per 100 000.[16] This reflects the environmental factors that lead to the similarly low incidence in Japanese women living in Japan. Jewish men are the only racial group with a higher incidence (2.3 per 100 000), irrespective of whether they are living in Israel[17] or in the USA.[18] This may be the result of a genetic predisposition, but possibly prescribed dietary practices play a role.

GYNAECOMASTIA

It is usually assumed that gynaecomastia is a necessary prerequisite for development of male breast cancer, although gynaecomastia is common but not always associated with mammary malignancy. In a study of boys aged 10–16 attending summer camps in the USA, who underwent a medical examination, gynaecomastia was present in 39%, reaching a peak of 65% in boys aged 14.[19]

A postmortem study of 447 men in the age group at risk showed gross breast enlargement in only four (1%), but histological evidence of gynaecomastia was found in 40%.[20] This was florid (type 1) in 21% and quiescent (type 2) in 79%. Nuttal examined a group of normal men aged 17–58 and found an increasing incidence of gynaecomastia with age so that, among those aged over 44, 47% had clinical evidence of breast enlargement.[21]

If there was a close relationship between gynaecomastia and malignancy, it would be expected that this would be an almost invariable accompaniment of the disease, but this is not the case. The reported incidence of gynaecomastia in various series of men with breast cancer is shown in Table 19.2.[4,6,8,11] What this shows clearly is that there is an under-representation of gynaecomastia compared with that expected in the population. Indeed these figures may be an overestimate because in some cases, the malignancy itself may have been responsible for swelling of the breast. At a histological level, Scheike examined 79 mastectomy specimens and found evidence of gynaecomastia in 21 (27%).[5] There were six cases (21%), with type 1 gynaecomastia and 15 (71%) with type 2, which is very similar to the proportions reported by Williams in the postmortem study of men without breast cancer.[20]

All these findings suggest that gynaecomastia is not a risk factor for development of male breast cancer. Those men with long-standing unilateral or bilateral breast swelling do not need to be under any kind of surveillance and can be reassured that they are not in a high-risk group.

Table 19.2 The incidence of gynaecomastia in male breast cancer patients

Breast cancer cases	Gynaecomastia cases No.	Reference
265	10 (4)	Treves and Holleb[4]
138	0	Ramantanis et al[8]
135	9 (7)	Carlsson et al[6]
169	43 (25)	Sasco et al[11]
707	**62 (9)**	**Total**

Values in parentheses are percentages

OCCUPATION

In a case-control study of 52 men with breast cancer and 52 controls matched for age, race, marital status and place of diagnosis, Mabuchi et al reported an increased frequency of the disease among men who worked in hot environments, such as blast furnaces, steel works and rolling mills.[18] It was postulated that a prolonged elevation of ambient temperature might lead to testicular failure.

McLaughlin et al examined occupational risk in 333 male cases reported to the Swedish Cancer Environment Registry and calculated the standard incidence ratio (SIR) from observed and expected numbers of cases within occupational groups.[22] Those with the highest risk (SIR = 7.6) were men who had worked in the soap and perfume industries. There was a sixfold increase in risk among journalists and mental health attendants. As in the study of Mabuchi, there was an increased risk in blast furnace workers and also for brewers, gardeners and business administrators.[18]

A Franco–Swiss case-control study of 91 cases and 255 controls, matched for age and year of diagnosis, found that, although the relative risk for those who worked in a high environmental temperature was elevated, this was not statistically significant.[23] Butchers were the only group with a significantly increased risk, and cases were more likely to be bachelors. After reports of an increased risk in men exposed to high electromagnetic fields,[24,25] Loomis conducted a case-control study of men working in electrical occupations.[26] There were 250 cases who died of breast cancer of whom four had worked in the electrical industry (odds ratio or OR = 0.9). However, three were less than 65 years old (OR = 2.2), i.e. twice the expected rate for this age group. Thus, although overall there appears to be no increase in risk, there may be an increased risk in younger men.

ENDOCRINOLOGY

As there is a hundredfold increase in risk of breast cancer for women compared with men, this would suggest that ovarian hormones play a role in the development of the disease. Any decrease in androgens, or increase in oestrogens, should lead to an increase in risk of male breast cancer. To some extent this is borne out by the available evidence.

In men taking therapeutic oestrogens for carcinoma of the prostate, bilateral breast cancer has been reported after a duration of 1–12 years.[27,28] Overall only 15 cases of breast cancer have been reported in men with prostatic cancer but in all cases oestrogen treatment had been documented.[28] Among trans-sexual men who had undergone castration followed, or preceded, by oral oestrogen, breast cancer occurred after 5–14 years.[29–31] When possible such individuals should be encouraged to undergo regular breast checks and keep oestrogen intake at the minimum necessary to maintain their persona.

Klinefelter's syndrome is characterized by testicular hypoplasia, aspermia and gynaecomastia, together with underdevelopment of secondary sexual features and increased gonadotrophin secretion. These individuals, who have the XXY karyotype, comprise 1–2 in 1000 of phenotypic males. In three series with a total of 147 cases of breast cancer, eight men were chromatin positive.[32–34] This would trans-late to an incidence of 33 cases of Klinefelter's syndrome in every 1000 cases of breast cancer so that there is at least a twentyfold increase in risk for men with this syndrome. At the very least these individuals should be under surveillance but a reasonable case could be made for prophylactic bilateral mastectomy.

Other conditions leading to testicular damage have been implicated in the aetiology of male breast cancer, in particular mumps. In their case-control study, Mabuchi et al found a significantly increased risk in men who had mumps after age 20, and a borderline increase in those who reported prior testicular injury.[18] Thomas et al conducted a case-control study of 227 cases and 300 controls selected by random digit dialling and, among other factors, examined the risk of various testicular insults and found a twelvefold increase in risk for men with undescended testis and a twofold increase in those who had had a congenital inguinal hernia or removal of one or both testes.[35] The age at which mumps was diagnosed was very important in terms of risk, having no effect up to age 14, slight increase at ages 15–19 (relative risk or RR = 1.6) and a greater risk after age 20 (RR = 2.5).

Thus conditions which lead to an increase in oestrogens in men, or a decrease in androgens, will lead to an increase in risk, but, as with the female disease, it is less certain that endogenous abnormalities of steroid metabolism are present in all cases of male breast cancer. The case-control studies that have measured serum testosterone and oestradiol are summarized in Table 19.3 and these show no significant reduction of testosterone among cases.[36–39]

Nirmul et al measured a variety of hormones in eight South African cases of male breast cancer (seven black, one Asian) and found an elevation of total oestradiol in comparison with eight healthy men matched for race and age.[38] However, there was elevation in both cases and controls which may have resulted partly from dietary causes. Calabresi et al also reported elevated levels of oestrone (E1), oestradiol (E2) and oestriol (E3) cases.[36] Of the three who underwent orchidectomy, there was a substantial

Table 19.3 Case-control studies of serum testosterone and oestradiol in male breast cancer

Mean testosterone (nmol/l)		Mean oestradiol (pmol/l)		
Cases	Controls	Cases	Controls	Reference
17	15	71	37	Calabresi et al[36]
23	17	95	67	Ribeiro et al[37]
18	12	223	101	Nirmul et al[38]
17	17	103	94	Casagrande et al[39]

diminution in E2, suggesting a testicular origin for circulating oestradiol. As total oestradiol includes a substantial proportion of protein-bound and therefore largely unavailable hormone, free oestradiol is a better index of available E2.

Nirmul et al found an elevated percentage of free E2, but Casagrande et al reported no difference between cases and controls.[39] In Casagrande's study the only significant risk factor was the weight of cases at age 30. Men weighing 80 kg or more had twice the risk of men weighing less than 60 kg, and as a result of a strong positive association between weight and E1. Together with a negative relationship with sex hormone-binding globulin (SHBG), it was suggested that weight indicated an increased lifetime exposure to biologically available oestrogen. However, at the time of sampling of blood there was no significant difference in weight of cases and controls so that their hormone profiles were similar.

Olsson et al reported a case of prolactinoma with bilateral gynaecomastia in whom bilateral breast cancer developed, and questioned whether hyperprolactinaemia could be a predisposing factor for male breast cancer.[40] In a subsequent study of 95 Swedish men with breast cancer, examining aspects of their past medical history showed that 9 (9%) had a previous skull fracture or concussion compared with only 1% of men with lung cancer.[41] In addition, significantly larger numbers of the cases were known to have taken drugs associated with hyperprolactinaemia, suggesting that prolonged exposure to elevated prolactin might promote male breast cancer.

Radiation

As exposure of the breasts to ionizing irradiation has been shown to increase the risk of cancer, it has been suggested that a similar situation occurs in men exposed to either radiotherapy or repeated fluoroscopies in tuberculosis sufferers.[42] The available evidence, summarized in Table 19.4, does suggest that

Table 19.4 Radiation and risk of male breast cancer

Radiation type	Relative risk	Reference
Fluoroscopy	2.4	Casagrande et al[39]
Chest radiograph	1.0	Casagrande et al[39]
Radiotherapy	7.2	Olsson and Ronstam[41]
Abdominal/ pelvic	0.5	Lenfant-Pejovic et al[23]

repeated prolonged diagnostic X-ray exposures may be harmful, but that limited numbers of plain chest radiographs are not associated with any increase in risk.[23,39,41]

Radiotherapy was once used to 'treat' unilateral gynaecomastia and thymic enlargement with subsequent malignancy being described after a substantial delay.[43,44] Sasco concluded that in combination, there was an increased risk of between 1.6 and 1.9, but that other upper body radiographs were not associated with any significant increase.[11]

Familial breast cancer

In the meta-analysis of case-control studies, a family history of either male or female breast cancer in first-degree relatives was associated with a relative risk of 2.5, which suggests a genetic basis for some male breast cancers.[11] However, a first-degree family history is not common, being reported in 4–7% of men with breast cancer.[39–42] Kozak et al reported breast cancer in an uncle and a nephew and reviewed the 10 reported families at that time, concluding that, because 60% had female relatives with breast cancer, there was a joint increase in risk for both sexes in some families.[45]

Anderson and Badzioch examined the effect of a diagnosis of male breast cancer on risk for female relatives compared with that of women with female relatives with the disease.[46] There was a twofold increase in risk for both groups. Female relatives of men with prostatic cancer exhibited a fourfold increase in risk of breast cancer, suggesting a joint susceptibility to the two malignancies.

Now that the breast cancer susceptibility genes BRCA-1 and BRCA-2 have been identified there has been extensive activity to determine their relationship with male disease. Serova et al tested 20 breast ovarian cancer families, and reported BRCA-1 mutations in 16, one of which contained a case of male breast cancer.[47] However, Stratton et al looked for evidence of linkage in 22 families with at least one affected male and found no evidence of BRCA-1 mutations in any of the cases.[48]

Wooster et al localized the BRCA-2 gene to chromosome 13q12–13 and reported that, in the families with this mutation, there was an increased risk of male disease.[49] After determining the complete coding sequence of BRCA-2 on chromosome 13q, Tavtigian et al found specific mutations in several families with male breast cancer.[50]

Anelli et al, using a combination of immuno-histochemistry, polymerase chain reaction (PCR), single strand conformation polymorphism and DNA sequencing, examined tumours from 35 men with breast cancer, to determine the incidence of mutations of the tumour-suppressor gene p53.[51] Point mutations were found in 12 (41%), and overexpression of p53 protein in 2 (6%). However, in a series of 10 male cases, Seth et al found point mutations of p53 in only two, of which one was a silent mutation.[52]

Clinical features

Presenting features of males with breast cancer in the larger published series are shown in Table 19.5. As with females the most common symptom is a painless lump, which alone or with other problems occurs in 75% of cases. Pain is associated with a lump in only 5%.[37,53] As a result of the paucity of breast tissue in the male, nipple involvement is a relatively early event, with retraction in 9%, discharge in 6% and ulceration in 6%. Ulceration was separate from the nipple in half the cases. Paget's disease was rare, being the presenting feature in only 1%, with a mean age of 60, similar to that of other men with breast cancer.[54,55] This feature was associated with axillary nodal metastases in 58%, prompting Satiani to suggest that, as this was a bad prognostic feature, any man with nipple changes should have a biopsy to exclude Paget's disease.[56]

It was very rare for a man to present with an axillary nodal metastasis in the absence of a palpable breast lump. In almost all cases it was the patient rather than his doctor who found the lump, underlining the need to make men aware that any breast or nipple symptoms

Table 19.5 Presenting features of males with breast cancer

Lump	Nipple inversion	Ulcer	Nipple discharge	Paget's disease	Other	Nil	Reference
105	4	7	8	5	3	–	Treves and Holleb[4]
182	10	17	11	2	28	5	Scheike[5]
158	7	20	7	–	5	3	Ribeiro et al[37]
147	44	30	20	–	–	–	Stierer et al[12]
314	40	–	22	3	–	–	Cutuli et al[10]
906	**105**	**74**	**68**	**10**	**36**	**8**	**Total**
(75)	**(9)**	**(6)**	**(6)**	**(1)**	**(3)**	**(–)**	**(%)**

require evaluation. It is the ignorance of this that is responsible for the delay in men seeking medical attention for nipple or breast problems, with the consequent worsening of their prognosis.

Stage at presentation

The rarity of male breast cancer, and therefore the low index of suspicion of both patients and their doctors, is in part responsible for the greater likelihood of men being diagnosed with more advanced disease. This is exemplified in Table 19.6 which gives the distribution of TNM stages in the larger reported series.[5,8,37,54]

It can be seen that 55% of men present with stage I/II disease and 45% with stage III/IV. This means that overall men will have a worse prognosis than women as a substantial proportion have advanced disease at the time of diagnosis. After adjusting for stage at presentation, however, the prognosis for both sexes is similar provided that optimal treatment is given.

Histology

As the male breast tissue is rudimentary, it does not usually undergo lobule formation. Thus the

Table 19.6 TNM stage at presentation of male breast cancer

I	II	III	IV	Reference
89	28	107	29	Scheike[5]
76	38	55	41	Ribeiro et al[37]
55	37	33	14	Ramantanis et al[8]
26	36	25	17	van Geel et al[54]
246	**139**	**220**	**101**	**Total**
(35)	**(20)**	**(31)**	**(14)**	**(%)**

predominant histological type of malignancy is invasive ductal. This type of cancer forms 87% of all male breast tumours, as is shown in the four large histopathological series summarized in Table 19.7.[4,5,8,55] Rare tumours are invasive papillomas (5%) and medullary (4%).

Lobular carcinoma of the male breast has been reported not only in cases of Klinefelter's syndrome,[57] but also in genotypically normal men with no prior history of oestrogen exposure or gynaecomastia.[58,59] This is, however, a very rare variant which may be

Table 19.7 Histopathological types of male breast cancer

Invasive ductal	Invasive papilloma	Mucoid	Medullary	Tubular	Lobular	DCIS	Reference
96	5	–	2	–	–	7	Treves and Holleb[4]
157	5	5	4	–	–	5	Scheike[5]
67	4	1	–	1	–	4	Heller et al[55]
113	9	–	14	–	–	–	Ramantanis et al[8]
443	**23**	**6**	**20**	**1**	**0**	**16**	**Total**
(87)	**(5)**	**(1)**	**(4)**			**(3)**	**(%)**

Table 19.8 Bloom and Richardson histological grade of male breast cancers

Grade I	Grade II	Grade III	Reference
44	129	50	Cutuli et al[10]
11	53	31	Stierer et al[12]
44	81	25	Visfeldt and Scheike[61]
99	**263**	**106**	**Total**
(21)	**(56)**	**(23)**	**(%)**

associated with lobular carcinoma in situ (LCIS). Ductal carcinoma in situ of the male breast is slightly more common, but comprises only 3% of all cases.

The recent large series reporting Bloom and Richardson grade[60] are shown in Table 19.8, which indicates that less than one-quarter of classified male tumours are grade III.[10,12,61]

Oestrogen receptors

As there is a relationship between Bloom and Richardson grade and oestrogen receptor (ER)

status, with grade III cancers being more likely to be ER negative, it would be expected that most male tumours would be ER positive. Large series have reported that about 80% of male breast cancers were ER positive, with 77% being progesterone receptor (PR) positive.[10,12] Not only were most tumours positive but the levels of measured ER/PR were also high. As about 60% of female tumours are ER positive this does imply that men are more likely to respond to endocrine therapy. When the binding specificity and properties of ER and PR were examined in male tumours, their characteristics were found to be similar to those in female cancers.[62] In studies that have measured other receptors it was found that, although c-erbB-2 proto-oncogene was present in 95% of male tumours, this did not have prognostic significance,[63] nor did cathepsin D expression.[64] Hatschek et al conducted an archival study of 85 male cancers and examined outcome in relation to DNA content and S phase, but without a relationship between S-phase fraction and outcome being found.[65]

Treatment

Although it is possible to obtain guidance from results of clinical trials of treatment in female disease, the rarity of male breast cancer means

Table 19.9 Five-year survival percentage after different primary treatments for operable male breast cancer

Total mast		Total + RT		Radical mastectomy		Radical + RT		Reference
Stage		Stage		Stage		Stage		
I	II	I	II	I	II	I	II	
				83	13			Crichlow[43]
				100	64			Donegan and Perez-Mesa[67]
63		58		67	82			Scheike[5]
					77	38		van Geel et al[54]
71	36			77	83			Ramantanis et al[8]
				91	63			Carlsson et al[6]
				88	55			Axelsson and Andersson[68]
67	**36**	**58**	**–**	**85**	**38**	**80**	**38**	**Total (%)**

that no prospective randomized trials have been conducted. The larger published series therefore need to be studied with care, because many have combined patients with disparate stages of disease treated in a variety of ways. For those with operable disease, mastectomy was the most frequent procedure, with only 10–13% being treated by local excision.[10,12,66] Those series in which outcome has been specified in relation to type of primary treatment are shown in Table 19.9.[5,8,43,54,67,68]

This suggests that there is a better survival in those who have more extensive local treatment, but it is not possible to be sure because frailer patients may have been selected for simple, rather than radical, mastectomy. It does assuredly show the significantly worse prognosis in those with axillary node involvement (stage II). Nowadays, most male patients receive postoperative radiotherapy, which was given to 62% of those in Cutuli's series[10] and 80% of those reported by Guinee et al.[66]

Both adjuvant tamoxifen[69] and chemotherapy[70] have been given to men with breast cancer and, as with women, tamoxifen is more frequently prescribed. This is logical in male disease because about 80% will have ER-positive tumours. Extrapolating from results of adjuvant trials in female breast cancer, it is likely that ER-positive cases have a better relapse-free survival if given endocrine therapy and patients with ER-negative tumours with nodal involvement will fare better if given chemotherapy.[71]

Outcome

In a French series comprising 397 cases, Cutuli examined the prognosis of men with T1, T2, and T3–4 tumours.[10] The results, which are shown in Fig. 19.1, demonstrate the inverse relationship between increasing T size and probability of survival, the 10-year relapse-free survival of those with T1 tumours being 74% compared with only 34% in those with T3–4 cancers.

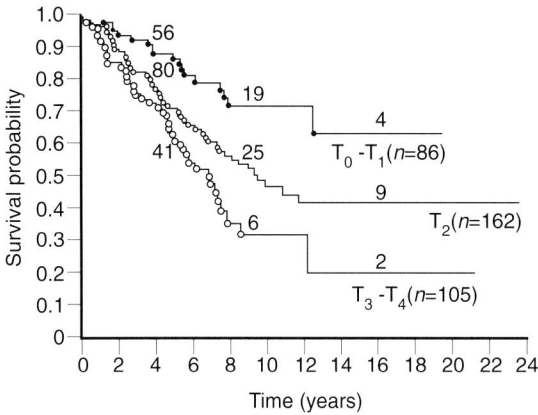

Fig. 19.1 Survival in relation to T size in males with breast cancer. (From Cutuli et al.[10])

Table 19.10 Clinical tumour size, axillary nodal histology and survival in males with breast cancer

Clinical tumour size (cm)	Number	Node positive (%)	5-year survival rate (%)
≤ 1	23	30	94
1.1–2	87	39	80
2.1–3	55	53	78
3.1–4	38	45	81
4.1–5	26	65	41
>5	28	71	39

From Guinee et al.[66]

Guinee et al analysed the outcome in relation to potential prognostic factors in 335 cases of male breast cancer.[66] The 5-year survival rate in relation to clinical size of primary tumour is shown in Table 19.10. This indicates the good survival of those with tumours up to 1 cm (94% alive), the similar survival for those with cancers 1.1–2, 2.1–3, 3.1–4, and the poor survival in those with lesions greater than 4.1 cm (40%). In addition, the incidence of axillary nodal involvement is shown in tumours of this size range. Even in those patients with tumours up to 1 cm, 30% had nodal involvement, rising to over 70% in those with cancers larger than 5.1 cm.

For patients with histologically negative nodes the 10-year survival rate was 84%, which fell to 44% in those with one to three involved nodes and 14% in the group with four or more positive nodes. In a multivariate analysis the presence of clinically palpable axillary nodes increased the risk of death from breast cancer twofold, as did a 3 cm difference in tumour diameter. The risk of dying was almost seven times greater in men with four or more involved nodes compared with those having negative nodes. These data underline the need to know the axillary nodal status in males with breast cancer. Axillary dissection should therefore form an intrinsic part of the surgical treatment, in order that those with a need for adjuvant treatment can be identified and also the most effective form of therapy can be selected.

In a recent study of male breast cancer, Willsher et al compared the outcome in 41 male patients compared with 123 female cases, matched for age, tumour size, grade and pathological nodal status.[72] The 5-year relapse-free survival rate of both groups was 50%. This adds further support to the view that the disease is the same in both sexes, when matched stage for stage. Delay in diagnosis, and hence increased tumour size and higher stage, are the reasons for a worse prognosis in some males with breast cancer.

Future work

It is likely that the improvements in adjuvant therapy which have occurred in female disease, will permeate through to the management of male breast cancer, with therapies being selected on a basis of the tumour type, grade, ER status and axillary nodal status. Local surgical treatment is likely to be by modified radical mastectomy rather than breast conservation. It is assumed that loss of the nipple will have no impact on the psychosocial adjustment of the male with breast cancer but no studies have been conducted on this topic. What is most important is that the concept of surgical minimalism does not spread to the treatment of invasive cancer in the male. The axilla should be dissected, in order to give the patient a more accurate assessment of his prognosis, which for some will be excellent.

For those with some nodal involvement (one to three) or tumours greater than 1 cm, some form of adjuvant treatment will be necessary. Among those with four or more nodes, a good case could be made for testing experimental by more aggressive therapies because these individuals have such a poor prognosis. To a large extent axillary nodal involvement is related to size of primary tumour and to delay in seeking medical advice. Probably the most important factor that could improve the prognosis for male breast cancer is prevention of ignorance. In the league of diseases that afflict males, breast cancer is in the fourth division but, nevertheless, knowledge that it can occur and the need for investigation of lumps could lead to the prevention of unnecessary deaths from this rare disease.

SYNOPSIS

- Male breast cancer is a rare disease, often with late presentation because men are unaware of the possibility of malignancy.
- There are wide international variations in incidence with European males comprising less than 1% of breast cancer cases rising to 15% in Zambia.
- Prior testicular injury, hepatic damage from bilharziasis, Klinefelter's syndrome or exposure to oestrogens increase risk but in most cases there is no detectable endocrine abnormality.
- Most male breast cancers are ductal in origin and most are oestrogen receptor positive.
- Treatment is by modified radical mastectomy and chest wall irradiation if the tumour is extensive with adjuvant tamoxifen for men with tumours larger than 1 cm diameter.
- Stage for stage the prognosis of breast cancer is similar in both males and females.

REFERENCES

1. Williams WR. Cancer of the male breast, based on the records of one hundred cases: with remarks. *Lancet* 1889; **ii**: 261–3.
2. Wainwright DIM. Carcinoma of the male breast. *Arch Surg* 1927; **14**: 836–60.
3. Sachs MD. Carcinoma of the male breast. *Radiology* 1941; **37**: 458–67.
4. Treves N, Holleb AJ. Cancer of the male breast. A report of 146 cases. *Cancer* 1955; **8**: 1239–50.
5. Scheike O. Male breast cancer. *Acta Pathol Microbiol Scand* 1975; **Suppl 251**: 1–33.
6. Carlsson G, Hafstrom L, Jonsson P. Male breast cancer. *Clin Oncol* 1981; **7**: 149–55.
7. Borgen PI, Wong GY, Vlamis V et al. Current management of male breast cancer: a review of 104 cases. *Ann Surg* 1992; **215**: 451–7.
8. Ramantanis G, Besbeas S, Garas JG. Breast cancer in the male: a report of 138 cases. *World J Surg* 1980; **4**: 621–4.
9. Gough DB, Donohue JH, Evans MM et al. A 50–year experience of male breast cancer: is outcome changing? *Surg Oncol* 1993; **2**: 325–33.
10. Cutuli B, Lacroze M, Dilhuydy JM et al. Male breast cancer: results of the treatments and prognostic factors in 397 cases. *Eur J Cancer* 1995; **31A**: 1960–4.
11. Sasco AJ, Lowenfels AB, Pasker De Jong P. Epidemiology of male breast cancer. A meta-analysis of published case-control studies and discussion of selected aetiological factors. *Int J Cancer* 1993; **53**: 539–49.
12. Stierer M, Rosen H, Weitensfelder W et al. Male breast cancer: Austrian experience. *World J Surg.* 1995; **19**: 687–93.

13. El-Gazayerli MM, Abdel-Aziz AS. On bilharziasis and male breast cancer in Egypt: a preliminary report and review of the literature. *Br J Cancer* 1963; **17:** 566–71.

14. Ojara EA. Carcinoma of the male breast in Mulaga Hospital in Kampala. *East Afr Med J* 1978; **55:** 489–91.

15. Bhagwandin SS. Carcinoma of the male breast in Zambia. *East Afr Med J* 1972; **49:** 176–9.

16. Waterhouse J, Muir C, Correa P, Powell JR, eds. *Cancer Incidence in Five Continents*, Vol 3. Lyon: IARC Science Publishers, 1976; 15.

17. Steinitz R, Katz L, Ben-Hur M. Male breast cancer in Israel: selected epidemiologic aspects. *J Med Sci* 1981; **17:** 816–21.

18. Mabuchi K, Bross DS, Kessler II. Risk factors for male breast cancer. *J Natl Cancer Inst* 1985; **74:** 371–5.

19. Nydick M, Bustos J, Dale JH et al. Gynaecomastia in adolescent boys. *JAMA* 1961; **178:** 449–54.

20. Williams MJ. Gynaecomastia. Its incidence and host characterisation in 447 autopsy cases. *Am J Med* 1963; **34:** 103–17.

21. Nuttal FQ. Gynaecomastia as a physical finding in normal men. *J Clin Endocrinol Metab* 1979; **48:** 338–40.

22. McLaughlin JK, Malker BR, Blot WJ et al. Occupational risks for male breast cancer in Sweden. *Br J Indust Med* 1988; **45:** 275–6.

23. Lenfant-Pejovic M-H, Mlika-Cabanne N, Bouchardy C et al. Risk factors for male breast cancer: a Franco-Swiss case-control study. *Int J Cancer* 1990; **45:** 661–5.

24. Tynes T, Andersen A. Electromagnetic fields and male breast cancer. *Lancet* 1990; **336:** 1596.

25. Demers PA, Thomas DB, Rosenblatt KA. Occupational exposure to electromagnetic fields and breast cancer in men. *Am J Epidemiol* 1991; **134:** 340–7.

26. Loomis DP. Cancer of breast among men in electrical occupations. *Lancet* 1992; **339:** 1482–3.

27. McClure JA, Higgins CC. Bilateral carcinoma of male breast after estrogen therapy. *JAMA* 1951; **146:** 7–9.

28. Schlappack OK, Braun O, Maier U. Report of two cases of male breast cancer after prolonged estrogen treatment for prostatic carcinoma. *Cancer Det Prev* 1986; **9:** 319–22.

29. Drelichman A, Amer M, Pontes E et al. Carcinoma of prostate metastatic to breast. *Urology* 1980; **16:** 250–5.

30. Symmers WSC. Carcinoma of breast in transsexual individuals after surgical and hormonal interference with the primary and secondary sex characteristics. *BMJ* 1968; **2:** 83–5.

31. Pritchard TJ, Pankowsky DA, Crowe JP et al. Breast cancer in a male-to-female transsexual. *JAMA* 1988; **259:** 2278–80.

32. Jackson AW, Muldal S, Ockey CH et al. Carcinoma of male breast in association with the Klinefelter syndrome. *BMJ* 1965; **1:** 223–5.

33. Nadel M, Koss LG. Klinefelter's syndrome and male breast cancer. *Lancet* 1967; **ii:** 366.

34. Harnden DG, Maclean N, Langlands AO. Carcinoma of the breast and Klinefelter's syndrome. *J Med Gen* 1971; **8:** 460–1.

35. Thomas DB, Jimenez LM, McTiernan A et al. Breast cancer in men: risk factors with hormonal implications. *Am J Epidemiol* 1992; **135:** 734–48.

36. Calabresi E, De Guili A, Becciolini P et al. Plasma estrogens and androgens in male breast cancer. *J Steroid Biochem* 1976; **7:** 605–9.

37. Ribeiro GG, Phillips HU, Skinner LG. Serum oestradiol-17β, testosterone, luteinising hormone and follicle-stimulating hormone in males with breast cancer. *Br J Cancer* 1980; **41:** 474–7.

38. Nirmul D, Pegogaro RJ, Jialal I et al. The sex hormone profile of male patients with breast cancer. *Br J Cancer* 1982; **48:** 423–7.

39. Casagrande JT, Hanisch R, Pike MC et al. A case-control study of male breast cancer. *Cancer Res* 1988; **48:** 1326–30.

40. Olsson H, Alm P, Kristofferson U et al. Hypophyseal tumor and gynecomastia preceding bilateral breast cancer development in a man. *Cancer* 1984; **53:** 1974–7.

41. Olsson H, Ranstam J. Head trauma and exposure to prolactin-elevating drugs as risk factors for male breast cancer. *J Natl Cancer Inst* 1988; **80:** 679–83.

42. Schottenfeld D, Lilienfeld AM, Diamond H. Some observations on the epidemiology of breast cancer among males. *Am J Public Health* 1963; **53:** 890–7.

43. Crichlow RW. Carcinoma of the male breast. *Surg Gynecol Obstet* 1972; **134:** 1011–19.

44. Lowell DM, Martineau RG, Luria SB. Carcinoma of the male breast following radiation. *Cancer* 1968; **22:** 581–6.

45. Kozak FR, Hall JG, Baird PA. Familial breast cancer in men. *Cancer* 1986; **58:** 2736–9.

46. Anderson DE, Badzioch MD. Breast cancer risks in relatives of male breast cancer patients. *J Natl Cancer Inst* 1992; **84:** 1114–17.

47. Serova O, Montagna M, Torchard D et al. A high incidence of BRCA-1 mutations in 20 breast-ovarian cancer families. *Am J Hum Genet* 1996; **58:** 42–51.

48. Stratton MR, Ford D, Neuhasen S et al. Familial male breast cancer is not linked to the BRCA-1 locus on chromosome 17q. *Nature Genet* 1994; **7:** 103–7.

49. Wooster R, Neuhausen SL, Mangion J et al. Localization of a breast cancer susceptibility gene (BRCA2) to chromosome 13q12–13. *Science* 1994; **265:** 2088–90.

50. Tavtigian SV, Simard J, Rommens J et al. The complete BRCA-2 gene and mutations in chromosome 13q-linked kindreds. *Nat Genet* 1996; **12:** 333–7.

51. Anelli A, Anelli TF, Youngson B et al. Mutations of the p53 gene in male breast cancer. *Cancer* 1995; **75:** 2233–8.

52. Seth A, Mariano J, Metcalf R et al. Relative paucity of p53 gene mutations in male breast carcinomas. *Int J Oncol* 1993; **2:** 739–44.

53. Yap HY, Tashima CK, Blumenschein GR et al. Male breast cancer. A natural history study. *Cancer* 1979; **44:** 748–54.

54. van Geel AN, van Slooten EA, Mavrunac M et al. A retrospective study of male breast cancer in Holland. *Br J Surg* 1985; **72:** 724–7.

55. Heller KS, Rosen PP, Schottenfeld D et al. Male breast cancer: a clinicopathologic study of 97 cases. *Ann Surg* 1978; **188:** 60–5.

56. Satiani B, Powell BW, Matthews WH. Paget's disease of the male breast. *Arch Surg* 1977; **112:** 587–92.

57. Sanchez AG, Villanueva AG, Redondo C. Lobular carcinoma of the breast in a patient with Klinefelter's syndrome. *Cancer* 1986; **57:** 1181–3.

58. Nance KVA, Reddick RL. In situ and infiltrating carcinoma of the male breast. *Hum Pathol* 1989; **20:** 1220–2.

59. Michaels BM, Nunn CR, Roses DF. Lobular carcinoma of the male breast. *Surgery* 1994; **115:** 402–5.

60. Bloom HJG, Richardson WW. Histological grading and prognosis in breast cancer. *Br J Cancer* 1957; **11:** 359–77.

61. Visfeldt J, Scheike O. Male breast cancer. 1. Histologic typing and grading of 187 Danish cases. *Cancer* 1973; **32:** 985–90.

62. Duffy MJ, Duffy GJ. Multiple steroid receptors in male breast cancer. *Clin Chim Acta* 1978; **85:** 211–14.

63. Blin N, Kardas I, Welter C et al. Expression of the c-erbB2 proto-oncogene in male breast cancer: lack of prognostic significance. *Oncology* 1993; **50:** 408–11.

64. Rogers S, Day CA, Fox SB. Expression of cathepsin D and estrogen receptor in male breast carcinoma. *Hum Pathol* 1993; **24:** 148–51.

65. Hatschek T, Wingren, Cartensen J et al. DNA content and S-phase fraction in male breast carcinomas. *Acta Oncol* 1994; **33:** 609–13.

66. Guinee VF, Olsson H, Moller T et al. The prognosis of breast cancer in males. A report of 335 cases. *Cancer* 1993; **71:** 154–61.

67. Donegan WL, Perez-Mesa CM. Carcinoma of the male breast. *Arch Surg* 1973; **106:** 273–9.

68. Axelsson J, Andersson A. Cancer of the male breast. *World J Surg* 1983; **7:** 281–7.

69. Ribeiro G, Smudeh R. Adjuvant tamoxifen for male breast cancer. *Br J Cancer* 1985; **65:** 252–4.

70. Patel HZ, Buzdar AU, Hortobagyi GN. Role of adjuvant chemotherapy in male breast cancer. *Cancer* 1989; **64:** 1583–5.

71. Scottish Breast Cancer Trials Group and ICRF Breast Unit, Guy's Hospital. Adjuvant ovarian ablation versus CMF chemotherapy in premenopausal women with pathological stage II breast cancer: the Scottish Trial. *Lancet* 1993; **341:** 1293–8.

72. Willsher PC, Leach IH, Ellis IO et al. A comparison outcome of male breast cancer with female breast cancer. *Am J Surg* 1997; **173:** 185–8.

20

Unusual presentations

And I will show you something different

TS Eliot

Paget's disease of the nipple • Bilateral breast cancer

PAGET'S DISEASE OF THE NIPPLE

Although Velpeau was the first to describe an eczematous disease of the nipple,[1] it was Sir James Paget's clear description in 1874 that gave the condition its eponymous title:[2]

> I believe it has not yet been published that certain chronic affections of the skin of the nipple and areola are very often succeeded by the formation of scirrhous cancer in the mammary gland. I have seen about 15 cases in which this has happened and the events were in all of them so similar that one description may suffice.
>
> The patients were all women various in age from 40 to 60 or more years, having in common nothing remarkable but their disease. In all of them the disease began as an eruption on the nipple and areola. In the majority it had the appearance of a florid, intensely red, raw surface, very finely granular, as if nearly the whole thickness of the epidermis were removed: like the surface of a very acute diffuse eczema, or like that of an acute balanitis.

It was Paget's hypothesis that chronic inflammation on the nipple might predispose to malignancy because he had seen male patients with chronic balanitis who subsequently developed penile cancer. Histogenetic studies have changed our perception of Paget's disease but it is a rare serious problem for which mastectomy may still be necessary.

Presentation

Paget's disease comprises about 2% of all cases of breast cancer. The red raw appearance of the nipple and areola described by Paget's disease can resemble either eczema or psoriasis. It may be associated with a serous exudate and itching or burning. The nipple may become inverted. An example is shown in Fig. 20.1.

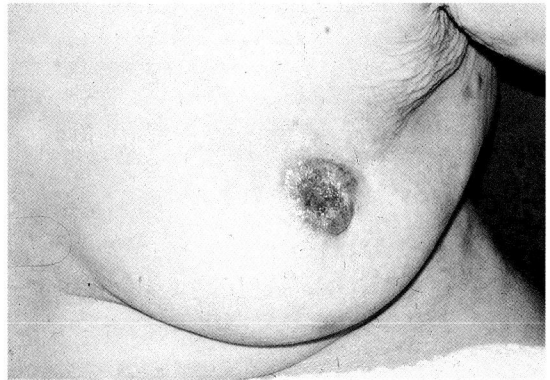

Fig. 20.1 Paget's disease of the nipple.

Table 20.1 Presenting features and underlying histology in Paget's disease

Cases	Paget's disease alone		Paget's disease + lump		Microscopic evidence	Reference
	DCIS	IBC	DCIS	IBC		
23	6	1	–	11	5	Kay[3]
53	18 (1)	2	2	30	–	Nance et al[4]
209	63	33	7	86	20	Ashikari et al[5]
35	14	9	–	11	–	Chaudary et al[6]
Total (%)	34	15	3	48		

DCIS, ductal carcinoma in situ; IBC, invasive breast cancer.

True Paget's disease is nipple pathology preceding any palpable lump but most series have included cases with palpable lumps and others in whom microscopic evidence of Paget's disease was found after mastectomy for a palpable cancer. Those series that correlated clinical presentation and underlying histology are summarized in Table 20.1.[3–6]

Omitting cases that were found on microscopic examination of the nipple, approximately equal proportions presented with and without a lump. When there was nipple erosion without a lump, one-third of cases had an invasive breast cancer (IBC) and two-thirds had ductal carcinoma in situ (DCIS) alone. In contrast, when there was a palpable lump only 6% had DCIS and the remainder were IBC.

In the absence of a lump the main clinical dilemma is making the diagnosis and not dismissing the nipple eruption as being part of a generalized eczema or psoriasis. In a patient with known skin disease who has Paget-like changes on the nipple, a short course of topical steroids may clear the eczema. However, caution has to be exercised because Paget's disease may heal spontaneously. In a series of 58 patients treated in Nottingham, there was healing in 10 (17%).[7] Thus it is safest to carry out a biopsy under local anaesthesia taking a small wedge of representative skin.

Histogenesis

The histological description of Paget's disease was given originally by Darier in 1889.[8] The pathognomic feature is the presence of large clear (ballooned) cells within the epidermis, as shown in Fig. 20.2. For many years the origin of Paget's cells was in dispute. Darier believed that they were epidermal cells that had undergone dyskeratosis. After examining specimens of Paget's disease from Indian patients, Orr and Parish concluded that the cells were part of a general epidermal disorganization and were non-malignant degenerated melanocytes.[9]

Cheatle and Cutler proposed that they were premalignant epidermal cells[10] whereas Willis postulated that they were malignant cells that had arisen within the nipple skin.[11] In contrast, Muir[12] and Inglis[13] suggested that Paget's cells were derived from mammary epithelium that had migrated. Sadly all these distinguished pathologists based their theories on morphology, a blunt instrument, only much later sharpened by the advent of immunohistochemistry.

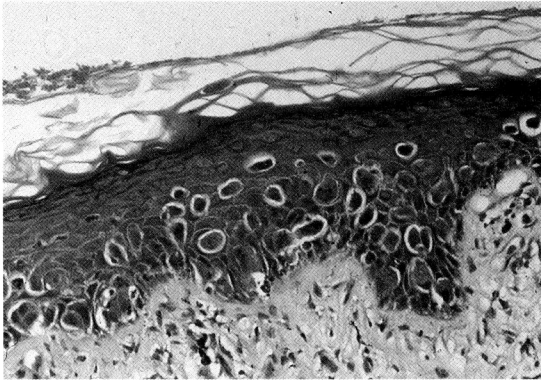

Fig. 20.2 Histological appearance of Paget's disease of the nipple showing characteristic ballooned cells.

Table 20.2 Immunohistochemical characterization of mammary Paget's disease (MPD) and extramammary Paget's (EPD)

Antibody	MPD	EPD	Reference
Casein	14/16	4/4	Bussolati and Pich[14]
CEA	7/7	16/16	Nadji et al[15]
CEA	0/6	2/7	Vanstapel et al[16]
HMFG	6/6	5/7	
Keratin 8	13/13	–	Chaudary et al[6]
Keratin 10	0/13		
Keratin 19	13/13 (weak)		
p53	4/12	0/5	Kanitakis et al[17]
Keratin 8	25/25		
Keratin 19	0/25		
c-erbB-2	24/25		
c-erbB-2	6/6	8/28	De Potter et al[18]
nm23	5/6	8/28	
GCDFP-15	2/6	11/28	
pS2	2/6	13/28	
p53	3/6	11/28	

Immunohistochemistry

As polyclonal and monoclonal antibodies were raised against specific cellular antigens, this enabled pathologists to distinguish between cells of similar morphology but different origin. Bussolati and Pich used a polyclonal antibody against human casein together with an immunoperoxidase technique to examine 16 cases of mammary Paget's disease (MPD) and four with the extramammary form (EPD).[14] As is shown in Table 20.2, there was staining in most of MPD cases and in all EPD specimens. The Paget's cells could not be distinguished from basal epidermal cells. Nadji et al investigated the presence of carcinoembryonic antigen (CEA) in seven MPD and 16 EPD cases.[15] There was staining of all Paget's cells and Nadji postulated that they were derived from apocrine or eccrine glands within the skin.

Using antibodies against CEA and human milk fat globule (HMFG) membrane antigen, Vanstapel et al examined both MPD and EPD.[16] All the mammary cases were positive for anti-HMFG, positive for polyclonal CEA but negative for monoclonal CEA. As some of the EPD stained with anti-HMFG it was postulated that the cells were eccrine. Chaudary et al used a panel of antibodies raised against cytokeratins 8, 10 and 19.[6] The Paget's cells stained strongly for keratin 8, less strongly for 19, and not at all for keratin 10. This phenotype was consistent with a mammary luminal cell origin, and was unlike that of keratinocytes.

There was no p53 protein expression found in EPD but staining of some MPD specimens in the study of Kanitakis et al who concluded that MPD cells arose from an underlying adenocarcinoma.[17] De Potter et al showed similar results to those of Chaudary et al and also reported that almost all MPD cells stained with c-erbB-2 antibody.[18] They postulated that epidermal keratinocytes released a chemotactic factor which attracted cells over-producing c-erbB-2 into the epidermis.

The immunotypes of 34 cases of MPD and 28 of EPD were determined by Nakamura et al, using a panel of antibodies recognizing c-erbB-2, nm23 (a marker of low metastatic potential), ps2 (an oestrogen-related protein), p53 and GCDFP-15 (derived from gross cyst disease fluid).[19] There was ubiquitous expression of c-erbB-2 in MPD but in only 28% of EPD. The marker nm23 was present in most cases of MPD and 28% of EPD cases. Gross cystic disease protein was found in similar proportions of MPD and EPD.

Cohen et al compared the immunostaining of 20 cases of MPD with the underlying invasive or non-invasive carcinoma, using antibodies to cytokeratins, epithelial membrane antigen, CEA, κ-casein, α-lactalbumin.[20] There was a similar immunoprofile in 18 of 20 (90%) cases strongly suggesting a similar origin for Paget's cells and the underlying carcinoma in most cases of MPD.

Table 20.3 Axillary nodal involvement in patients with Paget's disease and a palpable lump

Number	Node positive	Reference
12	8	Culberson and Hom[22]
16	11	Kay[3]
12	8	Ridenhour et al[23]
13	10	Rissanen and Holsti[24]
18	9	Nance et al[4]
113	74	Ashikari et al[5]
38	25	Kister and Haagensen[25]
11	5	Chaudary[6]
233	**150 (64%)**	**Total**

Prognosis

Paget's disease encompasses at least two groups of patients whose prognosis is very different. If associated with DCIS the outlook is excellent with an almost 100% cure rate. However, even in the absence of a lump there will be an underlying invasive cancer in almost one-third of cases. Taking just those patients with Paget's disease and an impalpable invasive cancer, there was axillary nodal involvement in 40% of cases.[5,6,21] As Table 20.3 shows, this rises to 64% if there is a palpable lump.

It was customary to define prognosis in MPD in relation to the presence or absence of a palpable lump, but it is more realistic to divide cases into DCIS and IBC and in the latter group to relate outcome to nodal status. Maier et al reported that, in a series of premenopausal women with Paget's disease the 5-year survival for the node-negative cases was 55% whereas none of the node-positive cases survived for 5 years.[26] In the postmenopausal woman the 5-year survival rates were 96% and 33% respectively.

Others have reported a 10-year overall survival rate of 44–79% in the node-negative cases and 10–20% in the node-positive cases.[5,6,27]

This suggests that invasive cancer presenting as Paget's disease does not carry a good prognosis and it is best to be circumspect about prognosis until full histological information is available.

Surgery

After obtaining a histological diagnosis of Paget's disease, in the absence of a palpable lump most surgeons would order mammography because this might give an indication of the underlying pathology. Unfortunately this is not always useful. In a series of 48 cases of Paget's disease, without a lump, Dixon et al reported that no mammographically suspicious lesion was seen in 43%.[28]

It is essential that a tissue diagnosis is obtained because other rare lesions such as a nipple adenoma or basal cell carcinoma may masquerade as MPD. Although basal cell carcinoma typically has a raised indurated pearly edge, it may look like Paget's disease. Treatment is by wide local excision of affected skin, not by mastectomy.[29] Adenoma of the nipple may cause nipple discharge, crusting and sometimes an associated lump, with or without a burning sensation, all of which can be symptoms and signs of MPD. The lesion is entirely benign but treatment is by excision and it is sometimes necessary to remove the nipple.[30]

There are no randomized trials to guide us in selecting treatment for Paget's disease which means that strongly held opinions cannot be countered with solid evidence. Erring on the side of safety, a mastectomy probably carries the best chance of cure, particularly if the disease is non-invasive. As a result of the uncertainty about the nature of the underlying malignancy, it has been the policy at Guy's Hospital to recommend a modified radical mastectomy. In part this was because in a series of 35 cases, 20% had a cancer away from the areola, 70% of which were in the upper outer quadrant.[6] Thus a cone excision of the nipple and areola will not necessarily succeed in removing the underlying cause.

In a series of ten cases treated by cone excision, recurrence occurred in four, of whom one had Paget's disease in the scar but three had invasive cancer (two with nodal involvement) and so the authors suggested that a mastectomy rather than breast conservation should be the treatment of choice. Fourquet et al treated 20 patients with MPD by radiotherapy alone (17) or cone excision (three cases).[31] After a median follow-up of 7.5 years relapse occurred in three cases (15%), each of which had Paget's disease without invasive disease.

Stockdale et al reported a series of 28 patients with MPD, treated by irradiation, of whom nine (32%) had an associated palpable lump.[32] After a median follow-up of 5 years, there was a recurrence in three of 19 (16%) of those without a palpable lump or mammographic abnormality. Of the nine with a lump or mammographic abnormality, relapse occurred in eight (89%), and death from breast cancer in five (56%). This suggests a very limited role for radiotherapy in patients with Paget's disease and a lump. Some selected cases may be successfully treated by a combination of cone excision and radiotherapy, but modified radical mastectomy with recon-

struction may give the best chance of long-term control with some preservation of body image.

BILATERAL BREAST CANCER

Some 1.5% of breast cancer cases present with bilateral synchronous disease and, every year thereafter, about 1% of the others will develop metachronous lesion. Synchronous breast cancers are defined as those diagnosed within 6 months of each other, metachronous as cancers presenting more than 6 months after a first primary has been diagnosed. As a result of their increased risk breast cancer patients are advised to undergo regular follow-up examinations and mammograms. This ties up substantial resources. If those at increased risk of bilateral disease could be identified, a better targeted follow-up regimen might be implemented. Alternatively women at high risk could be advised to undergo bilateral mastectomy.

Synchronous breast cancers

When Leis et al reviewed the literature on bilateral disease in 1965 they reported a range of incidence of synchronous cancers from 0.1 to 2% (mean 0.8%).[33] In more recent studies synchronous breast cancers were diagnosed in 1.7%,[34,35] the reason for the increase being the detection of impalpable contralateral lesions by mammography. De la Rochefordière et al reported a large series of 149 patients with synchronous bilateral cancers and showed that there were more positive correlations between the two tumours than would have been expected by chance alone.[36]

Cancers were more likely to be of the same histological grade, similar ER and PR status, with an over-representation of lobular carcinomas which comprised 6% of cases. Breast conservation therapy had been used in over half the cases. At a median follow-up of 68 months the overall survival rate was 86%. After matching for maximum stage there was a similar survival for simultaneous bilateral and unilateral cases.

The standard treatment was bilateral mastectomy but, because of the major potential

Table 20.4 Risk factors for contralateral breast cancer derived from case-control and cohort studies

Number	Follow-up (months)	Young age	Lobular cancer	Adjuvant chemotherapy	Breast RT	Reference
136/4550	52	1	2.0	0.56	1.2	Bernstein et al[42]
655/1189	>60	1.6	–	–	1.33	Boice et al[43]
77/1624	95	1.3	–	0.54	–	Solin et al[38]
282/4748	80	1.4	1.7	0.5	–	Prior and Waterhouse[39]
234/234	35	1.7	1.5	0.6	1.9	Adami et al[40]

RT, radiotherapy.

psychological impact of this change in body image, attempts have been made to treat bilateral disease by conservation therapy. When there are synchronous cancers, the problem of midline overlap is less problematic but nevertheless a large field is required.

Kopelson et al reported 11 synchronous cases treated by irradiation focusing on the problem of the large amount of normal tissue that has to be included in the radiation fields.[37] Irradiation of the internal mammary chain will also spill over onto the anterior pericardium and lung so that to reduce morbidity electrons need to be used. Another series of 11 simultaneous bilateral cases was treated by irradiation at Fox Chase Cancer Center.[38] The 5-year relapse-free survival rate was 74% in the bilateral cases and 72% in matched patients with unilateral disease. No serious complications of bilateral breast irradiation were reported.

Magnitude of risk

In a population-based survey from the Birmingham Regional Cancer Registry, Prior and Waterhouse reported the incidence of contralateral breast cancers in 21 969 patients followed for more than 90 000 women years.[39] A total of 399 contralateral cancers was diagnosed, and this represented a threefold increase in risk compared with the normal population. After exclusion of synchronous lesions the relative risk fell to 2.4, but this was not evenly distributed with age of patients. The relative risk (RR) of those aged 15–44 at diagnosis of first tumour was 5.3, for those 45–59, it was 3.0 and among those aged over 60 it was unity.

Similar results were found by Adami et al in a population-based case-control study of 1351 Swedish breast cancer cases and an equal number of controls.[40] The overall relative risk for the breast cancer cases was 3, but in women aged under 50 it was 10, compared with 2 in those aged over 50 years. A Danish study of 56 237 breast cancer cases, of whom 1840 developed non-simultaneous cancers, found an overall relative risk of 2.8.[41] After 10 years of follow-up those who had been irradiated had a higher risk than the non-irradiated (RR = 2.6 vs 2.0).

After these early findings, several case-control and cohort studies have used multivariate analyses to determine risk factors for contralateral breast cancer, and these are outlined in Table 20.4. Bernstein et al conducted a prospective cohort study of 4550 breast cancer cases participating in the Cancer and Steroid Hormone (CASH) study.[42] There were 136 metachronous cancers and the significant risk factors were prior benign breast biopsy (RR = 1.7), and invasive lobular primary tumour (RR = 2). Those who received adjuvant chemotherapy had a diminished relative risk of 0.56. There was no significant effect of breast irradiation.

In a case-control study from Connecticut, Boice et al compared 655 women with metachronous cancers and 1189 matched controls who had breast cancer but no second primary.[43] The main objective was to examine the influence of breast irradiation on contralateral risk. Of those who survived 10 years there was a small but significant increase in risk in those who had received breast radiotherapy (RR = 1.33). This risk was found only in women aged under 45 at the time of first treatment (RR = 1.6).

Healey et al, from the Joint Centre for Radiation Therapy Boston, followed 1624 women with unilateral breast cancer treated by breast conservation including radiotherapy.[44] Contralateral cancers were found in 77 and there was an increased risk among younger women. Other factors such as the presence of lobular carcinoma in situ (LCIS), vascular invasion and tumour stage were of borderline significance. Adjuvant chemotherapy was shown again to be protective against contralateral disease.

A cohort of 4748 women with unilateral invasive breast cancer treated at the Institut Curie were followed for a median of 80 months and 282 developed metachronous contralateral tumours.[45] This represented a 4% cumulative rate at 5 years. In a multivariate analysis the significant risk factors were age less than 55 (RR = 1.4) and lobular carcinoma (RR = 1.7). Adjuvant chemotherapy led to a diminution in risk (RR = 0.5).

Cook et al conducted a nested case-control study of 234 metachronous contralateral cases and a similar number of control patients matched for age, stage and year of diagnosis.[46] Premenopausal women had an increased risk as did those with a family history (1.96), but the effect of family history was found in both younger and older women. There was an increased risk in women with lobular compared with ductal cancers (RR = 1.5). Within the first 3 years of treatment, radiotherapy increased risk and chemotherapy decreased incidence of contralateral cancer, but after this time no significant effect was seen, although this may have been the result of relatively short follow-up.

Histological subtypes

To determine whether a contralateral breast cancer is a new primary lesion or a metastasis

Table 20.5 Comparative histological type of first and second tumours in patients with metachronous bilateral breast cancers

First tumour			Second tumour			
DCIS	IDC	ILC	DCIS	IDC	ILC	Reference
8	44	4	3	49	7	Michowitz et al[47]
–	34	10	–	40	6	Sterns and Fletcher[48]
–	43	13	–	45	9	Gogas et al[35]
0	28	3	4	27	3	Awad et al[49]
8 (4)	**149 (80)**	**30 (16)**	**7 (4)**	**161 (83)**	**25 (13)**	**Total***

DICS, ductal carcinoma in situ; IDC, invasive ductal carcinoma; ILC, invasive lobular carcinoma.

* Values in parentheses are percentages.

from the first tumour may sometimes be impossible. If the two tumours are of different type or grade, or when there is in situ disease around the second tumour, this is indicative of it being a second primary. If the two cancers appear to be of the same type and when there is no in situ change in the second breast, the contralateral cancer may be a metastasis. In the absence of any evidence of other metastases the patient is given the benefit of the doubt and the second cancer treated on its own merits, or demerits.

In terms of the comparative histology of primary and contralateral metachronous tumours, results from four series are summarized in Table 20.5.[35,47–49] This shows that, although most of the bilateral cancers are of ductal type, there is an over-representation of lobular lesions in this group, which comprise 15% of first and 13% of second tumours.

To compare aspects of the biological behaviour of primary and metachronous tumours Silvestrini et al measured the [³H]thymidine labelling index ([³H]dTLI) and steroid receptors in 25 cases.[50] There was no relationship between the ER/PR profile or the [³H]dTLI of the primary and the metachronous cancers. However, those tumours that were steroid receptor negative were more rapidly proliferating, with a higher [³H]dTLI.

Contralateral breast biopsy

In the absence of clinical or radiological evidence of a contralateral cancer, is it justifiable to perform a mirror image biopsy? This procedure was routine at Memorial Sloan Kettering in New York, and over a 12-year period Urban et al performed 954 contralateral biopsies, finding cancers in 119 (12.5%).[51] This apparently high pick-up rate would suggest that mirror image biopsy should be more widely used. However, when the patients were divided into three groups on a basis of index of suspicion (suspected, equivocal or normal), the results alter in their significance as shown in Table 20.6.

Among those with suspected contralateral cancers, 71% proved to have invasive disease

Table 20.6 Results of mirror image biopsy

	Number	Invasive cancer (%)	In situ cancer (%)
Suspicious	28	20 (71)	2 (7)
Equivocal	625	30 (5)	44 (7)
Normal	301	5 (2)	18 (6)

From Urban et al.[51]

and 7% had in situ carcinoma. There were 30 (5%) invasive cancers in the equivocal group and only 2% in the normal cases. Thus, combining the equivocal and normal cases, 926 biopsies were performed to pick up 35 invasive and 62 non-invasive cancers (some of which were LCIS). Hence over 90% of patients had an unnecessary operation.

More recently, Smith et al reported results from 95 mirror image biopsies from patients without clinical or radiological evidence of contralateral disease.[52] Invasive cancers were found in two cases (2%), and LCIS in three others. Histology of the primary tumour did not identify a group at increased risk of a positive contralateral biopsy. Thus, even in patients with invasive lobular carcinoma, mirror image biopsy is not justified as part of the routine management.

Family history

The relationship of a family history of breast cancer to development of bilateral breast cancer can be explored in two ways: first, the impact of a family history of bilateral breast cancer on risk of developing the disease and second the effect of a family history on likelihood of bilateral tumours. Anderson reported an eightfold increase in risk of breast cancer for women with a first-degree relative with bilateral disease developing before age 50.[53] In contrast, a

Table 20.7 Family history of bilateral breast cancer and relative risk of disease

Feature	Unilateral	Bilateral
Diagnosis < 50 years	1	5.5
Diagnosis < 40 years	2.4	10.5
< 3 years between cancers	–	1.6

From Ottman et al.[56]

Swedish case-control study of 1330 breast cancer cases and paired controls found that the risk of breast cancer was 1.7 for those with a family history of unilateral cancer and 2.2 in those who had relatives with bilateral disease.[54] The risk was not significantly affected by age at onset in the relative.

In an analysis of 4735 cases in the CASH study, they were compared with 4688 population controls.[55] The overall relative risk for a woman with a first-degree relative with unilateral disease was 2.3, but only 1.6 for those who had a relative with bilateral cancers. In the premenopausal woman the relative risks were 2.7 and 1.5, whereas for postmenopausal women they were 2.5 for unilateral and 2.4 for bilateral disease.

In a study of 295 cases (82 bilateral and 213 unilateral) and 229 controls, Ottman et al examined the risk in sisters in terms of numbers of affected relatives, age at diagnosis, bilateral versus unilateral, and temporal separation of metachronous tumours.[56] The results are given in Table 20.7. For those with a family history of unilateral breast cancer diagnosed before the age of 50, there was no significantly increased risk whereas those who had a relative with bilateral disease were at a fivefold increased risk. This rose to 10.5 for those with relatives with bilateral disease diagnosed before age 40, and 2.4 for those with unilateral disease. For those whose relatives had bilateral cancers

diagnosed less than 3 years apart, the relative risk was 6.3 and this fell to 3.9 when the cancers were more than 3 years apart, although this was a non-significant trend.

In terms of a family history and risk of bilateral disease, it is apparent that this can be a significant actor. Sakamoto et al reported a threefold increase in family history in Japanese women with bilateral as compared with unilateral disease.[57] In a series of patients treated at Guy's Hospital, 54 bilateral cases were compared with 208 women with unilateral cancers.[58] In the unilateral group 13% gave a first-degree history, compared with 28% of the bilateral cases (RR = 2.2).

As more becomes known about the genetics of breast cancer so certain individuals with pathological mutations can be identified. The first germline mutation described was *BRCA-1*, and Ford et al estimated risks of unilateral and bilateral breast cancer in 35 families carrying *BRCA-1* mutations.[59] The lifetime risk for unilateral disease was 90% and for bilateral disease 60%. Kinoshita et al used PCR single-strand conformation polymorphism (PCR-SSCP) to look for *p53* mutations in 38 bilateral and 62 unilateral breast cancers.[60] There were *p53* mutations in 26% of the unilateral cases and 50% of the bilateral cancers. Among those with metachronous lesions, 56% had *p53* mutations.

Hence some subgroups of women with a family history are at very high risk of bilateral disease. If a *BRCA-1* or *BRCA-2* mutation is found in a patient with unilateral disease, bilateral mastectomy should be considered as an appropriate option and, because of the strong possibility of a field susceptibility, unilateral breast conservation treatment should be undertaken with great caution.

Prognosis

There is some confusion in the literature with regard to the prognosis of patients with bilateral disease in terms of both synchronous versus metachronous cancers and bilateral versus unilateral lesions. This has arisen because of heterogeneity of patient groups and

Table 20.8 Five-year survival of patients with bilateral and unilateral breast cancer

Synchronous (%)	Metachronous (%)	Unilateral (%)	Reference
40	70	–	McCredie et al[61]
72	68	84	Schell et al[62]
70	70	100	Burns et al[63]
–	74	68	Fisher et al[64]
44	56	–	Fraschia et al[65]
60	54	–	Holmberg et al[66]
65	–	65	Graham et al[34]
71	61	–	Gustafsson et al[67]

lack of adjustment for age, stage and interval between cancers, with sometimes an insufficiently rigorous statistical analysis. Studies are summarized in Table 20.8.[34,61-67] McCredie et al compared the survival of women with metachronous and synchronous cancers and found that the latter group fared worse.[61] For those aged less than 50 the survival after the second primary was better than that for women aged over 50 (72% vs 56%).

In a study that included only those cases with stage I and II disease, Schell et al examined the outcome for 39 women with synchronous cancers, 87 with metachronous disease and 1856 with unilateral lesions.[62] At 5 years the unilateral group had a better survival than both bilateral groups and the synchronous cases fared worse than those with metachronous cancers. After 20 years of follow-up, however, there was no significant difference in survival of the three groups. Using data from the Alberta Cancer registry, Burns et al reported that the survival of metachronous cases was better than that of women with synchronous or unilateral disease, when calculated from the time of diagnosis of the first cancer.[63] When starting from the date of diagnosis of the second, the survival of the three groups was similar.

In the NSABP Protocol 4 there were 66 metachronous cases with no significant differ-

ences in axillary nodal status between the first and second tumours or in the 5-year survival, and it was concluded that a second cancer had no impact on survival.[64] Fracchia et al compared node-negative unilateral and bilateral cases and reported 10-year relapse-free survival rates of 84% and 71% respectively.[65] Those with synchronous disease had the worst prognosis, and Fracchia et al concluded that bilateral breast cancer placed a patient in a state of 'double jeopardy'.

Holmberg et al reported a relative 8-year survival rate of 69% for unilateral cases and 53% for those with metachronous bilateral cancers.[66] This difference was not statistically significant. However, after a very rigorous analysis, adjusting for age, stage and tumour type, it emerged that the relative hazard of death from breast cancer was significantly elevated in bilateral cases (RR = 1.6), a 60% increase in risk. When the interval between cancers was considered, the relative hazard was 2 in the first and second years, 1.82 at 5 years, 1.6 at 10 years, 1.2 at 20 years and 1.0 at 30 years. In contrast, Graham et al found that although their patients with metachronous cancers appeared to have a better prognosis than that of women with unilateral disease from time of presentation, if dated from the second cancer there was no difference in survival of those with synchronous, metachronous or unilateral disease.[34]

In a series of 95 bilateral cancers Gustafsson et al found a significantly better distant relapse-free survival (DRFS) for metachronous cases.[67] In addition, the interval between cancers significantly affected outcome: those with cancers less than 5 years apart had a 5-year DRFS of 58%, whereas those with cancers diagnosed more than 5 years later had a DRFS of 95%. However, De la Rochefordière et al found no relationship between interval between cancers and survival.[36] Using a multivariate analysis of factors for distant relapse, Healey et al reported that a contralateral breast cancer led to a significantly increased likelihood (RR = 1.7) of developing distant metastases.[44]

Treatment

As the risk of metachronous contralateral breast cancer remains constant with time, the more effective that primary treatments become, the longer patients will survive and the greater the proportion who will develop a new primary. This will be the case for both breasts in those treated by conservation therapy. As a benefit of primary therapy, however, there will be an approximately 40% reduction in contralateral cancers in women given adjuvant tamoxifen.[68]

Other than a few women with mutations such as *BRCA-1*, *BRCA-2* and *p53*, those at increased risk cannot be accurately identified. Thus all breast cancer patients with retained breasts have to be followed carefully to pick up new lesions either clinically or radiologically.

There is some evidence of second cancers being smaller and of lower stage.[45] Prevention or early diagnosis of second primaries is essential if late mortality from breast cancer is to be reduced.

Treatment of the contralateral cancer will, in part, be determined by size but also by the success of previous therapy. Some who have had a mastectomy will want the same on the second side, others will wish to conserve the breast. Women who have had prior radiotherapy as part of breast conservation can be safely treated by contralateral irradiation, provided that midline overlap of fields is avoided. With care and accurate knowledge of prior treatment, sequential irradiation can be given without undue morbidity and with good cosmetic outcome.[44] Those few who have confirmed pathological mutations should be offered bilateral mastectomy because removal of all mammary epithelium is essential when a tumour-suppressor gene is defective.

SYNOPSIS

- Bilateral breast cancer carries a higher risk of mortality than unilateral disease.
- Synchronous cancers are worse than metachronous lesions.
- The longer the time interval, the better the prognosis.
- Incidence of contralateral cancers will be reduced by tamoxifen.
- Mortality from contralateral disease may be reduced by clinical and radiological detection of early cancers.

REFERENCES

1. Velpeau A. On disease of the mammary areola preceding cancer of the mammary region. (Transl. H Mitchell.) London: Sydenham Society, 1856.
2. Paget J. On disease of the mammary areola preceding cancer of the mammary gland. *St Bart's Hosp Rep* 1874; **10**: 87–9.
3. Kay S. Paget's disease of the nipple. *Surg Gynecol Obstet* 1966; **123**: 1010–14.
4. Nance FC, DeLoach DH, Welsh RA, Becker WF. Paget's disease of the breast. *Ann Surg* 1970; **171**: 864–74.
5. Ashikari R, Park K, Huvos AG, Urban JA. Paget's disease of the breast. *Cancer* 1970; **26**: 680–5.
6. Chaudary MA, Millis RR, Lane EB et al. Paget's disease of the nipple: a ten year review including clinical, pathological and immunohisto-

chemical findings. *Breast Cancer Res Treat* 1986; **8:** 139–46.

7. Masters RK, Robertson JFR, Blamey RW. Healed Paget's disease of the nipple. *Lancet* 1993; **341:** 253.

8. Darier J. Sur une nouvelle forme de psorospermose cutanée: la maladie de paget du mamelon. *CR Soc Biol* (Series 9) 1889; **1:** 294–7.

9. Orr JW, Parish DJ. The nature of the nipple changes in Paget's disease. *J Pathol Bacteriol* 1962; **84:** 201–8.

10. Cheatle GL, Cutler M. Paget's disease of the nipple: review of the literature: clinical and microscopical study of 17 breasts by means of whole serial sections. *Arch Pathol* 1931; **12:** 435–66.

11. Willis RA. *Pathology of Tumours*, 4th edn. London: Butterworth, 1967.

12. Muir R. Pathogenesis of Paget's disease of the nipple and associated lesions. *Br J Surg* 1935; **22:** 728–37.

13. Inglis K. Paget's disease of the nipple, with special reference to changes in the ducts. *Am J Pathol* 1946; **22:** 1–33.

14. Bussolati G, Pich A. Mammary and extramammary Paget's disease. *Am J Pathol* 1975; **80:** 117–24.

15. Nadji M, Morales AR, Girtanner RE et al. Paget's disease of the skin. A unifying concept of histogenesis. *Cancer* 1982; **50:** 2203–6.

16. Vanstapel M-J, Gatter KC, De Wolf-Peeters C, Millard PR et al. Immunohistochemical study of mammary and extramammary Paget's disease. *Histopathology* 1984; **8:** 1013–23.

17. Kanitakis J, Thivolet J, Claudy A. P53 protein expression in mammary and extramammary Paget's disease. *Anticancer Res* 1993; **13:** 2429–34.

18. De Potter CR, Eeckhout L, Schelfhout AM et al. Keratinocyte induced chemotaxis in the pathogenesis of Paget's disease of the breast. *Histopathology* 1994; **24:** 349–56.

19. Nakamura G, Shikata N, Shoji T et al. Immunohistochemical study of mammary and extramammary Paget's disease. *Anticancer Res* 1995; **15:** 467–70.

20. Cohen C, Guarner J, De Rose PB. Mammary Paget's disease and associated carcinoma. *Arch Pathol Lab Med* 1993; **117:** 291–4.

21. Aktan AÖ, Gökoz A, Göksel H. Paget's disease without a palpable mass in the breast. *Br J Surg* 1990; **77:** 226–7.

22. Culberson JD, Horn RC. Paget's disease of the nipple. *Arch Surg* 1956; **72:** 224–7.

23. Ridenhour CE, Perez-Mesa C, Hori JM. Paget's disease of the nipple. *Cancer Bull* 1969; **21:** 15–16.

24. Rissanen PM, Holsti P. Paget's disease of the breast. *Oncology* 1969; **23:** 209–16.

25. Kister SJ, Haagensen CD. Paget's disease of the breast. *Am J Surg* 1970; **119:** 606–9.

26. Maier WP, Rosemond GP, Harasym EL et al. Paget's disease in the female breast. *Surg Gynecol Obstet* 1969; **128:** 1253–63.

27. Paone JF, Baker RR. Pathogenesis and treatment of Paget's disease of the breast. *Cancer* 1981; **48:** 825–9.

28. Dixon AR, Galea MH, Ellis IO et al. Paget's disease of the nipple. *Br J Surg* 1991; **78:** 722–3.

29. Davis AB, Patchefsky AS. Basal cell carcinoma of the nipple: case report and review of the literature. *Cancer* 1977; **40:** 1780–1.

30. Vianna LL, Fentiman IS. Adenoma of the nipple: a diagnostic dilemma. *Br J Hosp Med* 1993; **50:** 639–42.

31. Fourquet A, Campana F, Vielh P et al. Paget's disease of the nipple without detectable breast tumor: conservative management with radiation therapy. *Int J Radiat Oncol Biol Phys* 1987; **13:** 1463–5.

32. Stockdale AD, Brierley JD, White WF et al. Radiotherapy for Paget's disease of the nipple: a conservative alternative. *Lancet* 1989; **ii:** 664–5.

33. Leis HP, Mersheimer WL, Black M, De Chabon A. The second breast. *N Y State J Med* 1965; **65:** 2460–8.

34. Graham MD, Yelland A, Peacock J et al. Bilateral carcinoma of the breast. *Eur J Surg Oncol* 1993; **19:** 259–64.

35. Gogas J, Markopoulos CH, Skandalakis P, Gogas H. Bilateral breast cancer. *Am Surg* 1993; **59:** 733–5.

36. De la Rochefordière A, Asselain B, Scholl S et al. Simultaneous bilateral breast carcinomas: a retrospective review of 149 cases. *Int J Radiat Oncol Biol Phys* 1994; **30:** 35–41.

37. Kopelson G, Munzendnrider JE, Doppke K, Wang CC. Bilateral breast cancer: radiation therapy results and technical considerations. *Int J Radiat Oncol Biol Phys* 1981; **7:** 335–41.

38. Solin LJ, Fowble BL, Schultz DJ, Goodman RL. Bilateral breast carcinoma treated with definitive irradiation. *Int J Radiat Oncol Biol Phys* 1989; **17:** 263–71.

39. Prior P, Waterhouse JAH. Incidence of bilateral tumours in a population-based series of breast cancer patients. *Br J Cancer* 1978; **37:** 620–34.

40. Adami H-O, Bergström R, Hansen J. Age at first primary as a determinant of the incidence of bilateral breast cancer. *Cancer* 1985; **55**: 643–7.

41. Storm HH, Jensen OM. Risk of contralateral breast cancer in Denmark 1943-80. *Br J Cancer* 1986; **54**: 483–92.

42. Bernstein JL, Thompson WD, Risch N, Holford TR. Risk factors predicting the incidence of second primary breast cancer among women diagnosed with a first primary breast cancer. *Am J Epidemiol* 1992; **136**: 925–36.

43. Boice JD, Harvey EB, Blettner M et al. Cancer in the contralateral breast after radiotherapy for breast cancer. *N Engl J Med* 1992; **326**: 781–5.

44. Healey EA, Cook EF, Orav EJ et al. Contralateral breast cancer: clinical characteristics and impact on prognosis. *J Clin Oncol* 1993; **11**: 1545–52.

45. Bröet P, De la Rochefordière A, Scholl SM et al. Contralateral breast cancer: annual incidence and risk parameters. *J Clin Oncol* 1995; **13**: 1578–83.

46. Cook LS, White E, Schwartz SM et al. A population-based study of contralateral breast cancer following a first primary breast cancer (Washington United States). *Cancer Causes Control* 1996; **7**: 382–90.

47. Michowitz M, Noy S, Lazebnik N, Aladjem D. Bilateral breast cancer. *J Surg Oncol* 1985; **30**: 109–12.

48. Sterns EE, Fletcher WA. Bilateral cancer of the breast: A review of clinical, histologic, and immunohistologic characteristics. *Surgery* 1991; **110**: 617–22.

49. Awad AT, El-Husseini G, Anwar M et al. Bilateral primary breast cancers: a clinicopathological study of the second primary. *Int Surg* 1996; **81**: 57–60.

50. Silvestrini R, Valentinis B, Daidone MG et al. Biological characterisation of primary and metachronous lesions in breast cancer patients. *Eur J Cancer* 1992; **28A**: 2006–10.

51. Urban JA, Papachristou D, Taylor J. Bilateral breast cancer. Biopsy of the opposite breast. *Cancer* 1977; **40**: 1968–73.

52. Smith BL, Bertagnolli M, Klein BB et al. Evaluation of the contralateral breast. The role of biopsy at the time of treatment of breast cancer. *Ann Surg* 1992; **216**: 17–21.

53. Anderson DE. A genetic study of human breast cancer. *J Natl Cancer Inst* 1972; **111**: 301–8.

54. Adami H-O, Hansen J, Jung B, Rimsten Ä. Characteristics of familial breast cancer in Sweden: absence of relation to age and unilateral versus bilateral disease. *Cancer* 1981; **48**: 1688–95.

55. Sattin RW, Rubin GL, Webster LA et al. Family history and breast cancer. *JAMA* 1985; **253**: 1908–13.

56. Ottman R, Pike MC, King M-C et al. Familial breast cancer in a population-based series. *Am J Epidemiol* 1986; **123**: 15–21.

57. Sakamoto G, Sugano H, Kasumi F. Bilateral breast cancer and familial aggregations. *Prev Med* 1978; **7**: 225–9.

58. Chaudary M, Millis RR, Bulbrook RD, Hayward JL. Family history and bilateral breast cancer. *Breast Cancer Res Treat* 1985; **5**: 201–5.

59. Ford D, Easton DF, Bishop DT et al. Risks of cancer in BRCA-1 mutations. *Lancet* 1994; **343**: 692–5.

60. Kinoshita T, Ueda M, Enomoto K et al. Comparison of p53 gene abnormalities in bilateral and unilateral breast cancer. *Cancer* 1995; **76**: 2504–9.

61. McCredie JA, Inch WR, Alderson M. Consecutive primary carcinomas of the breast. *Cancer* 1975; **35**: 1472–7.

62. Schell SR, Montague ED, Spanos WJ et al. Bilateral breast cancer in patients with initial stage I and II disease. *Cancer* 1982; **50**: 1191–4.

63. Burns PE, Darbs K, May C et al. Bilateral breast cancer in northern Alberta: risk factors and survival patterns. *Can Med Assoc J* 1984; **130**: 881–6.

64. Fisher ER, Fisher B, Sass R et al. Pathologic findings from the National Surgical Adjuvant Breast Project (Protocol No. 4). XI. Bilateral breast cancer. *Cancer* 1984; **54**: 3002–11.

65. Fracchia AA, Robinson D, Legaspi A et al. Survival in bilateral breast cancer. *Cancer* 1985; **55**: 1414–21.

66. Holmberg L, Adami HO, Ekbom A et al. Prognosis in bilateral breast cancer. Effects of time interval between first and second primary tumours. *Br J Cancer* 1988; **58**: 191–4.

67. Gustafsson A, Tartter PI, Brower ST, Lesnick G. Prognosis of patients with bilateral carcinoma of the breast. *J Am Coll Surg* 1994; **178**: 111–16.

68. Early Breast Cancer Trialists' Collaborative Group. Systemic treatment of early breast cancer by hormonal, cytotoxic or immune therapy. *Lancet* 1992; **339**: 1–15.

21

Rarer problems

The most heterogeneous ideas are yoked by violence together.

Samuel Johnson

Mucinous carcinoma • Tubular carcinoma • Medullary cancer

MUCINOUS CARCINOMA

Mucinous carcinomas are a relatively rare special type comprising 1–2% of all breast cancers.[1] Variously termed colloid, gelatinous, myxomatous, mucinous and mucoid, these cancers all contain mucin derived from epithelium.[2] They usually occur in women aged over 60 years and are associated with a good prognosis, provided that stringent diagnostic criteria have been applied. Mucin may be detected in various tumours and Saphir described four separate types: true mucoid, infiltrating ductal carcinoma with mucoid features, signet ring cell carcinoma and intracystic papilloma with mucoid features.[2] Nowadays most pathologists restrict the term mucinous to pure mucoid and mixed mucoid lesions. The latter is defined as a tumour in which at least 10% of the carcinoma is of mucoid type, but this is mixed with an infiltrating component of a different type usually ductal not otherwise specified (NOS).[3]

Presentation

The diagnosis of mucinous carcinoma may be suspected on palpation because, as described by Halsted in 1915, there is a 'delicate swish or crush of a jelly-like structure under tension'.[4] In four successive cases Halsted was surprised by the 'swish' sensation on clinical examination of what proved to be mucinous carcinomas. However, in the series of 102 cases reported by Norris and Taylor this clinical sign was never elicited.[5] The mean ages at diagnosis and mean tumour sizes from four series are given in Table 21.1.[5–8] In all studies those with pure mucoid cancers were slightly older than those with mixed tumours. The mean tumour diameter was significantly less in pure lesions in the Guy's Hospital[8] and large Danish series,[6] but the reverse was seen in the two other studies. Thus, unless Halsted's 'swish' sign can be demonstrated, it is unlikely that most mucinous cases will be suspected preoperatively, or that pure and mixed cases can be distinguished clinically. Even when a core needle biopsy suggests pure mucoid, this should not be taken as confirmation since full tumour examination is necessary before so designating a cancer.

Another potential source of diagnostic confusion is the mucocele-like tumour. This lesion is a multilobulated, well-circumscribed mass, comprising mucin-filled cysts. Mucocele-like tumours may be associated with atypia or ductal carcinoma in situ (DCIS),[9] and have been described as precursors of mucinous carcinomas.[10] An example is shown in Fig. 21.1.

Table 21.1 Comparative clinical features of patients with pure and mixed mucinous cancers						
Pure mucinous			**Mixed mucinous**			
Number	Age (years)	Size (cm)	Number	Age (years)	Size (cm)	Reference
62	55	3.6	40	47	3.3	Norris and Taylor[5]
95	69	2.0	112	68	2.6	Rasmussen[6]
58	61	3.9	24	59	3.4	Andrea et al[7]
24	62	2.2	49	63	3.2	Fentiman et al[8]

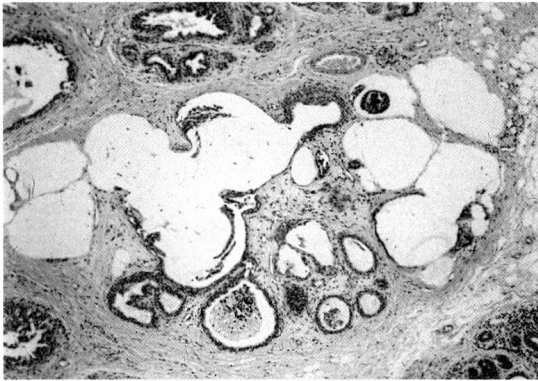

Fig. 21.1 Photomicrograph of mucocele-like tumour.

In a series of 53 cases reported by Hamele-Bena et al, 25 were benign and 28 malignant.[11] Mean age of both malignant and benign cases was 48 years, and the only non-histological distinguishing feature was that the malignant lesions were more likely to contain coarse calcifications and be detected mammographically. Of the benign cases, only one developed a breast relapse and there were no distant recurrences or deaths from metastatic breast cancer.

Mammography

It is likely that there is a morphological continuum with all mixed tumours starting as pure lesions with the non-mucoid component developing at a later stage. Thus the earlier the diagnosis is made the better the outcome. As a result of mammographic screening, more pure mucinous lesions are being diagnosed.[8] Cardenosa et al reported the mammographic appearance of seven impalpable pure mucoid cancers.[12] None of the lesions had associated microcalcification. Most were poorly defined, lobulated masses.

In a series of 19 mammographically detected pure mucoid lesions, however, 75% appeared as well-defined lobulated opacities and 40% had associated calcification.[13] As this can be the radiological appearance of benign lesions, it was suggested that, if there was any blurring of the margins of a mass, magnification views should be taken.

It is the rarity of spiculation in pure mucinous tumours that can lead to false-negative diagnosis. Chopra et al examined the value of both mammography and ultrasonography in the diagnosis of mucinous cancers.[14] Of 15 cases, 86% had poorly defined opacities and 71% were lobulated, with only 14% having microcalcification. Less commonly, the lesions were well defined. All seven cases examined ultrasonically were found to have a mass lesion, which in most (86%) was hypoechoic. None showed distal attenuation.

To avoid misinterpretation of pure mucinous cancers as benign, therefore, mammographic opacities that do not have fully distinct margins

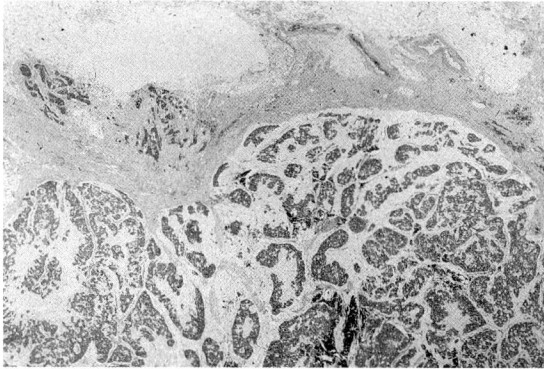

Fig. 21.2 Photomicrograph of mixed mucinous carcinoma.

Table 21.2 Axillary nodal status of patients with operable pure and mixed mucinous carcinomas

Pure mucinous node +ve	Mixed mucinous node +ve	Reference
3/95 (3)	37/112 (33)	Rasmussen[6]
21/140 (15)	16/35 (46)	Komaki et al[21]
10/35 (29)	15/23 (65)	Scopsi et al[19]
14/53 (26)	9/22 (41)	Andrea et al[7]
3/21 (14)	18/39 (46)	Fentiman et al[8]
51/344	**95/231**	**Total**
(15)	**(41)**	**(%)**

Values in parentheses are percentages.

should be investigated further by a combination of magnification/compression views and ultrasonography.

Histopathology

Mucinous carcinomas have also been categorized not only as pure and mixed but also, by Capella et al, according to growth pattern.[15] Type A tumours comprise more pleomorphic malignant cells than type B tumours; they are arranged in small groups with abundant extracellular mucin and usually with no intracellular mucin. In type B tumours the cells are more monomorphic, more prominent and arranged in larger groups, with less extracellular mucin but containing occasional intracellular mucin. A high proportion of type B tumours is found to be argyrophylic. A few tumours have an intermediate pattern (type AB). Others have tried with variable success to divide these lesions on the basis of morphology or argyrophilia.[16–19]

Adequate sampling of carcinomas with a mucoid appearance is essential and strict diagnostic criteria should be adhered to. It has been recommended that, if 90% of the carcinoma is of one histological type, the tumour should be so designated,[3] but this does not appear to be applicable to mucoid carcinomas.

A further criterion for the diagnosis of pure mucoid carcinoma is that a minimal proportion of the volume of the tumour should consist of mucin: 30% has been suggested by Rasmussen,[6] and 50% by Silverberg.[20] A mixed mucinous carcinoma is shown in Fig. 21.2.

As shown in Table 21.2, all the series indicate that patients with mixed mucinous lesions are more likely to have axillary nodal metastases.[6–8,19,21] Overall, 41% of those with operable mixed mucinous cancers had nodal metastases compared with 15% of those with pure lesions. Thus, although pure mucoid lesions are said to have a good prognosis, some have associated nodal metastases. This may be related to differentiation of the tumour because Pereira et al found that patients with grade II pure mucoid carcinomas fared significantly worse than those with grade I tumours.[22] It has been suggested that the presence of axillary nodal metastases in a pure lesion is an indication of inadequate sampling of the tumour.[23] However, some axillary nodal metastases have a mucoid

Table 21.3 Ten-year overall survival of patients with pure and mixed mucinous breast cancers

Pure mucinous (%)	Mixed mucinous (%)	Reference
85	60	Norris and Taylor[5]
90	66	Komaki et al[21]
80	20	Andrea et al[7]
75	40	Scopsi et al[19]
100	60	Fentiman et al[8]

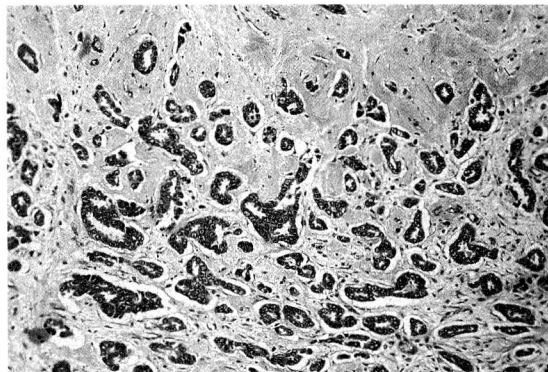

Fig. 21.3 Photomicrograph of a tubular carcinoma.

appearance indicating that the mucoid component does have a metastatic potential.

Prognosis

Clayton suggested that lower cellularity (≤10%) and more mucin production denoted a more favourable prognosis.[24] Argyrophilic tumours are more cellular so this type may have a higher malignant potential.[17] However, Rasmussen et al reported fewer lymph node metastases in patients with argyrophilic tumours but no difference in prognosis.[18] It would therefore appear that the most important prognostic feature is the presence or absence of a mixed pattern.

Studies comparing survival of patients with pure and mixed cancers are summarized in Table 21.3.[5,7,8,19,21] Although there is a consistently better prognosis for pure cases, the 10-year overall survival rate ranges from 75% to 100%. The probable explanation is variations in sampling. In the Guy's Hospital study,[8] which reported a 100% overall survival rate, even when only an extremely small proportion of the infiltrating tumour was not surrounded by mucoid stroma it was excluded from the category and the original diagnosis was changed from pure to mixed mucoid in four cases.

In mixed lesions the percentage of the mucoid component was found to be a significant prognostic feature, with an increasing proportion of mucoid element being associated with a more favourable outcome.[8] Nevertheless, even when 90% or more of the infiltrating carcinoma was mucoid the survival rates did not match that of the pure tumours. This is in agreement with one study which found that, when patients were divided into those with pure mucoid, mixed and minimal mucoid component, survival rates were better in those with tumours having a proportionally greater gelatinous element.[25]

TUBULAR CARCINOMA

A tubular carcinoma is a highly differentiated invasive cancer with regular cells arranged in well-defined tubules, one layer thick with an abundant fibrous stroma.[26] Figure 21.3 shows an example of tubular carcinoma. These lesions have acquired an aura of sanctity which cannot be sustained after close examination of their behaviour. As more are diagnosed by screening, so there is more lobbying for a policy of minimal treatment. Although some of these lesions carry an excellent prognosis if treated properly, others will metastasize to axillary

Table 21.4 Clinical features of patients with tubular carcinomas

Number	Mean age (years)	Duration (months)	Lump (%)	Mammography (%)	Reference
33	44	5.4	100	–	Taylor and Norris[27]
35	51	–	94	6	Carstens et al[28]
12	50	11	100	–	Cooper et al[29]
17	56	–	59	41	Lagios et al[30]
16	53	–	100	–	Peters et al[31]
90	48	2	100	–	Deos and Norris[32]
13	–	–	31	69	Leibman et al[33]
20	59	–	35	65	Elson et al[34]
40	54	–	–	–	Winchester et al[35]

nodes and elsewhere. If all small tubular carcinomas are regarded as being almost benign and undertreated, some will cause unnecessary deaths. It is essential that stringent diagnostic criteria are adopted before a lesion is dubbed tubular.

Presentation

Originally most tubular carcinomas presented as lumps, with or without signs of local invasion, such as skin tethering, but the proportion of impalpable lesions is increasing as a result of the more widespread introduction of screening. Table 21.4 shows the clinical features reported in several series.[27-35] The mean age at diagnosis was 53 years which was 2–7 years earlier than that of patients with other infiltrating cancers.[29,31,32]

In addition, those with pure tubular lesions were younger than those with mixed cancers, suggesting that, with time, there may be a change towards more aggressive behaviour. Up to 50% of tubular carcinomas are now being diagnosed at an impalpable stage, the usual mammographic finding being a spiculated mass, sometimes with microcalcification.

In one series of 17 cases with tubular carcinomas, 40% gave a first-degree family history of breast cancer,[30] but this has not been reported by others. In the same study, six cases (38%) developed contralateral breast cancer, three before diagnosis of the tubular cancer, two synchronously and one subsequently. This high incidence might result partially from increased use of mammography in those with breast cancer, leading to pick-up of impalpable tubular tumours. Other series reported an incidence of contralateral cancers of 12–26%.[30-35] In the last study 62% of cases had a prior contralateral invasive or non-invasive cancer.

Histology

Many well-differentiated breast cancers have a tubular component, but the criteria for establishing a lesion as pure tubular have not been defined. Those studies that have described the proportion of the cancer with a tubular component, together with axillary nodal status, are given in Table 21.5.[28,31-36] Overall, 15% of cases had axillary nodal involvement and this proportion did not bear any relationship to the percentage tubular component of the cancer.

In a series of 336 patients from Guy's Hospital with breast cancers 1 cm or less in

Table 21.5 Tubular component and axillary nodal status

Tubular component (%)	Involved axillary nodes*	Reference
>75	6/36 (17)	Carstens et al[28]
>75	3/22 (14)	Oberman and Fidler[36]
>50	4/52 (8)	Peters et al[31]
>50	18/114 (16)	Deos and Norris[32]
>90	0/9	Leibman et al[33]
>75	4/14 (29)	Elson et al[34]
>90	9/44 (20)	Winchester et al[35]
	(15)	**Mean**

* Values in parentheses are percentages.

diameter, 13 had tubular lesions: eight palpable and five impalpable.[37] Of the palpable lesions, 25% were node positive as were 20% of those with impalpable lesions. This underlines the need for axillary surgery, even in patients with small, apparently well-differentiated cancers.

Green et al compared the outcome of 90 women with pure tubular cancer and 17 with tubulolobular carcinoma, treated at the Memorial Sloan-Kettering Cancer Center.[38] Both groups were of similar age (mean 42 years) and tumour size (1.2 cm), but of the pure cases 20% were multifocal compared with 29% of those with tubulolobular lesions. As Table 21.6 shows, among those with pure tubular cancers, there was a small percentage (7%) with nodal involvement when the tumour was unifocal, but this rose to 33% in those with multifocal cancers. In contrast one-third of the tubulolobular cases had nodal involvement in the absence of multifocality and 60% were node positive when multifocal disease was present. This illustrates the need for accurate pathological characterization of tubular carcinomas.

Treatment

Most of tubular cancers diagnosed will be suitable for breast conservation therapy and this should include both tumourectomy and axillary surgery for the reasons discussed previously. The need for breast irradiation has been questioned and two trials are on-going to examine this. The BASO-II (British Association of Surgical Oncology) trial includes patients with completely excised grade I or tubular carcinomas measuring up to 2 cm in diameter. Cases are randomized into a 2 × 2 factorial design trial. The four options are: no further treatment; breast irradiation; tamoxifen; or breast irradia-

Table 21.6 Multifocality and axillary nodal involvement in pure tubular and tubulolobular carcinomas

Multifocality	Pure tubular carcinoma (%)		Tubulolobular carcinoma (%)	
	Node negative	Node positive	Node negative	Node positive
Absent	93	7	67	33
Present	67	33	40	60

From Green et al.[38]

Table 21.7 Survival of patients with pure and mixed tubular carcinomas

Follow-up (years)	Pure tubular (%)	Mixed tubular (%)	Reference
10	100	68	Taylor and Norris[27]
6	100	74	Peters et al[31]
5	90	82	Deos and Norris[32]

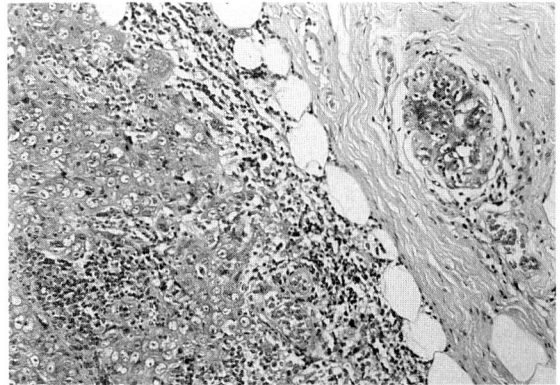

Fig. 21.4 Photomicrograph of a medullary carcinoma.

tion and tamoxifen. The EORTC Breast Cancer Co-operative Group are running a trial of similar design. Until results are available, patients with tubular carcinomas suitable for breast conservation should receive radiotherapy as an intrinsic part of primary treatment.

As these cancers are well differentiated they are likely to be oestrogen dependent. However, in a series of 25 patients with tubular carcinomas who had oestrogen receptors (ER) measured by the dextran charcoal method, five (20%) were ER negative.[35] Thus, although tamoxifen may benefit those who are node negative, there are some with ER-negative tumours for whom chemotherapy may be a more effective option.

Prognosis

Taking tumours with over 80% tubular component as pure lesions, Winchester et al reported a 5-year disease-free survival rate of 88%.[35] The survival rates of those with 100% tubular component and others with mixed tubular lesions are given in Table 21.7.[27,31,32] Although two series show no relapses in the pure tubular group, the third reported a 90% 5-year survival. Mixed tubular lesions had a worse prognosis. Unless complete sampling of the lesion has been performed, some patients will be mislabelled as having good prognosis disease, whereas they may be at risk of relapse and in need of adjuvant therapy.

MEDULLARY CANCER

Medullary cancer of the breast is an enigmatic lesion, which can cause problems in histopathological diagnosis and uncertainty as to whether it carries a better or worse prognosis than other invasive cancers. The macroscopic and microscopic features were described by Moore and Foote in 1949.[39] Grossly, the tumours were soft and well circumscribed, with a tendency to appear expansive rather than infiltrative at the margins. The cut surfaces bulged and the tumours were homogeneous, grey, and glistening with scattered old and new haemorrhages. On microscopy the growing edge was well circumscribed. The tumour cells were arranged in cords with a loose connective tissue stroma and a surrounding infiltration of small round cells comprising lymphocytes and plasma cells. An example is shown in Fig. 21.4.

Presentation

There are no specific clinically distinguishing features of medullary carcinoma, although patients may be slightly younger than those with other invasive cancers, with a slightly higher likelihood in a family carrying the

290 DETECTION AND TREATMENT OF BREAST CANCER

BRCA-1 mutation.[40] They are no more nor less likely to give a family history of breast cancer. On examination the lump may appear soft and fairly well circumscribed, and there may be a disparity between tumour size and axillary nodal status. Black et al reported that 37% of medullary cancers were over 4 cm in diameter, but of those patients with tumours measuring 4.5–7 cm, only 33% had axillary nodal metastases.[41]

Imaging

Meyer et al described the mammographic and ultrasonic appearance of 24 medullary carcinomas.[42] Mammographically the lesions were rounded, with uniform density and lobulated margins. Like some benign lesions, one-third displayed a partial or complete halo sign. On ultrasonography all had a hypoechoic internal echo with enhancement. None produced attenuation of signal. As some have fine spiculation at the tumour margins, compression/magnification may be helpful in making a preoperative diagnosis of medullary carcinoma.

Histology

Although many breast cancers have a lymphoplasmacytic reaction around them, it is necessary to be rigorous in making a diagnosis of medullary carcinoma. Ridolfi et al reviewed 192 cases from Memorial Hospital, New York, and divided them into typical and atypical variants based on morphology.[43] The criteria are shown in Table 21.8. Using this classification, the 10-year survival rate of the typical cases was 84% compared with only 63% in patients with atypical medullary cancers.

Although these are clear criteria, their application has sometimes been suboptimal. When 30 medullary cancers diagnosed over a 10-year period were subsequently reviewed, only nine (30%) met the criteria.[44] Of the other 21, 7 were deemed atypical and 14 were diagnosed as nonmedullary. In a French double-blind study, 16 tumours previously diagnosed as medullary, atypical or infiltrating duct cancer were sent

Table 21.8 Criteria for histological diagnosis of typical and atypical medullary carcinoma

Feature	Typical	Atypical
Syncytial growth pattern (%)	>75	<75
Completely circumscribed	Yes	No
Lymphatic infiltration	Moderate/ marked	Mild/ negligible
Nuclear grade	1–2	3
Microglandular features	No	Yes
In situ component	No	Yes

twice to nine pathologists.[45] There was very low interobserver and intraobserver agreement (κ value < 0.5). The only feature on which there was any agreement was the presence or absence of an in situ component.

Gaffey et al asked six pathologists to classify 53 tumours previously diagnosed as medullary.[46] Three different sets of criteria were used: those of Ridolfi,[43] Wargotz and Silverberg,[47] and Pedersen et al.[48] The best agreement was reached with regard to nuclear grade and the least concerning tumour margin. The classification of Pedersen et al achieved the most reproducible results, with a consensus diagnosis in 96% of cases, and 17% being reclassified as atypical medullary.

In an immunohistochemical study Hsu et al examined the lymphoid stroma of 10 typical and 10 atypical medullary cancers.[49] In typical medullary cancers the lymphoid infiltrate mostly comprised IgA plasma cells, and the malignant cells contained both IgA and secretory component. In contrast, around the atypical tumours the plasma cells were predominantly of IgG type, and the cancer cells contained very little IgA or secretory component. It was postulated that this functional differentiation of tumour cells in typical

Table 21.9 Comparison of axillary nodal status of patients with typical medullary, atypical medullary and non-medullary cancers

Typical node –ve	Atypical node –ve	Non-medullary node –ve	Reference
77	70	71	Ridolfi et al[43]
54	48	35	Rapin et al[54]
66	71	49	Fisher et al[55]
67	43	31	Reinfuss et al[56]
66	**58**	**47**	**Mean**

medullary cancers might contribute to a better prognosis.

Using a similar technique, Larsimont et al searched for keratin 19 staining in 12 typical, 4 atypical and 29 undifferentiated high-grade carcinomas with lymphoid response.[50] None of the typical medullary carcinomas expressed keratin 19 and this was similar to the lack of staining in a subclass of luminal cells from the terminal ductal–lobular unit.[51] Larsimont et al suggested that medullary carcinomas were derived from luminal precursor cells.

Not only do medullary cancers not express keratin 19, they are also lacking in steroid receptors. In a series of 20 cases who had receptor assays performed on medullary tumours, 75% were negative and the remainder were only weakly positive.[52] Of those tested for progesterone receptors only one was weakly positive. This is also manifest at a functional level. Patel et al reported a series of 6 premenopausal and 16 postmenopausal patients, with metastatic medullary cancers, who were treated with endocrine ablative or additive therapy.[53] The premenopausal cases were treated by bilateral oophorectomy and most of the postmenopausal patients with bilateral adrenalectomy. Only one postmenopausal case had a brief response. These results suggest that there is only a minor, if any, role for adjuvant tamoxifen in patients with medullary cancer.

The incidence of axillary nodal metastases in patients with medullary cancers is shown in Table 21.9. This summarizes series that have compared typical, atypical, and nonmedullary cancers.[43,54–56] In almost all the studies there was a lower incidence of lymph node involvement in typical cases, with the highest in those with non-medullary tumours. Overall, two-thirds of cases with typical medullary cancers had negative axillary nodes, compared with 58% of atypical cases and 47% of those with non-medullary carcinomas.

Prognosis

As it can be difficult to make a diagnosis of typical medullary carcinoma, in many studies there has been a dilution of true cases with atypical and non-medullary variants. For this reason there was doubt about whether typical medullary carcinomas carried a better prognosis than other cancers. As Table 21.10 clearly shows, in those studies that have rigorously separated typical from atypical and non-medullary carcinomas, there is a very good prognosis for patients having true medullary lesions with 82–92% being alive 10 years after diagnosis.[43,54–56]

Despite being of high histological grade and without oestrogen receptors, these tumours carry a better prognosis than atypical or non-medullary cancers. Rapin et al consequently

Table 21.10 Ten-year survival in patients with typical medullary, atypical medullary and non-medullary cancers

Typical (%)	Atypical (%)	Non-medullary (%)	Reference
85	70	60	Ridolfi et al[43]
92	62	61	Rapin et al[54]
82	65	70	Fisher et al[55]
85	65	50	Reinfuss et al[56]

suggested that systemic adjuvant therapy could be avoided provided that tumour and lymph nodes were removed.[54] Fisher et al examined the outcome for 336 cases with typical and 273 with atypical medullary cancers who participated in eight protocols of the National Surgical Adjuvant Breast and Bowel Projects (NSABP).[55]

For node-negative cases the survival rate of those with typical medullary cancers was significantly better than for atypical medullary tumours (85% vs 75%). For those who were node positive but not given adjuvant therapy, the survival of women with typical, atypical and non-medullary cancers was similar but, among those receiving adjuvant therapy (melphalan and fluorouracil), patients with typical medullary cancers fared better (10-year survival rate of 60% vs 42%).

This does indicate a benefit for node-positive cases given adjuvant chemotherapy and this should be considered for both pre- and postmenopausal patients with true medullary carcinomas. For node-negative cases, because of the good prognosis and the absence of hormone sensitivity, adjuvant therapy, either tamoxifen or chemotherapy, can be avoided.

SYNOPSIS

MUCOID CARCINOMA

* A diagnosis of pure mucinous carcinoma should be made only after a thorough histological examination of a completely excised tumour.
* If there is a mixed component the good prognosis is lost and approximates to that of patients with invasive ductal carcinoma (NOS).
* Pure mucinous cancers have to be distinguished from mixed lesions and mucocele-like tumours.
* Although there may be rare axillary metastases in patients with pure mucinous carcinoma, the overall survival rate is almost 100% at 10 years.

TUBULAR CARCINOMA

* Pure tubular carcinoma should be diagnosed only after stringent histological characterization.
* Tubular carcinomas may be multifocal and are then more likely to metastasize to axillary lymph nodes.
* Axillary nodal dissection and radiotherapy should be part of standard treatment and be omitted only in the context of randomized clinical trials.

MEDULLARY CARCINOMA

* Typical medullary carcinomas have a syncitial growth pattern, are well circumscribed, and have a moderate or marked lymphatic infiltration; based on these features they can be distinguished from atypical lesions.
* These cancers do not express keratin 19, nor do they contain oestrogen receptors.
* Despite the apparent lack of differentiation, typical medullary cancers carry a good prognosis with a 10-year survival rate of over 85%.

REFERENCES

1. Azzopard, JG. In: *Problems in Breast Pathology.* Bennington JL ed. London: WB Saunders, 1979: 294–6.
2. Saphir O. Mucinous carcinoma of the breast. *Surg Gynecol Obstet* 1941; **72**: 908–14.
3. NHSBSP. *Pathology Reporting in Breast Cancer Screening*, 2nd edn. Sheffield: National Co-ordinating Group for Breast Screening Pathology, 1995.
4. Halsted WS. A diagnostic sign of gelatinous carcinoma of the breast. *JAMA* 1915; **64**: 1653.
5. Norris HJ, Taylor HB. Prognosis of mucinous (gelatinous) carcinoma of the breast. *Cancer* 1965; **18**: 879–81.
6. Rasmussen BF. Human mucinous breast carcinomas and their lymph node metastases. *Pathol Res Precept* 1985; **180**: 377–82.
7. Andrea S, Cunha F, Bernardo M et al. Mucinous carcinoma of the breast: a pathologic study of 82 cases. *J Surg Oncol* 1995; **58**: 162–7.
8. Fentiman IS, Millis RR, Smith P et al. Mucoid breast carcinomas: histology and prognosis. *Br J Cancer* 1997; **75**: 1061–5.
9. Ro JY, Sneige N, Sahin AA et al. Mucocele-like tumor of the breast associated with atypical duct hyperplasia or mucinous carcinoma. A clinicopathological study of seven cases. *Arch Pathol Lab Med* 1991; **115**: 137–40.
10. Fisher CJ, Millis RR. A mucocele-like tumour of the breast associated with both atypical ductal hyperplasia and mucoid carcinoma. *Histopathology* 1992; **23**: 59–71.
11. Hamele-Bena D, Cranor ML, Rosen PP. Mammary mucocele-like lesions (MLL): benign and malignant. *Am J Surg Pathol* 1996; **9**: 1081–5.
12. Cardenosa G, Doudna C, Eklund GW. Mucinous (colloid) breast cancer: clinical and mammographic findings. *AJR* 1994; **162**: 1077–9.
13. Ruggieri AM, Scola FH, Schepps B, Esparza AR. Mucinous carcinoma of the breast: mammographic findings. *Breast Dis* 1995; **8**: 353–61.
14. Chopra S, Evans AJ, Pinder SE et al. Pure mucinous breast cancer – mammographic and ultrasound findings. *Clin Radiol* 1996; **51**: 421–4.
15. Capella C, Eusebi V, Mann B, Azzopardi JG. Endocrine differentiation in mucoid carcinoma of the breast. *Histopathology* 1980; **4**: 613–30.
16. Ferguson DJP, Anderson TJ, Wells CA, Battersby S. An ultrastructural study of mucoid carcinoma of the breast: variability of cytoplasmic features. *Histopathology* 1986; **10**: 1219–30.
17. Coady AT, Shousha S, Dawson PM et al. Mucinous carcinoma of the breast: further characterization of its three subtypes. *Histopathology* 1989; **15**: 617–26.
18. Rasmussen BB, Rose C, Thorpe SM et al. Argyrophilic cells in 202 human mucinous breast carcinomas. *Am J Clin Pathol* 1985; **84**: 737–40.
19. Scopsi L, Andreola S, Pilotti S et al. Mucinous carcinoma of the breast. *Am J Surg Pathol* 1994; **18**: 702–11.
20. Silverberg SG, Kay S, Chitale AR, Levitt SH. Colloid carcinoma of the breast. *Am J Clin Pathol* 1971; **55**: 355–63.
21. Komaki K, Sakamoto G, Sugano H et al. Mucinous carcinoma of the breast. *Jpn J Cancer* 1988; **61**: 989–96.
22. Pereira H, Pinder SE, Sibbering DM et al. Pathological prognostic factors in breast cancer. IV: Should you be a typer or a grader? A comparative study of two histological prognostic features in operable breast carcinoma. *Histopathology* 1995; **27**: 219–26.
23. Rasmussen BB, Rose C, Christensen I. Prognostic factors in primary mucinous breast carcinoma. *Am J Clin Pathol* 1987; **87**: 155–60.
24. Clayton F. Pure mucinous carcinomas of breast. *Hum Pathol* 1986; **17**: 34–8.
25. Melamed MR, Robbins GF, Foote FW. Prognostic significance of gelatinous mammary carcinoma. *Cancer* 1961; **11**: 699–704.
26. World Health Organization. *Histological Typing of Breast Tumours*, 2nd ed. International histological classification of tumours #2. Geneva: WHO, 1981: 19.
27. Taylor HB, Norris HJ. Well-differentiated carcinoma of the breast. *Cancer* 1970; **25**: 687–92.
28. Carstens PHB, Huvos AG, Foote FW et al. Tubular carcinoma of the breast: a clinicopathologic study of 35 cases. *Am J Clin Pathol* 1972; **58**: 231–8.
29. Cooper HS, Patchefsky AS, Krall RA. Tubular carcinoma of the breast. *Cancer* 1978; **42**: 2334–42.
30. Lagios MD, Rose MR, Margolin FR. Tubular carcinoma of the breast. Association with multicentricity, bilaterality, and family history of mammary carcinoma. *Am J Clin Pathol* 1980; **73**: 25–30.
31. Peters GN, Wolff M, Haagensen CD. Tubular carcinoma of the breast. Clinical pathologic

correlations based on 100 cases. *Ann Surg* 1981; **193:** 138–49.

32. Deos PH, Norris HJ. Well-differentiated (tubular) carcinoma of the breast. A clinico-pathologic study of 145 pure and mixed cases. *Am J Clin Pathol* 1982; **78:** 1–7.

33. Leibman AJ, Lewis M, Kruse B. Tubular carcinoma of the breast: mammographic appearance. *AJR* 1993; **160:** 263–5.

34. Elson BC, Helvie MA, Frank TS et al. Tubular carcinoma of the breast: mode of presentation, mammographic appearance, and frequency of nodal metastases. *AJR* 1993; **161:** 1173–6.

35. Winchester DJ, Sahin AA, Tucker SL, Singletary SE. Tubular carcinoma of the breast. Predicting axillary nodal metastases and recurrence. *Ann Surg* 1996; **223:** 342–7.

36. Oberman HA, Fidler WJ. Tubular carcinoma of the breast. *Am J Surg Pathol* 1979; **3:** 387–95.

37. Fentiman IS, Hyland D, Chaudary MA, Gregory WM. Prognosis of patients with breast cancers up to 1 cm in diameter. *Eur J Cancer* 1996; **32A:** 417–20.

38. Green I, McCormick B, Cranor M, Rosen PP. A comparative study of pure tubular and tubulolobular carcinoma of the breast. *Am J Surg Pathol* 1997; **21:** 653–7.

39. Moore OS, Foote FW. The relatively favourable prognosis of medullary carcinoma of the breast. *Cancer* 1949; **2:** 635–42.

40. Pedersen L, Holck S, Schiedt T. Medullary carcinoma of the breast. *Cancer Treat Rev* 1988; **15:** 53–63.

41. Black CL, Morris DM, Goldman LI, McDonald JC. The significance of lymph node involvement in patients with medullary carcinoma of the breast. *Surg Gynecol Obstet* 1983; **157:** 497–9.

42. Meyer JE, Amin E, Lindfors KK et al. Medullary carcinoma of the breast: mammographic and US appearance. *Radiology* 1989; **170:** 79–82.

43. Ridolfi RL, Rosen PP, Port A et al. Medullary carcinoma of the breast. A clinicopathological study with 10 year follow-up. *Cancer* 1977; **40:** 1365–85.

44. Rubens JR, Lewandrowski KB, Kopans DB et al. Medullary carcinoma of the breast. Over-diagnosis of a prognostically favourable neoplasm. *Arch Surg* 1990; **125:** 601–4.

45. Rigaud C, Theobald S, Noël P et al. Medullary carcinoma of the breast. A multicentre study of its diagnostic consistency. *Arch Pathol Lab Med* 1993; **117:** 1005–8.

46. Gaffey MJ, Mills SE, Frierson HF et al. Medullary carcinoma of the breast: interobserver variability in histopathologic diagnosis. *Modern Pathol* 1995; **8:** 31–8.

47. Wargotz ES, Silverberg SG. Medullary carcinoma of the breast: a clinicopathologic study with appraisal of current diagnostic criteria. *Hum Pathol* 1988; **19:** 1340–6.

48. Pedersen L, Zedeler K, Holck S et al. Medullary carcinoma of the breast, proposal for a new simplified histopathological definition. *Br J Cancer* 1991; **63:** 591–5.

49. Hsu S-M, Raine L, Nayak RN. Medullary carcinoma of breast: an immunohistochemical study of its lymphoid stroma. *Cancer* 1981; **48:** 1368–76.

50. Larsimont D, Lespagnard L, Degeyter M, Heimann R. Medullary carcinoma of the breast: a tumour lacking keratin 19. *Histopathology* 1994; **24:** 549–52.

51. Bartek J, Durban EM, Hallowes RC, Taylor-Papadimitriou J. A subclass of luminal epithelial cells in the human mammary gland defined by antibodies to cytokeratins. *J Cell Sci* 1985; **75:** 17–33.

52. Ponsky JL, Gliga L, Reynolds S. Medullary carcinoma of the breast: an association with negative hormonal receptors. *J Surg Oncol* 1984; **25:** 76–8.

53. Patel JK, Nemoto T, Dao TL. Is medullary carcinoma of the breast hormone dependent? *J Surg Oncol* 1983; **24:** 290–1.

54. Rapin V, Contesso G, Mouriesse H et al. Medullary breast carcinoma. A re-evaluation of 95 cases of breast cancer with inflammatory stroma. *Cancer* 1988; **61:** 2503–10.

55. Fisher ER, Kenny JP, Sass R et al. Medullary cancer of the breast revisited. *Breast Cancer Res Treat* 1990; **16:** 215–19.

56. Reinfuss M, Stelmach A, Mitus J et al. Typical medullary carcinoma of the breast: a clinical and pathological analysis of 52 cases. *J Surg Oncol* 1995; **60:** 89–94.

22

Non-epithelial cancers

Scarce sir. Mighty scarce.

Mark Twain

Sarcoma • Lymphoma

SARCOMA

Although mesenchymal malignancy of the breast is rare, stromal proliferation is common, as a component of fibroadenomas. It may be both difficult for the pathologist to categorize a breast sarcoma and problematic for the surgeon whose experience of such lesions may be limited. Principles of management are complete excision of the lesion and avoidance of nodal surgery, because, when these tumours disseminate, it is via veins rather than lymphatics. No clinical trial results are available to guide our decisions.

The most common lesion is the phyllodes tumour but only one in seven of these is malignant. Of the 'classic' sarcomas, angiosarcoma and stromal sarcoma are the most common, with fibrosarcoma and malignant fibrous histiocytoma (MFH) being diagnosed less frequently. Rarer tumours include liposarcoma, leiomyosarcoma, rhabdomyosarcoma and osteosarcoma, usually being reported as single cases.

Phyllodes tumour

In 1838 Müller described a carnose (fleshy) tumour of the breast which he regarded as benign but named cystosarcoma because of the fleshiness of the lesion.[1] This old term was an incitement to surgical excess which was partly diminished when Azzopardi proposed the nomenclature of phyllodes tumour.[2] Even so, phyllodes tumour encompasses a spectrum of lesions which range from benign tumours to very aggressive variants that can metastasize and kill.

A phyllodes tumour is a fibroepithelial neoplasm which arises in periductal connective tissue and has a very cellular stromal component and integral ductal elements. Azzopardi divided phyllodes into three types: benign, borderline and malignant. The criteria for histological typing are given in Table 22.1. There are four features: stromal cellularity, tumour margins, mitotic rate (based on number of mitoses per 10 high-power fields, hpf), and nuclear pleomorphism.

Presentation

Behaviour of phyllodes tumours can only partly be predicted on a basis of their histological appearance or clinical features. In only one series was there a relationship between age, size and malignancy.[3] There were 22 benign cases (mean age 34, mean tumour size 3.6 cm), eight borderline (age 38, size 5.7 cm) and four malignant (age 44, size 16.8 cm). Others have found

Table 22.1 Histological typing of phyllodes tumours

Feature	Benign	Borderline	Malignant
Stromal cellularity	Low	Moderate	High
Tumour margins	Pushing	Borderline	Infiltrative
Mitotic rate (per hfp)	< 5	5–9	≥ 10
Nuclear pleomorphism	Mild	Moderate	Severe

that age and tumour size were no guide to future recurrence or metastasis.[4,5]

Using incidence data from the Los Angeles County Tumor Registry, Bernstein et al studied the epidemiology of malignant phyllodes tumours.[6] There were 154 cases diagnosed between 1972 and 1989 with a mean annual age-adjusted incidence rate of 2 per one million women. Overall, the peak incidence occurred between ages 45 and 49, but this varied with age and ethnic background, and showed an increasing incidence with time.

Table 22.2 shows that the highest rate was seen in Hispanic women, but that the disease was diagnosed significantly later than in Asian women (46 vs 33 years). Among white women the average age at diagnosis was 54 years. Hispanic women born in Mexico or Central America had a threefold increase in risk of being diagnosed with a phyllodes tumour, and it was postulated that acquired infections during lactation might play a role in the aetiology of this disease.

Table 22.2 Age at diagnosis and ethnicity in patients with phyllodes tumours

Ethnic group	Mean age	Age-adjusted incidence rate per million	
		1972–81	1982–89
Hispanic	46	1.5	3.9
White	54	1.6	2.4
Black	49	1.1	1.6
Asian	33	0.5	2.6
All	50	1.5	2.6

From Bernstein et al.[6]

Histogenesis

It is likely that both fibroadenomas and phyllodes tumours are derived from intralobular fibroblasts because both express functional dipeptidyl peptidase IV.[7] When sequential samples from a benign phyllodes tumour were subjected to cytogenetic analysis and fluorescent in situ hybridization (FISH), there were additional copies of chromosome 1q,i(1)(q10), present in both.[8] Furthermore one copy of chromosome 21 was deleted in both specimens. In another contemporary cytogenetic study of a borderline phyllodes tumour, it was also found that two copies of i(1)(q10) were present.[9]

Noguchi et al carried out clonal analysis of cells from three fibroadenomas and four phyllodes tumours excised sequentially from the same patient.[10] In all cases the same allele of the androgen receptor (AR) gene was inactivated. As there is a low probability that the same allele of the AR gene would be spontaneously inactivated in all the lesions, the like-

Table 22.3 Local relapse after excision of phyllodes tumours

Follow-up (years)	Benign	Borderline	Malignant	Reference
9	2/22 (9)	2/8 (25)	3/4 (75)	Kario et al[3]
4	6/92 (6)	0/12	0/2	Bartoli et al[11]
4	5/22 (23)	3/12 (25)	9/25 (36)	Ciatto et al[4]
8	15/189 (8)	10/58 (17)	8/39 (21)	Zurrida et al[12]
4	2/24 (8)	1/6 (17)	0/3	Stebbing and Nash[5]

Values in parentheses are percentages.

lihood is of a clonal origin with phyllodes tumours evolving from fibroadenomas.

Histology and outcome

Classification of a phyllodes tumour as benign is not a guarantee that local relapse will not occur. As Table 22.3 shows, there may be similar local relapses in this group than in tumours diagnosed as malignant, possibly because surgery is likely to be more radical in such cases.[3–5,11,12] The only discordant series was that of Kario et al in which there was a higher relapse rate in those with malignant tumours that were both substantially larger and associated with greater stromal overgrowth.[3]

In a large series of 106 cases from the Istituto Tumori, Milan, all of whom had tumours small enough for day surgery excision, the only relapses were seen in 6% of those with histologically benign lesions.[11] The multicentre Italian series of Ciatto et al indicated that tumour type bore little relationship to risk of local relapse,[4] as did that of Stebbing and Nash.[5] In the largest series of 286 cases relapse occurred in 8% of benign cases, 17% of borderline and 21% of malignant phyllodes tumours.[12]

Luckily distant metastases from malignant phyllodes tumours are rare. There were none in three series[3,5,11] and 3 of 25 (12%) in that of Ciatto et al.[4] Hawkins et al reviewed 33 patients treated at the Royal Marsden Hospital, to determine factors predicting for distant metastases from phyllodes tumours.[13] Distant metastases occurred in eight (24%), after a median interval

of 14 months, and seven (21%) died of their disease. The most significant variables predicting metastasis were: nuclear pleomorphism, stromal overgrowth, high mitotic count and infiltrating margin. When data from previous series were re-analysed in relation to these variables, the most significant prognostic indicator was stromal overgrowth.

Treatment

Surgery for phyllodes tumour will depend upon the clinical preoperative diagnosis and size of the lesion. If clinically suspected to be a fibroadenoma, many of these tumours will be enucleated. If a subsequent wide excision is performed to remove the leaf-like projections of a benign tumour, this will reduce the chance of local relapse. The recurrence rates after different types of surgery are shown in Table 22.4.[3–5,11,14] Enucleation alone is usually reserved for those with benign lesions, but even under these circumstances a relapse rate of between 2% and 60% was reported. After wide excision a local recurrence rate of 11–40% occurred. Mastectomy achieved the best local control with a relapse rate of between zero and 14%. Only one case in one series[14] had axillary nodal involvement and this was locally advanced with chest wall invasion. Thus axillary nodal dissection is redundant in patients with phyllodes tumours.

The role of radiotherapy is speculative. Several case reports have suggested that phyllodes tumours are radioresistant, when

Table 22.4 Local relapse after different types of surgery for phyllodes tumour

Enucleation	Wide excision	Mastectomy	Reference
–	7/30 (23)	0/4	Kario et al[3]
BE 1/47 (2)	4/38 (11)	1/7 (14)	Bartoli et al[11]
BO –	0/12	–	Bartoli et al[11]
M –	–	0/2	Bartoli et al[11]
3/5 (60)	12/30 (40)	2/24 (8)	Ciatto et al[4]
–	–	3/36 (8)	Reinfuss et al[14]
1/10 (10)	3/17 (18)	0/6	Stebbing and Nash[5]

BE, benign; BO, borderline; M, malignant.
Values in parentheses are percentages.

radiotherapy was used to palliate metastatic disease.[15-18] In a series of 77 cases from the Swedish Cancer Registry, 24 (31%) received radiotherapy after either local excision or mastectomy.[19] Relapse occurred in 13 of 24 (54%) of those treated by excision and two of 53 (4%) of those who underwent mastectomy. Radiotherapy had no effect on local control, but as this was not a randomized trial the result could be biased. At present optimal treatment is complete excision with histologically confirmed clear margins, and for some patients this will necessitate a total mastectomy.

Angiosarcoma

The incidence of this rare tumour may be undergoing an iatrogenic increase, after surgery and radiotherapy as breast conservation therapy. Indeed, radiation may have been responsible for many of these sarcomas. In 1948, Stewart and Treves reported six cases with long-standing severe arm oedema in whom lymphangiosarcomas had developed on the arm or chest wall after radical mastectomy and gland field irradiation.[20] These tumours were aggressive and, even after local treatment by forequarter amputation, death from blood-borne metastases usually followed (Fig. 22.1).

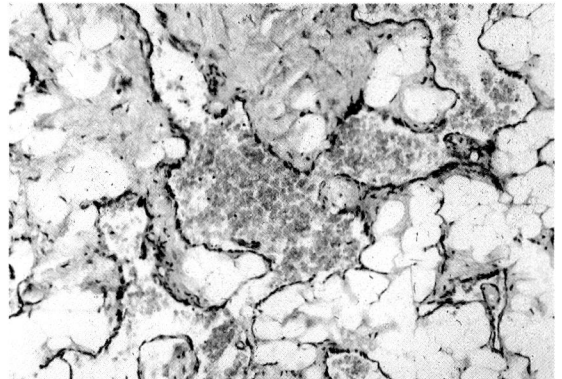

Fig. 22.1 Angiosarcoma of the breast.

As the combination of surgery and radiotherapy to the axilla came to be recognized as both unnecessary and also associated with severe morbidity, so it might have been hoped that angiosarcomas would become even more of a rarity.

Sadly, this has not proved to be the case. An increasing number of publications have described breast angiosarcomas following breast irradiation, and these are summarized in Table 22.5.[21-40] Up to 1996, 34 cases had been reported. The average age at diagnosis of angiosarcoma was 63 years (range 47–83) and the mean inter-

Table 22.5 Case reports of breast angiosarcoma after radiotherapy

Age (years)	Interval (years)	Treatment	Outcome	Reference
75	6	TM	A&W	Body et al[21]
73	4		DOD 10 months	Shaikh et al[22]
60	10	MRM	A&W	Givens et al[23]
67	7	MRM	A&W	Rubin et al[24]
54	6.5	TM	DOD 24 months	Badwe et al[25]
67	7	TM	A&W	Roukeema et al[26]
71	5	TM	A&W	Roukeema et al[26]
57	6	TM	A&W	Stokkel et al[27]
53	2.5	TM	DOD 6 months	Stokkel et al[27]
75	7	TM	A&W	Stokkel et al[27]
70	6.5	TM	D 1 month	Taat et al[28]
83	15	Inop.	DOD 4 months	Edeiken et al[29]
80	5	TM	A&W	Edeinken et al[29]
77	5	TM	A&W	Sessions and Smink[30]
58	6	TM	DOD 34 months	Wijnmaalen et al[31]
71	5	TM	A&W	Wijnmaalen et al[31]
59	7	TM	A&W	Wijnmaalen et al[31]
57	8	WE	LR 6 months	Choy et al[32]
71	4.5	TM	A&W	Slotman et al[33]
47	1	WE	A&W	Zucali et al[34]
72	5	TM	DOD 6 months	Zucali et al[34]
64	3	TM	LR 12 months	Zucali et al[34]
72	6	TM	LR 6 months	Buatti et al[35]
75	5	MRM	DOD 9 months	Fineberg and Rosen[36]
70	3.5	Nil	D 1 month	Fineberg and Rosen[36]
70	4	TM	A&W	Fineberg and Rosen[36]
79	6	TM	DOD 10 months	Provencio et al[37]
49	5	Inop.	DOD	Weber and Marchal[38]
49	6	WE	A&W	Weber and Marchal[38]
59	5	WE	A&W	Weber and Marchal[38]
59	4	TM	DOD 14 months	Molitor et al[39]
49	6.5	TM	DOD 19 months	Molitor et al[39]
66	4.5	TM	A&W	Molitor et al[39]
81	10	TM	A&W	Bolin and Lukas[40]

A&W, alive and well; DOD, died of disease; LR, local relapse.

val between original radiotherapy and diagnosis of sarcoma was 6 years (range 1–15). The most common presentation was a red, blue or violet lump, sometimes with ecchymosis, in the oedematous skin of an irradiated breast. Most cases were treated by total mastectomy (TM), a few by modified radical mastectomy (MRM) or wide excision (WE), and two were inoperable.

Table 22.6 Histological features and outcome in breast angiosarcoma

Feature	Group I	Group II	Group III
Number	13	7	20
Mean age	41	38	30
Endothelial tufting	Minimal	Present	Prominent
Papillary formation	Absent	Foci	Present
Solid and spindle cell foci	Absent	Absent/minimal	Present
Mitoses	Rare	Present	Numerous
Blood lakes	Absent	Absent	Present
Necrosis	Absent	Absent	Present
No. disease free (%)	10 (77)	3 (43)	2 (10)
No. died of disease (%)	1 (8)	2 (29)	14 (78)

From Donnell et al.[43]

After relatively short follow-up 18 (53%) were alive and well without recurrence. There were 11 cases (32%) who died of metastatic angiosarcoma and the average interval between diagnosis of angiosarcoma and death was 13.5 months (range 4–34). The incidence among women who have had radiotherapy as part of breast conservation is very low. The three cases from the Istituto Tumori Milan were derived from a total of 3295 patients treated over a 17-year period, representing an incidence of 0.09%.[39] Thus, although the association is real, its magnitude is not such as to cast a shadow over breast irradiation. It does, however, underline the need to monitor irradiated patients carefully and determine cytologically or histologically the nature of pigmented lesions developing within the irradiated field.

True mammary angiosarcomas comprise 0.04% of all breast malignancies and only 8% of sarcomas, so they may be initially misdiagnosed.[41] Liberman et al reviewed the records of 29 women with mammary angiosarcomas treated at the Sloan-Kettering Memorial Hospital between 1966 and 1991.[42] The mean age was 42 years (range 20–70), all had a palpable mass ranging from 1 to 8 cm, but only five (17%) had a bluish discoloration to the lesion. Mammography showed a non-calcified solitary mass in most and ultrasonography, performed in five cases, revealed a solid mass in three, multiple masses in one, and no demonstrable lesion in another. Magnetic resonance imaging (MRI) was performed in only one case and showed a mass with low signal density on T1–weighted images and higher signal intensity in T2-weighted images.

Histopathology and prognosis
Angiosarcomas had been regarded as carrying a dire prognosis until Donnell et al reported the relationship between histology and outcome in 40 cases.[43] All had breast parenchymal lesions comprising interanastomosing vascular channels, lined by hyperchromatic endothelial cells. Other features sought were endothelial tufting, papillary formation, solid and spindle cell foci, mitoses, blood lakes and necrosis, and the patients were divided into three groups based on these. The results, in Table 22.6, show that the group with the worst histological features were younger women (average age 30);

they had a significantly poorer prognosis, with 78% dying from metastatic disease, compared with only one case from the group with less aggressive histological findings.

Fibrosarcoma – malignant fibrous histiocytoma

Nomenclature for breast fibrosarcomas can be bewildering with cases being variously described as fibrosarcoma, stromal cell sarcoma, malignant fibrous histiocytoma and sometimes fibromatosis. Each comprises a different entity. The last condition, also known as extra-abdominal desmoid, is a progressive, non-encapsulated well-differentiated fibroblastic growth which may show infiltrative borders but which does not metastasize. Gump et al reported a series of 17 cases of fibromatosis, treated at Columbia-Presbyterian Hospital, New York, all of whom presented with a palpable mass usually associated with skin retraction.[44] The average age was 49 years (range 18–80) and the usual preoperative diagnosis was carcinoma. Treatment was by either local or wide excision. Of those who had local excision recurrence occurred in 25% compared with 20% in the wide excision group. No recurrence occurred after truly radical excision.

There may be a genetic predisposition to breast desmoids, particularly in those with Gardner's syndrome. Histological distinction between fibromatosis and fibrosarcoma can be problematic and it has been suggested that the diagnosis of fibromatosis should not be entertained unless there is a family history of fibromatosis, known Gardner's syndrome, history of breast trauma, skin/pectoral muscle involvement, or fibromatosis elsewhere.[45]

Fibrosarcoma

The typical histological appearance of a fibrosarcoma is a monomorphic population of spindle cells arranged in a herringbone fashion (see Fig. 22.2). Fletcher has described malignant fibrous histiocytoma (MFH) as a fashionable diagnosis for over 20 years and has questioned

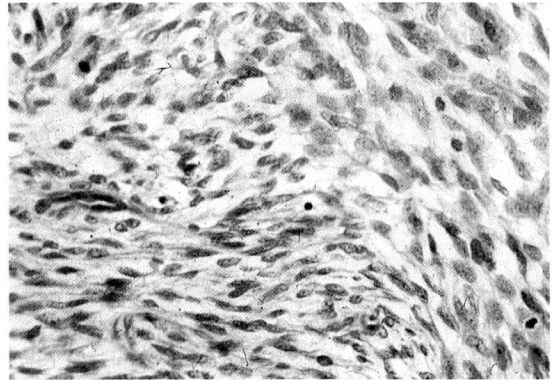

Fig. 22.2 Fibrosarcoma of the breast.

whether pleomorphic MFH is a cohesive histological entity.[46] He suggested that it represents a wide range of anaplastic tumours which with special staining can be shown to have a specific line of differentiation. The term stromal cell sarcoma was originally used to describe all breast sarcomas other than phyllodes and angiosarcoma, but has been redefined as being a rare variant of a non-specific type which is derived from intralobular stroma.[47]

Gutman et al reviewed a series of 60 patients with breast sarcomas treated at MD Anderson Hospital, Texas: 16 (27%) had stromal cell sarcoma, 10 (17%) fibrosarcoma and 6 (10%) malignant fibrous histiocytoma (MFH).[48] The comparative features of these cases are shown in Table 22.7. Patients with MFH were older than those with stromal cell and fibrosarcoma, and had a much worse disease-free and overall survival, with none surviving 10 years.

In a clinicopathological study of 32 cases reviewed at the Armed Forces Institute of Pathology, Washington DC, Jones et al classified the tumours as either low-grade fibrosarcoma–MFH (16) or high-grade fibrosarcoma–MFH (16).[49] High-grade sarcomas had marked atypia and a mitotic rate of 5 or more per high power field. Those with low-grade tumours were younger and had a better overall survival despite local recurrence occurring in 63%, as shown in Table 22.8.

Table 22.7 Comparative features of patients with stromal sarcoma, fibrosarcoma and malignant fibrous histiocytoma

Type of sarcoma	Number	Mean age (years)	Size (cm)	10-year DFS (%)	10 year OS (%)
Stromal sarcoma	16	50	8	25	35
Fibrosarcoma	10	48	9	30	40
MFH	6	65	6	0	0

From Gutman et al.[48]

Table 22.8 Comparative features of patients with low and high grade fibrosarcoma-mixed fibrous histiocytoma

Grade	Age	Mitoses (per hpf)	Local relapse rate (%)	Survival rate (%)
Low	45	2	63	100
High	64	12	44	69

From Jones et al.[49]

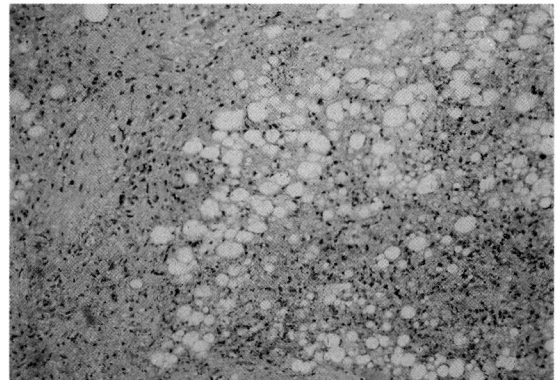

Fig. 22.3 Liposarcoma of the breast.

Liposarcoma

These rare cancers may arise either from mammary fat or within a phyllodes tumour. They are identified histologically by the presence of lipoblasts and it may be necessary to carry out special staining with alcein blue and colloidal iron for these to become apparent (see Fig. 22.3). Enzinger et al proposed the World Health Organization classification which comprises five subtypes: predominantly well differentiated, predominantly myxoid, predominantly round cell, predominantly poorly differentiated, and mixed.[50] This can be useful in predicting clinical behaviour as local relapse was reported in 53% of cases with well-differentiated and myxoid liposarcomas, but in 80% of those with round cell and poorly differentiated tumours.[51] However, these data were derived from a series of 103 liposarcomas from all sites. Those arising in the breast have a better prognosis.

Ii et al reviewed 42 cases from the literature[52] and subsequently Austin and Dupree reported 20 cases from the Armed Forces Institute of Pathology.[53] The features of these cases are summarized in Table 22.9. The mean age at

Table 22.9 Features of patients with mammary liposarcomas

Feature	Austin and Dupree[53]	li et al[52]
Number	20	42
Age (mean)	47	47
Male	2 (10)	1 (2)
Within phyllodes tumour	7 (35)	12 (29)
Local relapse	3 (15)	5 (12)
Distant metastases	3 (15)	11 (26)

Values in parentheses are percentages.

diagnosis was 47 years and 5% of cases were men. Overall, 31% of liposarcomas arose from phyllodes tumours. Local relapse occurred in only 13% and distant metastases in 23%.

Liposarcomas may appear to be encapsulated so that enucleation may be attempted. Wide local excision is necessary, which may sometimes mean total mastectomy for patients with large lesions. Axillary surgery is unnecessary unless there is direct invasion. Both radiotherapy and chemotherapy are speculative options and have no place in routine treatment of mammary liposarcoma.

Leiomyosarcoma

These sarcomas are rarely reported as breast primaries and no large series have accumulated. Less than a score of cases have been reported and these are shown in Table 22.10.[47,54–59] The mean age at diagnosis was 52 years (range 24–77), and 4 of 19 (21%) were male. The histological features were of a pleomorphic neoplasm with a focal spindle cell pattern. In the more recent cases mitotic rate (mitoses per 10 high-power fields) was measured and reported as between 3 and 29 mitoses/hpf.

Almost all patients were treated by either radical (RM) or total mastectomy (TM) with only three more recent cases having wide excision (WE). Local relapse was reported in 4 of 17 cases (24%) and occurred in 2 of 6 (33%) of those treated by RM, one of eight (12.5%) of TM cases and one of four (25%) of WE cases. Death from metastatic disease was reported in three patients (16%). Neither clinical nor histological features so far studied have any significant prognostic value in terms of local relapse or distant metastases.[59]

Osteogenic sarcoma

In 1700, Bonet described a breast tumour that consisted of cartilage and bone, which may have been the first recorded diagnosis of this rare and aggressive sarcoma.[60] Osteogenic sarcoma may present as a bone-hard mass which histologically shows pleomorphic spindle cells with abundant osteoid, often calcified. The calcified osteoid may take up ^{99m}Tc-labelled methylene diphosphonate used for bone scanning and this may suggest preoperatively the diagnosis of osteogenic sarcoma.[61,62] Typically patients complain of a breast lump that has recently increased in size, sometimes because a sarcoma has developed in a longstanding fibroadenoma. An example of a breast osteosarcoma is shown in Fig. 22.4.

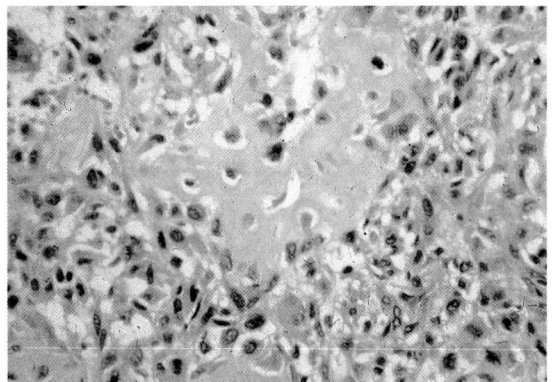

Fig. 22.4 Osteosarcoma of the breast.

Table 22.10 Reported cases of breast leiomyosarcoma

Age (years)	Sex	Size (cm)	Mitosis	Surgery	Outcome	Reference
35	F	19	–	RM	LR	Yamashina[54]
50	M	–	–	TM	–	Yamashina[54]
53	M	6	–	RM	–	Yamashina[54]
51	M	5	–	RM	LR	Yamashina[54]
77	F	8	–	TM	DF	Yamashina[54]
49	F	7	16	RM	DF	Yamashina[54]
40	F	5	–	TM	LR	Yamashina[54]
55	F	3	10	TM	DF	Yamashina[54]
53	M	4	15	RM	DF	Yamashina[54]
59	F	6	3	TM	DOD	Yamashina[54]
24	F	2	14	WE	DOD	Nielsen[55]
56	F	3	21	RM	DF	Yatsuka et al[56]
50	F	9	5	RM	DF	Yatsuka et al[56]
54	F	3	10	TM	DF	Callery et al[47]
56	F	2	10	TM	DF	Callery et al[47]
62	F	3	15	TM	DF	Yamashina[54]
50	F	5	4	WE	LR	Arista-Nasr et al[57]
58	F	4	10	WE	DF	Waterworth et al[58]
52	F	3	29	TM	DOD	Parham et al[59]

RM, radical mastectomy; TM, total mastectomy; WE, wide excision; DF, disease-free; LR, local relapse; DOD, died of disease.

Cases of osteogenic sarcoma with follow-up and outcome are shown in Table 22.11, indicating the generally poor prognosis of patients with this neoplasm.[63–73] The mean tumour diameter at presentation was 5 cm and most cases were treated by either radical or total mastectomy. Of these cases of osteogenic sarcoma, 73% died of metastatic disease, usually from pulmonary metastases.

Kaiser et al reported a case in whom the tumour was imaged with an echocontrast agent followed by colour ultrasonography, which showed disordered vascularization and a long washout time for the contrast, thereby delineat-ing the extent of the lesion.[73] As reported in other cases, there was elevation of alkaline phosphatase in the blood. As survival can be prolonged in patients with bone sarcomas given chemotherapy,[74] Kaiser et al administered doxorubicin and cisplatin and the patient remained disease free 18 months later.[73] There were reports of four other cases given combination chemotherapy.[68,72,75,76] One patient who received methotrexate, ifosphamide and cisplatin died of disease and another developed progression.[75] Two patients who were given high-dose methotrexate, bleomycin, cyclophosphamide, dactinomycin and doxorubicin

Table 22.11 Treatment and outcome of patients with osteogenic sarcoma of the breast

Size (cm)	Treatment	Outcome	Reference
5	RM	DOD	Fry[63]
12	RM	DOD	Carlucci and Wagner[64]
8	TM	DOD	Rottino and Howley[65]
2	WE	DWR	Jernstrom et al[66]
4	RM	DOD	Gonzalez-Licea et al[67]
3	RM	DOD	Aubrey and Andrews[68]
4	RM	DOD	Annani and Baumann[69]
3	RM	DF	Mertens et al[70]
2	TM	DOD	Watt et al[71]
7	RM	DOD	Mufarrij and Feiner[72]
3	WE	DF	Kaiser et al[73]

DOD, died of disease; DWR, died without relapse; DF, disease free.

remained disease free after 38 and 49 months.[76] This suggests that there may be a role for intensive chemotherapy in patients with osteogenic sarcoma of the breast.

LYMPHOMA

Primary breast lymphoma (PBL) has been estimated to account for 0.04–0.53% of all breast neoplasms.[77] The breast is the site of 2% of all extranodal lymphomas.[78] It was originally suggested by Adair and Hermann that there were two distinct variants of PBL: bilateral diffuse occurring in young puerperal women and unilateral disease affecting older patients.[79] Subsequent work indicated that histology of the former group was Burkitt's lymphoma, usually diagnosed in African patients,[80,81] and such cases comprise 20% of all PBL. The clinical course is rapid with involvement of the central nervous system, gastrointestinal tract and ovaries without lymph node invasion. The main type of PBL is more heterogeneous in behaviour but presents as a breast lump which may be suspected as a carcinoma, sometimes lobular because of the relatively soft texture of the tumour. Histologically, most cases of PBL prove to be B-cell lymphomas.

Classification of lymphomas can be complex and most recent series used the Rappaport system in which the categories are based on cytology and growth pattern.[82] Cytological categories are: lymphocytic well-differentiated; lymphocytic poorly differentiated; mixed histiocytic/lymphocytic; histiocytic; and poorly differentiated. Growth patterns are either diffuse or nodular. The more complex Kiel classification attempts to relate the malignant cells to their benign counterpart and avoids the questionable histiocytic terminology.[83] Lymphomas are divided into high and low grade and subdivided into multiple cell types within these two grades. Almost all cases of PBL are non-Hodgkin's lymphoma, with many series having no cases of Hodgkin's disease.

It was suggested that these lymphomas arise from mucosa-associated lymphoid tissues (MALTs),[84,85] and so an immunohistochemical study was conducted on nine cases of PBL treated at Guy's Hospital between 1974 and 1990.[86] All the patients were aged over 50 years and eight (89%) were B-cell lymphomas, the other being a histiocytic lymphoma. Of the B-cell cases seven (88%) were high grade and one was a follicular lymphoma. A panel of antibodies was used to stain for panleukocytic marker, T cells, B cells, low-molecular-weight keratin, follicular dendritic cells and transformed lymphocytes. Almost all the lymphomas were positive for panleukocyte antibody and B-cell marker, but negative for almost all other markers, indicating that the cells were centroblastic in origin and not derived from MALT. Similar results were reported in a Danish study of six cases.[77]

Staging

Most cases of PBL are stage IE and IIE, based on the Ann Arbor system.[87] This means that the disease is extranodal (E) without (I) or with (II) nodal involvement in one or more regions on the same side of the diaphragm. After a full history and clinical examination, subsequent investigations can be directed towards other potential sites of disease. All will require a full blood count, biochemical screen, chest radiograph and bone marrow biopsy, together with computed tomography scans of thorax and abdomen.

Treatment

After histological confirmation and staging of disease, the treatment will be similar to that of other lymphoma cases. If localized low-grade disease is present the breast and gland fields are irradiated. When localized disease is of high grade, first-line chemotherapy is used, comprising CHOP (cyclophosphamide, doxorubicin or Adriamycin, vincristine and prednisone), or a variant thereof.[88] If there is bulky residual disease after chemotherapy this can be backed up with external radiotherapy. For patients with stage III/IV lymphoma, chemotherapy comprises CHOP for high grade and chlorambucil in those with low-grade disease. Patients with PBL need management by specialized oncological teams and should not be treated by those whose expertise is in the field of breast cancer surgery.

SYNOPSIS

- Phyllodes tumours are most common in women in their late 40s and local relapse is unrelated to histological type, provided that complete excision has been performed.
- Angiosarcomas are rare lesions which are being seen more frequently as a result of breast irradiation occurring on average 6 years later.
- Fibrosarcomas frequently recur locally, particularly when of high grade.
- Breast lymphoma is rare with treatment being determined by histological type and grade.

REFERENCES

1. Müller J. *Uber den feineran Bau und die Forman der Krankhaften Geschwilste*. Berlin: G Reiner, 1838.
2. Azzopardi JG. Problems in breast pathology. In: *Major Problems in Pathology*, Vol 11. Bennington JL, ed. Philadelphia: WB Saunders, 1979.
3. Kario K, Maeda S, Mizuno Y et al. Phyllodes tumor of the breast: a clinico-pathologic study of 34 cases. *J Surg Oncol* 1990; **45**: 46–51.
4. Ciatto S, Bonardi R, Cataliotti L et al. Phyllodes tumor of the breast: a multicenter series of 59 cases. *Eur J Surg Oncol* 1992; **18**: 545–9.
5. Stebbing JF, Nash AG. Diagnosis and management of phyllodes tumour of the breast: experience of 33 cases at a specialist centre. *Ann R Coll Surg Engl* 1995; **77**: 181–4.
6. Bernstein L, Deapen D, Ross RK. The descriptive epidemiology of malignant cystosarcoma phyllodes tumors of the breast. *Cancer* 1993; **71**: 3020–4.
7. Atherton A, Monaghan P, Warburton MJ et al. Dipeptidyl peptidase 1V expression identifies a functional sub-population of breast fibroblasts. *Int J Cancer* 1992; **50**: 15–19.
8. Birdsall SH, Summersgill BM, Egan M et al. Additional copies of 1q in sequential samples from a phyllodes tumor of the breast. *Cancer Genet Cytogenet* 1995; **83**: 111–14.
9. Dal Cin P, Moreman P, De Wever I, Van Den Berghe H. Is i(1)(110Q) a chromosome marker in phyllodes tumor of the breast? *Cancer Genet Cytogenet* 1995; **83**: 174–5.
10. Noguchi S, Yokouchi H, Aihara T et al. Progression of fibroadenoma to phyllodes tumor demonstrated by clonal analysis. *Cancer* 1995; **76**: 1779–85.
11. Bartoli C, Zurrida S, Veronesi P et al. Small sized phyllodes tumor of the breast. *Eur J Surg Oncol* 1990; **16**: 215–19.
12. Zurrida S, Galimberti V, Bartoli C, Squicciarni P. The treatment of phyllodes tumor of the breast: experience of 286 cases [Abstr]. *Eur J Cancer* 1993; **Suppl 6**: S67.
13. Hawkins RE, Schofield JB, Fisher C et al. The clinical and histologic criteria that predict metastases from cystosarcoma phyllodes. *Cancer* 1992; **69**: 141–7.

14. Reinfuss M, Mitus J, Smolak K, Stelmach A. Malignant phyllodes tumours of the breast. A clinical and pathological analysis of 55 cases. *Eur J Cancer* 1993; **29A:** 1252–6.

15. Kessinger A, Foley JF, Lemon HM, Miller DM. Metastatic cystosarcoma phyllodes: a case report and review of the literature. *J Surg Oncol* 1972; **4:** 131–47.

16. Sheen-Chen S, Chou F, Chen W. Cystosarcoma phyllodes of the breast: a review of clinical, pathological and therapeutic options in 19 cases. *Int Surg* 1991; **76:** 101–4.

17. Al-Jurf A, Hawk JA, Crile G. Cystosarcoma phyllodes. *Surg Gynecol Obstet* 1978; **146:** 358–64.

18. Blichert-Toft M, Hansen JPH, Hansen OH, Schiodt T. Clinical course of cystosarcoma phyllodes related to histologic appearance. *Surg Gynecol Obstet* 1975; **140:** 929–32.

19. Cohn-Cedermark G, Rurqvist LE, Rosendahl I, Silfersward C. Prognostic factors in cystosarcoma phyllodes. A clinicopathologic study of 77 patients. *Cancer* 1991; **68:** 2017–22.

20. Stewart FM, Treves N. Lymphangiosarcoma in postmastectomy lymphedema. *Cancer* 1948; **1:** 64–81.

21. Body G, Sanvanet E, Calais G et al. Angiosarcoma cutane du sein après adenocarcinome mammaire operé et irradié. *J Gynecol Obstet Biol Reprod (Paris)* 1987; **16:** 479–83.

22. Shaikh NA, Beasconsfield T, Walker M, Ghilchik M. Post-irradiation angiosarcoma of the breast: a case report. *Eur J Surg Oncol* 1988; **14:** 449–51.

23. Givens SS, Ellerbroek NA, Butler JJ et al. Angiosarcoma arising in an irradiated breast. A case report and review of the literature. *Cancer* 1989; **64:** 2214–16.

24. Rubin E, Maddox WA, Mazur MT. Cutaneous angiosarcoma of the breast 7 years after lumpectomy and radiation therapy. *Radiology* 1990; **174:** 258–60.

25. Badwe RA, Hanby AM, Fentiman IS, Chaudary MA. Angiosarcoma of the skin overlying an irradiated breast. *Breast Cancer Res Treat* 1991; **19:** 69–72.

26. Roukeema JA, Leenen LPH, Kuizinga MC, Maat B. Angiosarcoma of the irradiated breast: a new problem after breast conserving surgery. *Neth J Surg* 1991; **43:** 114–16.

27. Stokkel MPM, Peterse HL. Angiosarcoma of the breast after lumpectomy and radiation therapy for adenocarcinoma. *Cancer* 1992; **69:** 2965–8.

28. Taat CW, van Toor BSJ, Slors JFM et al. Dermal angiosarcoma of the breast: a complication of primary radiotherapy? *Eur J Surg Oncol* 1992; **18:** 391–5.

29. Edeiken S, Russo DP, Knecht J et al. Angiosarcoma after tylectomy and radiation therapy for carcinoma of the breast. *Cancer* 1992; **70:** 644–7.

30. Sessions SC, Smink RD. Cutaneous angiosarcoma of the breast after segmental mastectomy and radiation therapy. *Arch Surg* 1992; **127:** 1362–3.

31. Wijnmaalen A, van Ooijen B, van Geel BN et al. Angiosarcoma of the breast following lumpectomy, axillary lymph node dissection, and radiotherapy for primary breast cancer: three case reports and a review of the literature. *Int J Radiat Oncol Biol Phys* 1993; **26:** 135–9.

32. Choy A, Barr LC, Serpell JW, Baum M. Radiation-induced sarcoma of the retained breast after conservative surgery and radiotherapy for early breast cancer. *Eur J Surg Oncol* 1993; **19:** 376–7.

33. Slotman BJ, van Hattum AH, Meyer S et al. Angiosarcoma of the breast following conserving treatment for breast cancer. *Eur J Cancer* 1994; **30A:** 416–17.

34. Zucali R, Merson M, Placucci M et al. Soft tissue sarcoma of the breast after conservative surgery and irradiation for early mammary cancer. *Radiat Oncol* 1994; **30:** 271–3.

35. Buatti JM, Harari PM, Leigh BR, Cassady JR. Radiation-induced angiosarcoma of the breast. *Am J Clin Oncol* (CCT) 1994; **17:** 444–7.

36. Fineberg S, Rosen PP. Cutaneous angiosarcoma and atypical vascular lesions of the skin and breast after radiation therapy for breast cancer. *Am J Clin Pathol* 1994; **102:** 757–63.

37. Provencio M, Bonilla F, Espana P. Breast angiosarcoma after radiation therapy. *Acta Oncol* 1995; **34:** 869.

38. Weber B, Marchal C. Three cases of breast angiosarcomas after breast-conserving treatment for carcinoma. *Radiotherapy Oncol* 1995; **37:** 250–2.

39. Molitor JL, Spielmann M, Contesso G. Angiosarcoma of the breast after conservative surgery and radiation therapy for breast carcinoma: three new cases. *Eur J Cancer* 1996; **32A:** 1820.

40. Bolin DJ, Lukas GM. Low-grade dermal angiosarcoma of the breast following radiotherapy. *Am Surg* 1996; **62:** 668–72.

41. Britt LD, Lambert P, Sharma R, Ladaga LE. Angiosarcoma of the breast. Initial misdiagnosis is still common. *Arch Surg* 1995; **130**: 221–3.

42. Liberman L, Dershaw DD, Kaufman RJ, Rosen PP. Angiosarcoma of the breast. *Radiology* 1992; **183**: 649–54.

43. Donnell RM, Rosen PP, Lieberman PH et al. Angiosarcoma and other vascular tumors of the breast: pathologic analysis as a guide to prognosis. *Am J Surg Pathol* 1981; **5**: 629–42.

44. Gump FE, Sternschein MJ, Wolff M. Fibromatosis of the breast. *Surg Gynecol Obstet* 1981; **153**: 57–60.

45. Payan HM, England DM. Fibrosarcoma mimicking breast fibromatosis. *Am J Med Genet Suppl* 1987; **3**: 257–62.

46. Fletcher CDM. Pleomorphic malignant fibrous histiocytoma: fact or fiction? A critical reappraisal based on 159 tumors diagnosed as pleomorphic sarcoma. *Am J Clin Pathol* 1992; **16**: 213–18.

47. Callery CD, Rosen PP, Kinne DW. Sarcoma of the breast. A study of 32 patients with reappraisal of classification and therapy. *Ann Surg* 1985; **201**: 527–32.

48. Gutman H, Pollock RE, Ross MI et al. Sarcoma of the breast: implications for extent of therapy. *Surgery* 1994; **116**: 505–9.

49. Jones MW, Norris HJ, Wargotz ES, Weiss SW. Fibrosarcoma-malignant fibrous histiocytoma of the breast. A clinicopathological study of 32 cases. *Am J Surg Pathol* 1992; **16**: 667–74.

50. Enzinger FM, Lattes R, Torlino H. *Histological Typing of Soft Tissue Tumours*. Geneva: WHO, 1969: 20.

51. Enzinger FM, Wisolow DJ. Liposarcoma. A study of 103 cases. *Virchows Arch [A]* 1962; **335**: 367–88.

52. Ii K, Hizawa K, Okazaki K et al. Liposarcoma of the breast – fine structural and histochemical study of a case and review of 42 cases in the literature. *Tokushima J Exp Med* 1980; **27**: 45–56.

53. Austin RM, Dupree WB. Liposarcoma of the breast: a clinicopathologic study of 20 cases. *Hum Pathol* 1986; **17**: 906–13.

54. Yamashina M. Primary leiomyosarcoma in the breast. *Jpn J Clin Oncol* 1987; **17**: 71–7.

55. Nielsen BB. Leiomyosarcoma of the breast with late dissemination. *Virchows Arch [A]* 1984; **403**: 241–5.

56. Yatsuka K, Mihara S, Isobe M et al. Leiomyosarcoma of the breast – a case report

and an electron microscopic study. *Jpn J Surg* 1984; **14**: 494–8.

57. Arista-Nasr J, Gonzalez-Gomez I, Angeles-Angeles A et al. Primary recurrent leiomyosarcoma of the breast. Case report with ultrastructural and immunohistochemical study and review of the literature. *Am J Clin Pathol* 1989; **92**: 500–5.

58. Waterworth PD, Gompertz RHK, Hennessy C et al. Primary leiomyosarcoma of the breast. *Br J Surg* 1992; **79**: 169–70.

59. Parham DM, Robertson AJ, Hussein KA, Davidson AIG. Leiomyosarcoma of the breast: cytological and histological features, with a review of the literature. *Cytopathology* 1992; **3**: 245–52.

60. Bonet T. Mammae osseae in virgine cum pectoris hydrope. In: *Sepulchretum Sine Anatomia Practica E-cadaveribus Morbo Denatis*, vol 2. Geneva: Cramer and Perachon, 1700: 522.

61. Savage AP, Sagor GR, Dovey P. Osteosarcoma of the breast: a case report with an unusual diagnostic feature. *Clin Oncol* 1984; **10**: 295–8.

62. Achram M, Issa S, Rizk G. Osteogenic sarcoma of the breast: some radiological aspects. *Br J Radiol* 1985; **58**: 264–5.

63. Fry HJB. Osteoclastoma (myeloid sarcoma) of the human female breast. *J Pathol Bacteriol* 1927; **30**: 529–36.

64. Carlucci GA, Wagner RF. Osteochondrofibrosarcoma of the breast. *Am J Surg* 1943; **61**: 271–6.

65. Rottino A, Howley CP. Osteoid sarcoma of the breast: a complication of fibroadenoma. *Arch Pathol* 1945; **40**: 44–50.

66. Jernstrom P, Lindberg AL, Meland ON. Osteogenic sarcoma of the mammary gland. *Am J Clin Pathol* 1963; **40**: 521–6.

67. Gonzalez-Licea A, Yardley JH, Hartmann WH. Malignant tumor of the breast with bone formation. Studies by light and electron microscopy. *Cancer* 1967; **20**: 1234–47.

68. Aubrey DA, Andrews GS. Mammary osteogenic sarcoma. *Br J Surg* 1971; **58**: 472–4.

69. Annani PA, Baumann RP. Osteosarcoma of the breast. *Virchows Arch [A]* 1972; **347**: 213–18.

70. Mertens HH, Langnickel D, Staedler F. Primary osteogenic sarcoma of the breast. *Acta Cytol* 1981; **26**: 512–16.

71. Watt AC, Haggar AM, Krasicky GA. Extraosseous osteogenic sarcoma of the breast: mammographic and pathologic findings. *Radiology* 1984; **150**: 34.

72. Mufarrij AA, Feiner HD. Breast sarcoma with giant cells and osteoid. A case report and review of the literature. *Am J Surg Pathol* 1987; **11**: 225–30.

73. Kaiser U, Barth P, Duda V et al. Primary osteosarcoma of the breast – case report and review of the literature. *Acta Oncol* 1994; **33**: 74–6.

74. Winkler K, Beron G, Kotz R et al. Neoadjuvant chemotherapy of osteogenic sarcoma: results of a cooperative German/Austrian study. *J Clin Oncol* 1984; **6**: 617–24.

75. Bernhards J, Hendrickx P, Maschek H et al. Primares osteogenes Sarkom der Mamma. *Tumordiagn u Ther* 1991; **12**: 173–6.

76. Rodier-Bruant C, Jacek D, Dufour P et al. Les ostéosarcomes mammaires. *Rev Fr Gynécol Obstét* 1991; **86**: 43–8.

77. Hansen TG, Ottessen GL, Pedersen NT, Andersen JA. Primary non-Hodgkin's lymphoma of the breast (PLB): a clinicopathological study of seven cases. *APMIS* 1992; **100**: 1089–96.

78. Freeman C, Berg JW, Cutler SJ. Occurrence and prognosis of extranodal lymphomas. *Cancer* 1972; **29**: 252–60.

79. Adair FE, Hermann JB. Primary lymphosarcoma of the breast. *Surgery* 1944; **16**: 836–53.

80. Bannerman RH. Burkitt's tumour in pregnancy. *BMJ* 1966; **2**: 1136–7.

81. Shepherd JJ, Wright DH. Burkitt's tumour presenting as bilateral swelling of the breast in females of childbearing age. *Br J Surg* 1967; **54**: 776–80.

82. Rappaport H. *Atlas of Tumor Pathology.* Section III, Fascicle 8, *Tumours of the haematopoetic system.* Washington DC: Armed Forces Institute of Pathology, 1966.

83. Gerard-Marchant R, Hamlin I, Lennert K et al. Classification of non-Hodgkin's lymphomas. *Lancet* 1974; **ii**: 1070–3.

84. Lamovec J, Jaucar J. Primary malignant lymphoma of the breast. Lymphoma of the mucosa associated lymphoid tissue. *Cancer* 1987; **60**: 3033–41.

85. Hugh JC, Jackson FI, Hanson J et al. Primary breast lymphoma. An immuno-histologic study of 20 new cases. *Cancer* 1990; **66**: 2602–11.

86. Bobrow LG, Richards MA, Happerfield LC et al. Breast lymphomas: a clinicopathologic review. *Hum Pathol* 1993; **24**: 274–8.

87. American Joint Committee for Cancer Staging and Reporting. *Manual for Staging of Cancer.* Chicago, 1978.

88. Miller TP, Jones SE. Initial chemotherapy for localised lymphomas of unfavourable histology. *Blood* 1983; **62**: 413–18.

23

Prevention

If we believe a thing to be bad, and if we have a right to prevent it,
it is our duty to try to prevent it and to damn the consequences.
                                        Alfred Milner

High-risk groups • Possible prevention methods

Examination of the epidemiological literature on breast cancer leaves one with a sense of unease about our present knowledge regarding the aetiology of this capricious disease. Our insight into the series of mutagenic events in mammary carcinogenesis is such that the processes might be occurring in a black box. What almost all the epidemiological research has indicated is the major promotional role of reproductive hormones and the protection achieved by differentiation during pregnancy and lactation. Although knowledge of causation is lacking, there is a potential opportunity to alter the evolution of breast cancer by hormonal manipulation or with differentiating agents and thereby reduce the incidence of the disease.

For prevention to be successful, high-risk groups must be identified and non-toxic and effective agents determined through prospective randomized trials. Some progress has been made in defining women with a two- to fourfold increase in risk, plus a few with a very high risk from mutations of *BRCA-1* and *BRCA-2*. A woman with a doubling of risk has a one in six chance of developing breast cancer, rising to one in four if she has a relative risk of 3. It is likely that, faced with this level of risk, many women would wish to participate in prevention

trials. At this time a variety of approaches is being evaluated in worldwide trials.

HIGH-RISK GROUPS

Guernsey project

The Guernsey project which was set up by Bulbrook and Hayward in the early 1960s is the longest running cohort study of breast cancer risk factors. The original aim was to determine whether measurement of the pattern of urinary excretion of steroid hormones could define a group of women with an increased risk of developing breast cancer. Prior work had indicated that a discriminant could be calculated, dichotomizing women with early breast cancer into good and bad prognostic groups.[1] Concentrations of 17–hydroxycorticosteroids (17–OHCS) in milligrams and aetiocholanolone in micrograms were measured in 24-hour urine specimens. From these values a discriminant was constructed:

Discriminant = 80 – 80[17–OHCS] (mg) + aetiocholanolone (µg).

Individuals with low levels of androgen excretion, resulting in a low discriminant, had a worse prognosis. Guernsey was chosen as the location of the study because of its stable population (income tax is significantly lower than in Britain), together with good medical services concentrated in one hospital and accurate population records. In the first study 5000 volunteers aged 35–55 were recruited and a 24-hour urine specimen collected from each. An aliquot was taken and stored at –20°C. After 27 breast cancers had been diagnosed among the volunteers, their urine specimens were assayed and compared with 187 volunteer controls. Among the cases there was a significantly lower aetiocholanolone excretion.[2]

This looked very encouraging but a subsequent analysis of results from 1445 women cast doubt on the prognostic value of urinary androgen estimation.[3] In a multivariate analysis, four variables emerged as significant: age at menarche, family history, age at first baby, and aetiocholanolone (log of daily excretion). The factors were additive and a woman with all four had a one in four chance of developing breast cancer. Such individuals were rare. One hundred per cent of the cancer cases had one risk factor, as did 90% of the controls; 82% of cancer cases and 55% of controls had two risk factors and 47% and 17% respectively had three risk factors. Four risk factors were present in 7% of cancers and 2% of controls. Hence aetiocholanolone could not be used as a sufficiently specific risk marker.

As it became possible to measure steroid hormones in blood rather than their metabolites in urine, so the second Guernsey study was set up to determine whether serum androgens were lower in women at risk. This proved to be the case with significantly lower levels of adrenal androgens compared with controls, but again without sufficient specificity to be of clinical value.[4] Shifting the approach towards the interaction between steroid hormone levels and mammographic parenchymal pattern (Wolfe grade) provided the initiative for the third Guernsey study. All participants gave urine and blood specimens and subsequently underwent mammography, both for screening purposes and to allow Wolfe grading to be performed.

Mammographic density

In the Wolfe grading system there are four categories which may define groups with different risks of breast cancer:[5]

Normal (N grade): a fatty-replaced breast
Prominent ducts (P)
P1 grade: prominent ducts occupying <25% of breast volume
P2 grade: prominent ducts occupying >25% of breast volume
Dysplastic (DY grade): prominent ducts with associated nodularity.

There was considerable controversy about the reproducibility of Wolfe grading, and the extent to which the grade was associated with increased risk. In an attempt to resolve these questions, Boyd et al critically reviewed 17 publications to assess whether they met methodological standards.[6]

Nine criteria were established: population assembly; lack of referral bias; blind reading of mammograms; interobserver variation; age; control for other risk factors; length of follow-up; examination frequency; and drop-out rate. With a maximum score of 9, the highest achieved was 7. As Table 23.1 shows, there was an association between rigour of methodology and relative risk of breast cancer in those with DY Wolfe grade. In those studies with the lowest scores (1–3) the mean relative risk was 0.9, whereas in those with the highest scores

Table 23.1 Relationship between methodological standards and breast cancer risk in studies of Wolfe grading

Score 1–3	Score 4	Score 6–7
RR = 0.9	RR = 3.3	RR = 4.4

From Boyd et al.[6]

Table 23.2 Relative risks of hyperplasia and neoplasia in relation to extent of parenchymal density on mammograms

Extent of density (%)	No hyper-plasia	Hyper-plasia	Carci-noma
0	1.0	1.0	1.0
< 10	2.1	8.0	4.7
10 to < 25	2.1	4.3	3.7
25 to 50	1.5	4.9	4.4
50 to < 75	1.8	7.3	2.4
≥ 75	3.1	12.2	9.7

From Boyd et al.[8]

Table 23.3 Wolfe grades of normal women participating in the third Guernsey study

Group	N (%)	P1 (%)	P2 (%)	DY (%)
Premenopausal	17	17	48	18
Postmenopausal	10	34	45	11
All	14	24	47	13

(6–7) there was a fourfold increase in risk of breast cancer for those women whose mammograms were graded as DY.

This being so, there should be a histological manifestation of atypia in breasts which are radiologically DY. Wellings and Wolfe correlated radiology and histology and reported that N breasts contained normal lobules and stroma.[7] There was moderate periductal and perilobular fibrosis in P1 which was more marked in P2 cases. DY breasts were more likely to contain high-grade atypical lobules and confluent fibrosis. In a more recent study, Boyd et al compared mammographic density with histology in 441 biopsied patients aged 40–49 years.[8] As shown in Table 23.2, there was a progressive rise in relative risk of hyperplasia and neoplasia with increasing density. Those without mammographic density had no hyperplasia or cancer, whereas there was an eightfold increase in relative risk of hyperplasia in those with 10% density. This rose to twelvefold among the women with more than 75% of the breast tissue appearing dense on mammograms. In parallel, the relative risk of cancer was 4.7 in those with less than 10% density and 9.7 among the women with more than 75%

density. Thus mammographic density (dysplasia) does appear to be associated with an increased risk of both premalignant and malignant disease.

Unfortunately, as with histological grading of tumours, there is a subjective element to Wolfe grading of mammograms with sometimes wide interobserver variations. This is susceptible to improvement. Toniolo et al asked two experienced radiologists to grade 100 mammograms on two separate occasions.[9] The intraobserver reliability was 0.68 and the interobserver variability 0.67. A consensus conference resulted in a reliability increase to 0.88. Although this is a great improvement, there will always be problems with a subjective assessment of radiological breast density.

To try and overcome this, Caldwell et al examined digitized mammograms and calculated fractal dimensions which were then compared with a Wolfe grading determined by three radiologists.[10] The weighted proportional agreement of the three doctors was 85% whereas that between fractal analysis and radiologists was 84%, suggesting that it may be possible to determine mammographic density by fractal analysis which could be automated.

Mammographic density may be insufficient to define an appropriate high-risk group. In the Guernsey study, 60% of normal women had P2/DY Wolfe grades, as shown in Table 23.3. Of the premenopausal women, 18% were DY compared with 11% of the postmenopausal.

Table 23.4 Relative risk of breast cancer in women with P2/DY Wolfe grades and other risk factors

Risk factor	Percentage of population	Relative risk
Nulliparity	7	2.1
Family history	5	2.1
Prior biopsy	11	1.9
Any	21	1.7

Table 23.5 Case-control studies of percentage free oestradiol (E2) in postmenopausal women

Percentage free E2

Cases	Controls	p value	Reference
2.2	1.5	<0.001	Siiteri et al[13]
2.2	1.7	<0.001	Moore et al[14]
1.9	1.5	NS	Reed et al[15]
2.1	1.96	<0.05	Langley et al[16]
1.7	1.5	<0.02	Jones et al[17]
1.2	1.2	NS	Bernstein et al[18]
1.3	1.4	NS	Pearce et al[19]

NS, not significant.

Cuzick et al re-analysed data from a case-control study to try and identify a higher risk group based on Wolfe grade and other factors.[11] Taking those women with P2/DY mammograms they examined the influence of nulliparity, family history and prior breast biopsy and, as Table 23.4 shows, all of these approximately doubled the relative risk of breast cancer. Thus a group that comprises nulliparous or previously biopsied women with P2/DY Wolfe grade has a doubling of risk and comprises 18% of the population – possibly an appropriate sized group for a prevention study.

As the major risk factor for developing breast cancer is the presence of Barr bodies in leukocytes, it is likely that female hormones play a central role in the genesis of the disease. This being so it was logical to look for abnormalities and particularly excess secretion of oestrogens in both women with breast cancer and those who were subsequently diagnosed with the disease. When Key and Pike reviewed the literature on plasma oestrogens and breast cancer risk, they concluded that there was no evidence of hyperoestrogenization in premenopausal women with breast cancer.[12] However, in 11 studies which measured plasma oestrogen levels in postmenopausal women, significantly elevated concentrations were reported in five, suggesting that there might be some excess stimulation in this age group.

Levels of oestradiol (E2) in the blood are only indirectly related to the free or biologically available oestrogen (free E2) because of differences in binding to sex hormone-binding globulin (SHBG) and serum albumin. In 1981, Siiteri et al reported that women with breast cancer had significantly elevated proportions of serum free E2,[13] after which a series of case-control studies examined this association and the results in postmenopausal women are summarized in Table 23.5.[13-19] Although most of studies have found a significantly elevated percentage of free E2, the centrifugal ultrafiltration dialysis method is very labour intensive, unsuitable for automation and subject to methodological problems, and so it does not constitute a workable technique for identifying high-risk groups within populations.

A nested case-control study was performed as part of the fourth Guernsey study in which serum concentrations of oestrogen (E2), testosterone (T) and SHBG were measured in 61 postmenopausal breast cancer cases and 179 age-matched controls.[20] Blood had been taken from the cases almost 8 years before diagnosis with timing of collection matched in the controls. There was a 31% higher geometric mean E2 concentration in the cases, and the odds ratio for breast cancer was 5.03 for those

Table 23.6 Odds ratios of breast cancer for increasing quartiles of oestrone (E1), oestradiol (E2), free oestradiol and sex hormone-binding globulin

Hormone	1	2	3	4	p value
Oestradiol	1.0	0.9	1.8	1.8	0.06
Oestrone	1.0	2.2	3.7	2.5	0.06
Free oestradiol	1.0	1.4	3.0	2.9	<0.01
SHBG	1.0	0.7	0.4	0.32	<0.01

From Toniolo et al.[21]

in the top third compared with the lowest third. Although there was some association between T and SHBG levels and risk, this disappeared after adjustment for E2 levels.

In a large cohort study of 14 291 women from New York City, Toniolo et al measured total oestrone (E1), E2, SHBG and free E2 in 130 cases and 251 control subjects.[21] As is shown in Table 23.6, when odds ratios (OR) were calculated for increasing quartiles of concentration, there was a non-significant trend for increased odds ratios with higher concentrations of both total E1 and E2. The trend was significant for free E2, and there was a reversed trend with SHBG so that, the more protein present, the less free E2 and the lower the risk of breast cancer.

Bone mineral content may be a surrogate measure for oestrogenization and so bone mineral content of the forearm was measured by single photon absorptiometry (SPA) in 4695 women who participated in the fourth Guernsey study.[22] In a nested case-control study of postmenopausal women, free E2 and SHBG were measured in 21 from the highest quintile of bone density and 23 from the lowest quintile. There was significant elevation of mean free E2 levels in the group with the highest bone density, so that the hyperostrogenization associated with increased risk of breast cancer

might be detectable by measuring bone mineral density, a considerably easier test than estimation of free E2 levels.

Some support for this approach came from the Osteoporotic Fractures Research Group who measured radial bone density with SPA in 6854 women aged over 65 and who, two years later, measured spinal and hip mineral density by dual photon absorptiometry (DPA).[23] Breast cancer was diagnosed subsequently in 97 participants and a multivariate analysis was conducted to adjust for age, obesity and family history of breast cancer. Mean bone densities of radius, hip and spine were significantly elevated in the cases. For those in the lowest bone density quartile the age-adjusted incidence rate per 1000 women-years was 2.5 compared with 6 in the highest quintile of bone density.

Further confirmation was provided by an analysis from the Framingham study in which posteroanterior hand radiography with radiogrametry was used to determine second metacarpal bone density in 1373 postmenopausal women.[24] Breast carcinoma subsequently developed in 91 of these subjects and a Cox's proportional hazards model was used to relate breast cancer risk to metacarpal bone density. The bone density results were split into quartiles. For those in the lowest quartile breast cancer developed in two of 1000 women-years, in the second, three of 1000, and in the third, three of 1000. However, in the quartile with the highest bone density, breast cancer occurred in seven of 1000 women-years – a threefold increase in risk. Hence relatively simple measurements of bone density may be able to detect a group with a two- to threefold increase in risk of breast cancer.

Family history

It is routine practice to enquire about a family history of breast cancer in all women complaining of breast problems or attending for well woman checks. About one in ten will have a relative with the disease but this does not as such mean that an individual is at increased risk. As breast cancer is a common disease, but only 5%

of cases are hereditary, there are many unnecessarily worried young women. A second-degree family history is insignificant unless there are substantial numbers of affected relations. Of those who have a mother or sister with the disease, even if there is early age at onset, less than a fifth will be at risk of a dominant gene mutation. Indeed, in a study of 80 women with breast cancer diagnosed before age 35, a mutation of BRCA-1 was found in only 10%.[25]

Those who carry mutations of BRCA-1, BRCA-2 and p53 are at significantly increased risk of breast cancer, as are heterozygotes with mutations of the ataxia–telangectasia gene. As these genes have been located, genetic testing is now a practical possibility for those deemed to be at risk. Such individuals have a first-degree relative with early-onset disease, several affected relatives, and a history of bilateral disease, or ovarian cancer and breast cancer. For a test to be meaningful a blood or tumour specimen has to be available from an affected relative when mutations at known loci can be sought. If a putative pathological mutation is found, then the same gene can be examined in DNA from the woman at risk.

Before conducting a genetic test the individual has to be informed that there is a 50% risk that she will have a mutation that gives a greater than 90% chance of developing breast cancer, predominantly in her premenopausal years.[26] About 10% of women with a mutation will not develop breast cancer but the reason for the lack of penetrance in these fortunate individuals is not yet known. Although at present there is no legal obligation to disclose results of genetic testing to insurance companies, it is likely that this will be challenged because one-sided knowledge could undermine the random distribution of unknown risks necessary for the insurance system to work.

To examine different approaches to conveying information before genetic testing for BRCA-1, Lerman et al conducted a prospective randomized trial of education alone or with counselling, and tested the knowledge gained by participants with that of similar women who were on a genetic waiting list.[27] There were 400

women in the trial, aged 18–75 years, all of whom had at least one first-degree relative with breast cancer, and were under the care of two hospitals in Washington DC.

At the start of the trial all participants completed a structured phone questionnaire which focused on knowledge of hereditary cancer, BRCA-1 test characteristics, with their perception of risks and benefits, and intention with regards to genetic testing. Next they were randomized to receive education, education and counselling, or serve as a 'waiting list control'. The intervention sessions were carried out and the telephone questionnaire was repeated one month later. The controls were also questioned 4–6 weeks after the baseline interview, and subsequently were called for education and counselling.

Education was derived from a structured protocol and comprised: review of individual risk, patterns of inheritance of susceptibility, benefits, limitations and risks of BRCA-1 testing, and limitation of surveillance options. The second group received the education component and, in addition, went on to non-directive counselling. This involved semi-structured discussion of cancer experience within the individual's family, expected impact of positive or negative BRCA-1 testing, anticipated outcome of not being tested, plus perception of personal ability both to deal with a positive test and to communicate the results to family and friends.

Both the educational and counselling approaches led to significant improvements in knowledge compared with the controls. Neither approach had any impact on the percentage (52%) of women wishing to be tested. The group who had additional counselling were significantly better informed about the limitations, risks and benefits, leading to a better understanding of the pros and cons of testing, but even this approach did not materially affect the proportion of women wishing to be tested.

Histological risk factors

'Benign breast disease' was coined as a catch-all nomenclature for non-malignant breast problems, which included a mixture of clinical, radiological and histological changes, some of which were variants of normality with others carrying an increased risk of subsequent breast cancer. This led to great imprecision in both diagnosis and thought which, in turn, caused distress to many women who had been told that they needed to be kept under surveillance because of an overestimated risk of malignancy.

When Webber and Boyd carried out a critical analysis of 36 cohort studies, they applied rigorous standards for classification, follow-up and data analysis to determine whether there was a true relationship between benign breast disease and cancer risk.[28] A positive association was reported in 22 studies and all these had substantially better methodological criteria than the 11 negative and 3 equivocal studies. For these reasons they concluded that there was real association between benign breast disease and cancer risk.

Definitive painstaking histopathological studies have been conducted by Page et al who reviewed 1600 benign biopsies from women, most of whom had been followed for at least 15 years.[29] Of the various components of fibrocystic change there was no increase in breast cancer risk in women with simple cysts or fibroadenomas, but there was a sixfold increase in risk in premenopausal women with atypical ductal hyperplasia, and a threefold increase in risk in postmenopausal women. Hyperplasia without atypia was not a risk factor in premenopausal women but led to a doubling of risk in postmenopausal cases. Subsequent work indicated that the four- to fivefold doubling of risk in women with atypical epithelial hyperplasia was doubled in those who also had a first-degree family history of breast cancer, although this group comprised only 39 from a total of 10 366 women.[30]

POSSIBLE PREVENTION METHODS

Diet

The widely differing international breast cancer incidence rates could be taken as evidence of either genetic or environmental factors at work.

The evidence from Japanese immigrants, however, strongly suggests a major environmental effect. Taking the relative risk of breast cancer of Japanese women as being unity, this rises to 3 in first-generation immigrants to San Francisco (Issei), rising to 4 in second-generation immigrants (Nisei) compared with 5.5 in white American women.[31]

When Armstrong and Doll examined environmental factors for various cancers diagnosed in 23 countries, the strongest correlation was found between risk and gross national product ($r = 0.83$), followed by total consumption of fat (0.79), meat (0.78) and animal protein (0.77).[32] This suggested that it was wealth rather than fat that was the major risk factor, with animal fat serving as a surrogate for wealth. Against this, Prentice et al carried out a multivariate analysis of international breast cancer incidence rates and diet: after adjusting for gross national product, height, weight and age at menarche, there was a consistent effect of dietary fat on risk.[33]

As a result of the inconsistency of the literature on dietary fat and breast cancer risk, Boyd et al conducted a meta-analysis of 23 published studies.[34] There was no significant increase in relative risk in cohort studies but a significantly increased relative risk of 1.21 in case-control studies. In the 19 studies that examined food intake the relative risk for meat was 1.2, milk 1.2, and cheese 1.2. Most of the studies showing a relationship between relative risk of breast cancer and dietary fat were European. One possible explanation for the absence of a clear effect is the relatively narrow range of animal fat consumption in Western women, all of whom might be consuming lipids in amounts above the threshold for enhancement of risk.

To escape from this problem of relative homogeneity of fat intake, Boyd et al, in Canada, have conducted a trial of the feasibility of dietary fat reduction in women deemed to be at increased risk of breast cancer because of mammographic parenchymal density.[35] Eligible women were aged over 30 years and had had a mammogram which showed more than 50% of the breast volume occupied by

Table 23.7 Alteration in food intake in Toronto Prevention Study

Component	Intervention		Controls	
	0 months	24 months	0 months	24 months
Energy (kcal)	1593	1530	1639	1643
Total fat (%)	33	23	33	34
Saturated fat (%)	12	8	12	12
Polyunsaturated fat	6	5	7	7
Monounsaturated fat	12	8	12	12
Protein (%)	18	19	17	18
Carbohydrate (%)	49	59	48	47

From Boyd et al.[35]

dense breast tissue (the equivalent of P2/DY Wolfe grades). In the first phase of the study, subjects were interviewed by a dietitian and after explanation of the trial were randomized either to a healthy diet based on Canada's Food Guide, although not specifically told to reduce dietary fat, or to enter the intervention group. Those in the latter group were advised how to reduce their fat intake to 15% of the daily calorie intake.

In the second phase of the trial, after explanation of the design, in order to improve compliance, those who were interested were asked to keep a dietary record of intake over 3 days, including a weekend day. Only those who kept adequate records were asked to participate. Between 1982 and 1990, 249 women entered the study in the intervention group and 248 in the control arm. Prognostic factors such as age, weight, height, parity and family history were equally balanced in the two groups. The majority (80%) of participants were premenopausal.

The mean dietary components before entry and 24 months later in the two groups are given in Table 23.7. This shows that there was a significant reduction in total fat and saturated

fat consumption in the intervention group, together with an increase in carbohydrate intake but no significant change in the control group. In phase I, 14% of the control group and 29% of the intervention group had dropped out of the study. In contrast with those recruited in phase II, only 9% of both groups had dropped out one year later. This encouraging compliance suggests that, once a true change in dietary intake has been achieved, it should be possible to assess the effects of long-term reduction in fat intake.

As a surrogate measure of breast cancer risk, after 817 women had entered the trial, the mammographic density was quantified by image analysis at baseline and after 2 years from allocation to either intervention (403) or control (414).[36] In the intervention group there was a significant reduction in area of breast glandular tissue and area of density. There was a significant association between weight loss and reduction in mammographic density, but after adjustment for this there remained a statistically significant reduction in density among those on a low-fat, high-carbohydrate diet. It remains to be determined whether this diminution in density is associated with either a reduction in incidence or earlier diagnosis of cancer, in the intervention group.

Part of the effect of altering diet may be to change endocrine function and thereby indirectly influence breast cancer risk. In an intervention study for women with fibrocystic breast disease, Rose et al instructed women to reduce their fat intake to 20% of calories and after 3 months found a significant reduction in serum E2 and E1.[37] Similar findings were reported by Bagga et al who persuaded 12 healthy premenopausal women to reduce their fat intake to 10% of calories and consume a high-fibre diet (35–45 g/day).[38] There were significant falls in both follicular and luteal levels of E1 and E2, but no effect on progesterone or SHBG.

Another potential protective mechanism may be via consumption of phyto-oestrogens in plant food. Although lignans in linseed and isoflavones in soya may be only weak oestrogens, with one-thousandth of the potency of E2, they are present in large quantities so that the urinary excretion may be 2000-fold that of oestrone glucuronide, the main oestrogen metabolite.[39] Thus, theoretically, phyto-oestrogens could compete with E2 at the receptor level inducing a functional hyperoestrogenic state.

Retinoids

The normal role of vitamin A (retinol) is in the synthesis of visual pigments and the maintenance of normal growth and differentiation of epithelial cells. The effect on differentiation suggested a potential for inhibition of carcinogenesis. However, excess intake of vitamin A is toxic and leads to skin desquamation and liver failure. To try and overcome this toxicity over 2300 retinol analogues (retinoids) have been synthesized. The two most promising first-line synthetic retinoids were tretinoin and isoretinoin. Of the recent analogues, 4–hydroxyphenylretinamide (HPR) (fenretinide) has been the most widely used.

Work with dimethylbenzanthracene (DMBA)-induced rat mammary cancers had shown that retinyl acetate induced a 50% reduction in tumours.[40] As retinoids inhibited progression of tumours rather than preventing their initiation, this would indicate the need for long-term administration.[41] That retinoids might be of value in humans was suggested by epidemiological studies which indicated a reduced intake of foods containing vitamin A in women with breast cancer.[42,43] Using both ER-positive and ER-negative human breast cancer cell lines, Wang and Phang reported that fenretinide treatment induced apoptotic death in both cell types in culture.[44] As part of the Guernsey project, serum retinol, β-carotene and retinol-binding protein were measured in a case-control study with no significant difference being found between levels in cases and controls.[45]

A prevention trial is now under way at the National Cancer Institute, Milan, which is seeking to find out whether fenretinide can reduce the incidence of contralateral disease in women with small node-negative breast cancers.[46] All participants have stage I disease, and almost 3000 cases have now been entered and receive either fenretinide 200 mg daily or placebo for 5 years. So far no effect on contralateral disease has been reported. In the placebo group, six ovarian cancers have been diagnosed whereas there have been none in those given fenretinide, implying that there may be an unexpected advantage for those who take retinoids.[47]

Exercise

The number of menstrual cycles to which the breasts are exposed is an important risk factor for malignancy, with a protective effect of late menarche, early menopause and pregnancies.[48] To start menstruation at puberty, a critical body mass has to be achieved in relation to height. If there is subsequent weight loss because of anorexia or increased exercise, amenorrhoea may occur and for menstruation to resume a weight gain of 10% more than that required to initiate menarche is necessary.[49] In addition, young women who take strenuous exercise such as ballet dancers and athletes may have altered menstrual function and breast cancer risk.

Frisch et al conducted a survey of 5398 female college alumni and compared cancer rates among those who had been athletes (2622) and non-athletes (2776).[50] About 70% of both groups responded and it emerged that the athletes had a substantially reduced risk of reproductive system cancers (4 vs 10 per 1000). There was also a significantly reduced lifetime risk of breast cancer (10 vs 16 per 1000) with an age-adjusted relative risk of 0.65.

Bernstein et al conducted an intervention study with 16-year-old college students to examine the relationship between moderate exercise and menstrual function.[51] There were 168 participants who kept bi-weekly menstrual calendars, daily exercise charts, and also provided two luteal phase early morning urine specimens. In those who took moderate exercise there was a significant trend towards anovular cycles, after adjustment for age at menarche and years since menarche. The relationship between anovular cycles and exercise was unrelated to weight and Bernstein et al postulated that long-term moderate exercise might reduce breast cancer incidence by 50%.

In a subsequent case-control study of 545 breast cancer patients aged 40 or younger and 545 age-matched controls, Bernstein et al determined lifetime physical exercise activity, taking participation as being over 2 hours per week.[52] After adjusting for other risk factors, such as family history, parity and age at menarche, there was a significant inverse relationship between number of hours of exercise per week and risk of breast cancer, as shown in Table 23.8. Those taking more than 5 hours of exercise per week had a greater than 50% reduction in risk of developing breast cancer.

Contrary results were reported from the Framingham study.[53] Data on exercise were available from 2307 women of whom 117 were diagnosed with breast cancer in 28 years of follow-up. There was a non-significant trend towards increasing breast cancer risk with increasing physical exercise and the relative

Table 23.8 Odds ratios of breast cancer in relation to number of hours of exercise per week

Hours of exercise per week	Odds ratio of breast cancer
0	1.0
0.1–0.7	0.95
0.8–1.6	0.65
1.7–3.7	0.80
≥ 5.6	0.42

From Bernstein et al.[52]

risk of the most active quartile was 1.6 compared with the least active ($p = 0.13$).

Recently, Gammon et al critically reviewed the 11 published studies on exercise and breast cancer, particularly in relation to assessment of physical activity.[54] Only two had used a validated instrument to measure physical activity and the reliability of the method of assessment was confirmed in only three studies. Of the three most recent studies one had shown that exercise increased risk[53] and two found that exercise was protective[52,55] and so it was concluded that there might be a protective effect of exercise in premenopausal women.

Ovarian suppression

An early menopause can reduce a woman's risk of developing breast cancer, and this risk may be further diminished by oophorectomy at a young age. This was demonstrated by Trichopoulos et al who compared 3581 breast cancer cases reported to the Connecticut Cancer Registry with a similar number of controls who were participating in the National Health Examination Study.[56] As Table 23.9 shows, there was a significant reduction in relative risk of breast cancer (RR = 0.36) in those who had a oophorectomy when aged less than 35.

Table 23.9 Age at oophorectomy and relative risk of breast cancer

Age at oophorectomy (years)	Relative risk
< 35	0.36
35–39	0.68
40–44	0.65
45–49	0.78
≥ 50	0.98

From Trichopoulos et al.[56]

Although surgical intervention is not a practical approach to breast cancer prevention, medical intervention to suppress ovarian function is now possible.

Gonadotrophin-releasing hormone agonists

Gonadotrophin-releasing hormone (GnRH) agonists are synthetic polypeptides which bind preferentially to luteinizing hormone-releasing hormone (LHRH) receptors in the hypothalamus, leading to a tonic rather than an intermittent stimulation of the pituitary gland.[57] This downregulates the receptors which become refractory to LHRH and so LH and follicle-stimulating hormone (FSH) release from the pituitary is inhibited and the plasma oestradiol level falls to castrated levels within 36 hours.

To examine the short-term and medium-term effects of a GnRH agonist in the premenopausal a study was run at Guy's Hospital in which 21 women with refractory or recurrent mastalgia were given depot injections of goserelin (3.6 mg) every 28 days for six cycles.[58] They had previously received danazol, bromocriptine or tamoxifen, and had either failed to respond or relapsed after cessation of treatment. Relief of breast pain, as measured on pain charts, was achieved in 81%, but in association with major

side effects. These included hot flushes (90%), headaches (57%), vaginal dryness (38%), loss of libido (38%), nausea/vomiting (29%), joint pains (29%) and depression/irritability (24%). As a result of side effects 14% asked for the treatment to be stopped.

Goserelin nevertheless appeared to be a very effective treatment under circumstances in which other agents were of little use, so a second study was conducted. In this, 40 women with previously untreated mastalgia were given goserelin and closely monitored for side effects, together with serial measurement of bone density using dual photon absorptiometry (DPA).[59] Bone mineral density was measured in the lumbar spine and hips in the cases and 23 controls matched for age, weight, height and menstrual status.

After six goserelin implants there was a 5% reduction in bone density compared with controls and this had not returned to the baseline level 12 months after stopping treatment. In addition, there was a significant increase in serum calcium, alkaline phosphatase and osteocalcin in the treated group. These short- and medium-term side effects indicate that GnRH agonists alone are too toxic for prevention studies.

Pike et al proposed a different approach in which a combination of GnRH agonist and oestrogen is used.[60] A mathematical model of incidence was developed based on the major risk factors:

$$I(T) = a[M(T)]^{4.5}$$

where I is incidence at age T, M(T) is the average mitotic rate of breast epithelial cells from birth to age T and a is age. Using this model Pike calculated the relative risks of breast cancer in those receiving GnRH agonists (GnRHA) for 5, 10 or 15 years, with or without added oestrogen, as shown in Table 23.10. The inhibition of mitosis by withdrawal of oestrogen could lead to a significant reduction in risk of breast cancer and also act as a form of contraception, provided that the oestrogen added back could abolish menopausal symptoms and not abolish libido.

Table 23.10 Predicted relative risks of breast cancer after different durations of GnRH agonists with or without oestrogen

Treatment	5 years	10 years	15 years
GnRHA	0.62	0.37	0.20
GnRHA + E2 (1.25 mg 26/28 days)	0.73	0.53	0.37
GnRHA + E2 (1.25 mg 21/28 days)	0.71	0.49	0.33
GnRHA + E2 (0.625 mg 26/28 days)	0.70	0.47	0.30
GnRHA + E2 (0.625 mg 21/28 days)	0.68	0.45	0.28

From Pike et al.[60]

As a result, a pilot study was started for premenopausal women with at least a fivefold increase in risk of breast cancer (mother or sister with bilateral disease or a personal diagnosis of lobular carcinoma in situ).[61] There was a two : one randomization to the treated or control groups. Participants received a depot injection of the GnRHA leuprolide acetate every 28 days, conjugated oestrogen for 6 days out of 7 and a progestin, medroxyprogesterone acetate, for 13 days every fourth cycle.

There were eleven treated cases and six controls with hot flushes being experienced by five of the treated group, abolished by increasing the dosage of conjugated oestrogen. Breast pain was reported less frequently by the treated group. No significant changes occurred in cholesterol levels or in the lumbar spine bone density, but there was a significant diminution in femoral neck bone density in the treated group (1.4% per year).

In a subsequent report with 14 women in the treated group and 7 controls, the baseline and one-year mammograms were reviewed blindly by two radiologists.[62] Films were graded from –2 to +2 using three criteria: change in appearance of fibrous septa, change in nodularity, and change in confluent areas of fibrous tissue. There was a significant reduction in density in those receiving GnRHA, indicating the possibility of a reduction in risk in this group, although this still remains speculative.

Progestins

Whether progestins have a primary role in breast cancer prevention is still contentious. Korenman suggested that women at increased risk of breast cancer had more anovulatory cycles.[63] This window of unopposed oestrogens occurs during the early postpubertal phase before regular menstrual cycles are established and could provide a more favourable state for cancer induction by environmental carcinogens. This argument was somewhat negated by the work of Bernstein et al suggesting that anovular cycles, resulting from increased exercise, reduces risk of breast cancer.[52]

Pike suggested that progestins should be used with GnRHA and oestrogen because of the probability of unopposed oestrogen causing endometrial hyperplasia and neoplasia.[60] He postulated a slight increase in risk of breast cancer with progestins because a previous study of oral contraceptive use had shown more malignancies in those taking progesterone-containing pills, together with a dose–response effect.[64] In a histopathological study of benign biopsies taken at various times in the menstrual cycle, maximum mitotic activity was seen in the luteal phase specifically on day 25.[65] Further work was carried out using [3H]thymidine labelling of benign tissue excised from women taking oral contraceptives with known date of last menstrual period and next period after surgery.[66] Those individuals taking a progestin-only formulation had the highest mitotic rate in their mammary epithelium.

In contrast, progestins such as medroxyprogesterone acetate, megestrol acetate and norethisterone have been found to exert an anti-cancer effect and induce remissions in advanced breast cancer cases.[67] Further evidence of an anti-cancer effect has been confirmed in vitro where the growth of the hormone-sensitive human cell line T47D was inhibited by gestodene, as was the synthesis of transforming growth factor β (TGF-β).[68]

Cohen et al postulated that a combination of progestin and melatonin might be preventative.[69] This was based on the observation that the number of menstrual cycles increased risk and that this has occurred because of the change from seasonal ovulation, partly controlled by melatonin. When a combination of melatonin and norethisterone was administered to 32 premenopausal women for 4 months, there was an additive effect with a significant fall in LH levels and inhibition of ovulation.[70] This might provide a non-toxic approach to breast cancer prevention, with an additional contraceptive benefit.

Tamoxifen

Tamoxifen has been scrutinized more closely than any other drug as a potential preventive agent for breast cancer, and major trials are now under way in both Europe and the USA. In January 1986, *The Lancet* published a paper by Cuzick, Wang and Bulbrook which outlined the theoretical basis for a tamoxifen trial.[71] They argued that this was a logical extension of breast screening and that, because of the evidence of the efficacy of tamoxifen in the established disease, without undue side effects, the agent could block the effect of more biologically available oestrogen in women at risk.

Proof that tamoxifen could prevent breast cancer came from adjuvant studies showing a substantial reduction in contralateral cancers in treated compared with control patients.[72,73] The subsequent meta-analysis of adjuvant therapy indicated a 39% reduction in contralateral breast cancers, predominantly in postmenopausal women.[74] The stage was set for a prevention trial.

In October 1986 a pilot study was started by Trevor Powles at the Royal Marsden Hospital, in which women with a family history of breast cancer were to receive tamoxifen 20 mg daily, or placebo, for 5 years.[75] As tamoxifen was regarded as an anti-oestrogen at that time there were concerns about the long-term effects on bone and plasma lipids, and so studies were instigated to examine these potential problems. Tamoxifen had been introduced originally as an oral contraceptive in the 1960s, but, because it stimulated rather than inhibited ovulation, it was put to one side. At that time the toxicity studies required before use in humans were less rigorous. When interest increased in use of the drug for treatment and prevention, the manufacturers, ICI, ran extended mutagenicity and carcinogenicity tests. There was no evidence that the agent was genotoxic, but when rats were given 35 mg/kg, 100 times the usual dose, some developed hepatocellular carcinomas. This cast a shadow over the use of tamoxifen for prevention and also for women with non-malignant conditions such as cyclical mastalgia.

To counter this, Fentiman and Powles reasoned that such results would be predictable if tamoxifen was regarded as a partial oestrogen agonist rather than an anti-oestrogen.[76] Administration of high doses of oestrogens to rodents resulted in several malignancies including liver cancers.[77] Furthermore, liver cancers had been reported in young women who had taken prolonged courses of oral contraceptives, but because this was a rare event no-one had suggested that they should be withdrawn from the market.[78] Following this no voices of dissent were raised and the pilot study continued.

Meanwhile, across the Atlantic, partly as a result of pressure from the women's health lobby, in less than one year, FDA authorization, ethical approval and financial support was obtained for a tamoxifen prevention trial to be run by the NSABP. In August 1992 the Milan trial was started, in which all eligible participants had had a prior hysterectomy. Back in the UK, the first volunteer entered the trial in late 1992, 7 years after the first protocol had been written.

Pilot study

Between 1986 and 1990, 435 women were recruited into the Royal Marsden Pilot Programme, of whom 217 received tamoxifen and 218 were given placebo.[79] Compliance with the randomized treatment was similar in both arms. When the side effects of the two groups were compared, the only significant difference was increased hot flushes reported by the tamoxifen group (33% vs 17%). There was a significant fall in cholesterol (18%), low-density-lipoprotein cholesterol (LDL-C), and apolipoprotein B levels in postmenopausal women taking tamoxifen. In the premenopausal women, tamoxifen caused significant falls in both cholesterol and LDL-C. More recent results have shown that there was a small but significant reduction in bone density of premenopausal women who had been taking tamoxifen for more than one year. The clinical significance of this in relation to risk of osteoporosis has yet to be determined.

New approaches

As pregnancy exerts a protective effect, Russo postulated that hormonally induced differentiation of the mammary gland might be of value.[80] In rodent model systems maximal susceptibility to carcinogens is found in the rapidly proliferating undifferentiated mammary glands of young females, whereas fully differentiated older breasts are protected against malignancy. It is possible that an oral contraceptive could be developed that would mimic the effect of pregnancy in young women and thereby give some protection against breast cancer.

Without invasive tests such as biopsy or fine needle aspiration cytology (FNAC), detection of atypical hyperplasia is not possible at present.

As most cancers start as intraductal malignancy, these cells might be detectable in nipple aspirates. Morphology may be of value but markers of premalignant change such as polymorphic epithelial mucins (PEMs) could be used to test cells in aspirates.[81] PEMs are glycoproteins synthesized by mammary epithelium and in breast cancers there is upregulation of aberrant glycoproteins.

As part of the process of malignant transformation involves the switching on of dominant oncogenes such as c-erbB-2,[82] or mutation of suppressor genes such as p53,[83] this raises the possibility of gene therapy to reverse the behaviour of cancer cells. This might be achieved with liposomes or using retroviruses and adenoviruses to transfect the malignant cells with non-mutated genetic material.

As more individuals with mutations of BRCA-1 and BRCA-2 are identified, so there will be more women asking for prophylactic mastectomy. Whether this is best achieved by total mastectomy or subcutaneous mastectomy is debatable, but it is likely that, if mutant breast epithelium is left behind, a cancer may develop in the remnant. If the aim is for total ablation or breast tissue at risk, this might be attained without removal of the stroma if the epithelial element could be specifically targeted. Use of a combination of mammary epithelial mucin, conjugated with a porphyrin moiety, might provide a means of fixation to the epithelium. Subsequent activation of the porphyrin by laser directed at the breast, in the manner of X-rays during mammography, could selectively destroy the potential killer cells.

SYNOPSIS

- High-risk groups, suitable for intervention studies, include those with a family history, mammographic density, higher bone mineral content, histological evidence of atypical hyperplasia and prior breast cancer.
- Reduction in fat intake is achievable and

does reduce mammographic density but with an as yet unknown effect on risk of breast cancer.

- Retinoids are of unproven effect on risk of breast cancer but may reduce the incidence of ovarian cancer.
- The protective effect of oophorectomy can probably be achieved with GnRH

analogues but with severe side effects necessitating add-back of oestrogens, which might negate any risk reduction.

- Tamoxifen reduces the incidence of contralateral cancers and so its potential as a preventive agent for various high-risk groups is being assessed worldwide in several randomized trials.

REFERENCES

1. Bulbrook RD, Hayward JL, Spicer CC et al. Abnormal excretion of urinary steroids by women with early breast cancer. *Lancet* 1962; **ii:** 1238–40.
2. Bulbrook RD, Hayward JL, Spicer CC. Relation between urinary androgen and corticoid excretion and subsequent breast cancer. *Lancet* 1971; **ii:** 395–8.
3. Farewell VT. The combined effect of breast cancer risk factors. *Cancer* 1977; **40:** 931–6.
4. Deshpande N, Hayward JL, Bulbrook RD. Plasma 17–hydroxycorticosteroids and 17–oxosteroids in patients with breast cancer and normal controls. *J Endocrinol* 1965; **32:** 167–77.
5. Wolfe JN. Risk for breast cancer development determined by mammographic parenchymal pattern. *Cancer* 1976; **37:** 2186–92.
6. Boyd NF, O'Sullivan B, Fishell E et al. Mammographic patterns and breast cancer risk: methodologic standards and contradictory results. *J Natl Cancer Inst* 1984; **72:** 1253–9.
7. Wellings SR, Wolfe JN. Correlative studies of the histological and radiological appearance of the breast parenchyma. *Radiology* 1978; **129:** 229–306.
8. Boyd NF, Jensen HM, Cooke G et al. Relationship between mammographic and histological risk factors for breast cancer. *J Natl Cancer Inst* 1992; **84:** 1170–9.
9. Toniolo P, Bleich AR, Beinart C et al. Reproducibility of Wolfe's classification of mammographic parenchymal patterns. *Prev Med* 1992; **21:** 1–7.
10. Caldwell CB, Stapleton SJ, Hodsworth DW et al. Characterisation of mammographic parenchymal pattern by fractal dimension. *Phys Med Biol* 1990; **35:** 235–47.
11. Cuzick J, Berridge BD, Whitehead D et al. Mammographic dysplasia as entry criteria for

breast cancer prevention trials. *Lancet* 1991; **337:** 1225.
12. Key TJA, Pike MC. The role of oestrogens and progestogens in the epidemiology and prevention of breast cancer. *Eur J Cancer* 1988; **24:** 29–43.
13. Siiteri PK, Hammond GL, Nisker JA. Increased availability of serum estrogens in breast cancer: a new hypothesis. In: *Banbury Report 8: Hormones and Breast Cancer.* Pike MC, Siiteri PK, Welsall CW, eds. New York: Cold Spring Harbor, 1981.
14. Moore JW, Clark GMG, Bulbrook RD et al. Serum concentrations of total and nonprotein-bound oestradiol and the percentage of unbound oestradiol in patients with breast cancer and in normal controls. *Int J Cancer* 1983; **43:** 2940–3.
15. Reed MJ, Noel CT, Dudley HAF et al. Plasma levels of estrone, estrone sulphate, and estradiol and the percentage of unbound estradiol in postmenopausal women with and without breast disease. *Cancer Res* 1983; **43:** 2940–3.
16. Langley MS, Hammond GL, Bardsley A et al. Serum steroid binding proteins and the bioavailability of estradiol in relation to breast diseases. *J Natl Cancer Inst* 1985; **75:** 823–9.
17. Jones LA, Ota DM, Jackson GA et al. Bioavailability of estradiol as a marker for breast cancer risk assessment. *Cancer Res* 1987; **47:** 5224–9.
18. Bernstein L, Ross RK, Pike MC et al. Hormone levels in older women: a study of postmenopausal breast cancer patients and healthy population controls. *Br J Cancer* 1990; **61:** 298–307.
19. Pearce S, Dowsett M, McKinna JA. Albumin-bound and nonprotein-bound oestradiol and testosterone in postmenopausal breast disease. *Eur J Cancer* 1991; **27:** 259–63.

20. Thomas HV, Key T, Allen DS et al. A prospective study of endogenous serum hormone concentrations and breast cancer risk in postmenopausal women on the island of Guernsey. *Br J Cancer* 1997; **76:** 901–5.

21. Toniolo PG, Levitz M, Zeleniuch-Jacquotte A et al. A prospective study of endogenous estrogens and breast cancer in postmenopausal women. *J Natl Cancer Inst* 1995; **87:** 190–7.

22. Fentiman IS, Wang DY, Allen DS et al. Bone density of normal women in relation to endogenous and exogenous oestrogens. *Br J Rheumatol* 1994; **33:** 808–15.

23. Cauley JA, Lucas FL, Kuller LH et al. Bone mineral density and risk of breast cancer in older women. The Study of Osteoporotic Fractures. *JAMA* 1996; **276:** 1404–8.

24. Zhang Y, Kiel DP, Kreger BE et al. Bone mass and the risk of breast cancer among postmenopausal women. *N Engl J Med* 1997; **336:** 611–17.

25. Langston AA, Malone KE, Thompson JD et al. BRCA1 mutations in a population-based sample of young women with breast cancer. *N Engl J Med* 1996; **334:** 137–42.

26. Ford D, Easton DF, Bishop DT et al. Risks of breast cancer in BRCA1–mutation carriers. *Lancet* 1994; **343:** 692–5.

27. Lerman C, Biesecker B, Benkendorf JL et al. Controlled trial of pre-test education approaches to enhance informed decision-making for BRCA1 gene testing. *J Natl Cancer Inst* 1997; **89:** 148–57.

28. Webber W, Boyd N. A critique of the methodology of studies of benign breast disease and breast cancer risk. *J Natl Cancer Inst* 1986; **77:** 397–404.

29. Page DL, Vander Zwaag R, Rogers LW. Relation between component parts of fibrocystic disease complex and breast cancer. *J Natl Cancer Inst* 1978; **61:** 1055–63.

30. Dupont WD, Page DL. Risk factors for breast cancer in women with proliferative breast disease. *N Engl J Med* 1985; **312:** 146–51.

31. Buell P. Changing incidence of breast cancer in Japanese-American women. *J Natl Cancer Inst* 1973; **51:**1479–83.

32. Armstrong B, Doll R. Environmental factors and cancer incidence and mortality in different countries with special reference to dietary practices. *Int J Cancer* 1975; **15:** 617–31.

33. Prentice R, Kakar F, Huisting S et al. Aspects of the rationale for the Women's Health trial. *J Natl Cancer Last* 1988; **80:** 802–14.

34. Boyd NF, Martin LJ, Noffel M et al. A meta-analysis of studies of dietary fat and breast cancer risk. *Br J Cancer* 1993; **68:** 627–36.

35. Boyd NF, Cousins M, Lockwood G, Tritchler D. Dietary fat and breast cancer risk: the feasibility of a clinical trial of breast cancer prevention. *Lipids* 1992; **27:** 821–6.

36. Boyd NF, Greenberg C, Lockwood G et al. Effects of a low-fat, high-carbohydrate diet on radiologic features of the breast: results from a randomized trial. *J Natl Cancer Inst* 1997; **89:** 488–96.

37. Rose DP, Boyar AP, Cohen C, Strong LE. Effect of a low fat diet on hormone levels in women with cystic breast disease: serum steroids and gonadotrophins. *J Natl Cancer Inst* 1987; **78:** 623–6.

38. Bagga D, Ashley JM, Geffrey SP et al. Effects of a very low fat, high fibre diet on serum hormones and menstrual function. Implications for breast cancer prevention. *Cancer* 1995; **76:** 2491–6.

39. Cassidy A, Bingham S, Setchell K. Biological effects of isoflavones present in soy in premenopausal women. Implications for the prevention of breast cancer. *Am J Clin Nutr* 1994; **60:** 333–40.

40. Moon RC, Grubbs CJ, Sporn MJ. Inhibition of 712–dimethylbenzantracene-induced mammary carcinogenesis by retinyl acetate. *Cancer Res* 1976; **36:** 2626–30.

41. McCormick DL, Burns FJ, Albert RE. Inhibition of rat mammary carcinogenesis by short dietary exposure to retinyl acetate. *Cancer Res* 1980; **40:** 1140–3.

42. Graham S, Mettlin C, Marshall J et al. Diet in the epidemiology of breast cancer. *Am J Epidemiol* 1982; **116:** 68–75.

43. Willett WC, Hunter DJ, Stampfer MJ et al. Dietary fat and fibre in relation to risk of breast cancer. *JAMA* 1992; **268:** 2037–44.

44. Wang TT, Phang JM. Effect of *N*-(4–hydroxyphenyl)retinamide on apoptosis in human breast cancer cells. *Cancer Lett* 1996; **107:** 65–71.

45. Wald NJ, Boreham J, Hayward JL et al. Plasma retinol β-carotene and vitamin E levels in relation to the future risk of breast cancer. *Br J Cancer* 1984; **49:** 321–4.

46. Veronesi U, Costa A. Chemoprevention of contralateral breast cancer with the synthetic retinoid Fenretinide. *Cancer Invest* 1978; **6:** 638–41.

47. De Palo G, Veronesi U, Camerini T et al. Can fenretinide protect women against ovarian cancer? *J Natl Cancer Inst* 1995; **87**: 146–7.

48. Henderson BE, Ross BK, Judd HL et al. Do regular ovulatory cycles increase breast cancer risk? *Cancer* 1985; **56**: 1206–9.

49. Frisch RE, McArthur JW. Menstrual cycles: fatness as a determinant of minimum weight for height necessary for their maintenance or onset. *Science* 1974; **185**: 949–51.

50. Frisch RE, Wyshak G, Albright NL et al. Lower lifetime occurrence of breast cancer and cancers of the reproductive system among former college athletes. *Am J Clin Nutr* 1987; **45**: 328–35.

51. Bernstein L, Ross RK, Lobo RA et al. The effects of moderate physical activity on menstrual cycle patterns in adolescence: implications for breast cancer prevention. *Br J Cancer* 1987; **55**: 681–5.

52. Bernstein LE, Henderson BE, Hanisch R et al. Physical exercise and reduced breast cancer risk in young women. *J Natl Cancer Inst* 1994; **86**: 1403–8.

53. Dorgan JF, Brown C, Barrett M et al. Physical activity and risk of breast cancer in the Framingham Heart Study. *Am J Epidemiol* 1994; **139**: 662–9.

54. Gammon MD, Britton JA, Teitelbaum SL. Does physical activity reduce the risk of breast cancer?: a review of the epidemiologic literature. *Menopause* 1996; **3**: 172–80.

55. Friedenreich CM, Rohan TE. Physical exercise and risk of breast cancer. *Eur J Cancer Prev* 1995; **4**: 145–51.

56. Trichopoulos D, MacMahon B, Cole P. Menopause and breast cancer risk. *J Natl Cancer Inst* 1972; **48**: 605–13.

57. Belchetz PE, Plant TM, Nakai Y et al. Hypophyseal responses to continuous and intermittent delivery of hypothalamic gonadotrophin releasing hormone. *Science* 1978; **202**: 631–7.

58. Hamed H, Chaudary MA, Caleffi M et al. LHRH analogue for the treatment of recurrent and refractory mastalgia. *Ann R Coll Surg Engl* 1990; **72**: 221–4.

59. Hamed H, Fogelman I, Gregory WM et al. Effect of goserelin on bone metabolism in patients with mastalgia. *Breast* 1993; **2**: 79–82.

60. Pike MC, Ross RK, Lobo RA et al. LHRH agonists and the prevention of breast and ovarian cancer. *Br J Cancer* 1989; **60**: 142–8.

61. Spicer DV, Pike MC, Pike A et al. Pilot trial of a gonadotropin hormone agonist with replacement hormones as a prototype contraceptive to prevent breast cancer. *Contraception* 1993; **47**: 427–44.

62. Spicer DV, Ursin G, Parisky YR et al. Changes in mammographic densities induced by a hormonal contraceptive designed to reduce breast cancer risk. *J Natl Cancer Inst* 1994; **86**: 431–6.

63. Korenman SG. Oestrogen window hypothesis of the etiology of breast cancer. *Lancet* 1980; **i**: 700–1.

64. Pike MC, Henderson BE, Krailo MD et al. Breast cancer in young women and use of oral contraceptives: possible modifying effect of formulation and age at use. *Lancet* 1983; **ii**: 926–30.

65. Fergusson DJP, Anderson TJ. Morphological evaluation of cell turnover in relation to the menstrual cycle in the 'resting' human breast. *Br J Cancer* 1982; **44**: 177–81.

66. Anderson TJ, Battersby S, King RJB et al. Oral contraceptive use influences resting breast proliferation. *Hum Pathol* 1989; **20**: 1139–44.

67. Lundgren S. Progestins in breast cancer treatment. A review. *Acta Oncol* 1992; **31**: 709–22.

68. Colletta AA, Wakefield LM, Howell FV et al. The growth inhibition of human breast cancer cells by a novel synthetic progestin involves the induction of transforming growth factor beta. *J Clin Invest* 1991; **87**: 277–83.

69. Cohen M, Small RA, Brzezinski A. Hypotheses: melatonin/steroid combination contraceptives will prevent breast cancer. *Breast Cancer Res Treat* 1995; **33**: 257–64.

70. Voordouw BC, Euser R, Verdonk RE et al. Melatonin and melatonin-progestin combinations alter pituitary-ovarian function in women and can inhibit ovulation. *J Clin Endocrinol Metab* 1992; **74**: 108–17.

71. Cuzick J, Wang DY, Bulbrook RD. The prevention of breast cancer. *Lancet* 1986; **i**: 83–6.

72. Cuzick J, Baum M. Tamoxifen and contralateral breast cancer. *Lancet* 1985; **ii**: 282.

73. Fornander T, Cedermark B, Mattson A et al. Adjuvant tamoxifen in early breast cancer. Occurrence of new primary cancers. *Lancet* 1989; **ii**: 1070–3.

74. Early Breast Cancer Trialists' Collaborative Group. Systemic treatment of early breast cancer by hormonal, cytotoxic, or immune therapy. *Lancet* 1992; **339**: 1–15, 71–84.

75. Powles TJ, Hardy JR, Ashley SE et al. A pilot study to evaluate the acute toxicity and feasibility of tamoxifen for prevention of breast cancer. *Br J Cancer* 1986; **60**: 126–33.

76. Fentiman IS, Powles TJ. Tamoxifen and benign breast problems. *Lancet* 1989; **ii:** 1070–1.

77. Wanless JR, Medcine D. Role of estrogens as promoters of hepatic neoplasia. *Lab Invest* 1982; **46:** 313–16.

78. Neuberger J, Forman D, Doll R, Williams R. Oral contraceptives and hepatocellular carcinoma. *BMJ* 1986; **292:** 1355–7.

79. Powles TJ, Tillyer CR, Jones AL et al. Prevention of breast cancer with tamoxifen – an update of the Royal Marsden Hospital Pilot Programme. *Eur J Cancer* 1990; **26:** 680–4.

80. Russo J, Russo IH. Hormonally induced differentiation: a novel approach to breast cancer prevention. *J Cell Biochem* 1995; **22:** 58–64.

81. Taylor-Papadimitriou J, Gendler SJ. Structure, biology and possible clinical applications of carcinoma associated mucins. *Int J Oncol* 1992; **1:** 9–16.

82. Borg A, Baldetrop B, Ferno M et al. C-erbB-2 amplification in breast cancer with a high rate of proliferation. *Oncogene* 1991; **6:** 137–43.

83. Levine AJ, Momand J, Finlay CA. The p53 tumour suppressor gene. *Nature* 1991; **351:** 453–6.

24

The future

We are passing from the sphere of history to the sphere of the present and partly to the sphere of the future.

VI Lenin

Prevention • Cancer detection • Treatment of the primary tumour • Axillary histology • Radiotherapy • Adjuvant therapy

Substantial improvements have been made in the management of breast cancer which have led to a documented better survival. Although not a matter for complacency, these advances have resulted from painstaking clinical research, rather than laboratory-based investigation. There has been a shift towards earlier diagnosis of symptomatic disease and the more widespread use of screening to detect asymptomatic breast cancer. In addition, clinical trials have defined the most appropriate forms of adjuvant therapy and mastectomy has been largely replaced by breast conservation therapy. For those with larger primary tumours (> 4 cm in diameter), primary systemic therapy with either cytotoxic chemotherapy or endocrine therapy may provide an opportunity to shrink the primary and enable breast conservation therapy to be carried out.

Subsequent work will probably examine new diagnostic and monitoring techniques, together with identification of high-risk groups, suitable for participation in prevention trials. Also, there will be studies seeking to determine less extensive, but equally effective, local treatments to tumour site, axilla and the rest of the breast, possibly avoiding axillary clearance and whole breast irradiation. New regimens of cytotoxic chemotherapy and endocrine treatment will be tested in adjuvant roles. Finally, both biological and gene therapy will be investigated as both primary and adjuvant treatment.

PREVENTION

At present, the main entry criteria for prevention trials are a first-degree family history of breast cancer, premalignant histological findings (lobular carcinoma in situ or atypical hyperplasia) or increased mammographic density. Largely these are factors that select a premenopausal risk group which, although vocal in asking for possible prevention, do not constitute a majority of the at-risk women because two-thirds of breast cancer cases are postmenopausal. It would be more effective in population terms if a postmenopausal high-risk group could be identified. Such a possibility exists.

Two studies have measured bone mineral density (as a surrogate of oestrogen exposure), and shown that those with higher bone density were at increased risk of subsequent breast cancer.[1,2] As Table 24.1 shows, there was a two- to threefold increase in risk among those in the highest quartile of bone density. As an increas-

Table 24.1 Relative risks of breast cancer in women with bone density in the lowest and highest quartiles

Study	Lowest quartile	Highest quartile	Reference
OFRG*	RR 1	2.4	Cauley et al[1]
Framingham	RR 1	3	Zhang et al[2]

*Osteoporotic Fractures Study Group

ing proportion of women are concerned about their risk of osteoporosis as well as breast cancer, a simple non-invasive measure of bone density would be acceptable to many. Those whose bone density fell within the highest quartile for their age could then be asked if they wished to participate in a prevention trial. If tamoxifen were the agent used in such a trial, participants could be reassured that this would not lead to an increase in risk of bone demineralization because the agent is osteoprotective.[3]

Of the drug prevention trials that are currently under way, the agents in use are tamoxifen and the retinoid fenretinide. Although tamoxifen has been subjected to more scrutiny than any other potential preventive drug there are still reservations about risk of endometrial cancer, possible hepatotoxicity and genotoxicity. For this reason great interest has been shown in tamoxifen analogues that might have different properties, which would make them more attractive candidates for preventive agents in healthy women.

Toremifine is a triphenylene analogue which has a similar profile of oestrogen antagonist/agonist properties as tamoxifen.[4] Both tamoxifen and toremifine reduce total serum cholesterol, low-density-lipoprotein cholesterol, and apolipoprotein B levels, but toremifine induces a greater rise in high-density-lipoprotein cholesterol.[5] This suggests that toremifine might be more effective than tamoxifen in reducing the risk of coronary heart disease. In addition, in the Sprague–Dawley rat model system, tamoxifen in high dosage induced hepatocellular carcinomas in all treated rats whereas none of the rats treated with high dose toremifine developed liver cancers.[6] When the two agents were administered to female Fischer rats, DNA adducts were detected in those given tamoxifen but not in those who received toremifine.

The efficacy and toxicity of tamoxifen and toremifine were compared in a double-blind randomized trial of 415 women with advanced breast cancer who had tumours that were either oestrogen receptor (ER) positive or ER unknown.[7] Tamoxifen was given at a dose of 40 mg/day and toremifine at 60 mg/day. The response rates and duration of response were similar in both groups but more patients taking tamoxifen suffered toxicity (44% vs 39%) and more discontinued treatment because of problems (4% vs 1%). Minimal toxicity is desirable in a preventive agent and so it is likely that toremifine may replace tamoxifen in the next round of prevention trials.

CANCER DETECTION

Although quality assurance can improve the technical aspects of mammography, nevertheless there is some agreement that this imaging method cannot detect all breast cancers, particularly in premenopausal women. Work is being conducted with both magnetic resonance imaging (MRI) and positron emission tomography (PET) to determine whether these techniques can complement the existing imaging systems. Both MRI and PET are expensive, however, and neither is generally available. It would be very useful if a more accessible method could be found and one such possibility is the measurement of breast electrical activity.

At a cellular level, there are alterations in the pattern of direct junctional intercellular communication between human mammary epithelium, stromal cells and malignant cells.[8] In particular there is loss of selectivity of

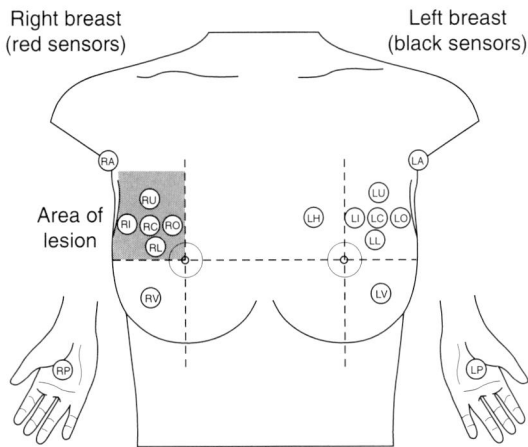

Fig. 24.1 Measurement of skin electropotentials over breast lesions using a Biofield device.

communication by breast cancer cells. There may be changes in the electrical resistance of gap junctions in the cell membranes of malignant cells, leading to an altered electropotential over tumours.[9] These electrical changes could possibly be apparent at a macroscopic level and Weiss et al found that skin sensors over breast cancers could detect an increased surface electric potential.[10] As this could be of great clinical interest as a non-invasive detection technique, a multi-centre prospective double-blind trial comprising 661 women was

conducted in eight European centres.[11] All the participants had a palpable lesion or a mammographic abnormality that was going to be excised. The Biofield device is shown in Fig. 24.1. Sensors were placed over the palpable lump or the involved quadrant, in those with impalpable lesions, and a mirror image array was set up on the contralateral breast. After a 10-minute equilibration, the test was performed and this took 1 minute.

The test results were sent to the study statistician. All histology was then reviewed by one reference pathologist, without knowledge of the test result and the histological report was also sent to the statistician. At the end of the study the results were collated. A pattern recognition algorithm was used, based upon an artificial neural network combining electrical variables and patient age to generate a neural net index for each patient. There was a significant relationship between the neural net index and the likelihood of the lesion being malignant. Using an intermediate threshold of 0.42, the overall neural net scores in relation to histological diagnosis are given in Table 24.2.

In women aged over 50, almost all the lesions were positive with the Biofield test, using an intermediate threshold, possibly because of the high prevalence of malignant and proliferative lesions in this age group. In women aged under 50, the Biofield test was positive in 35% of those with benign lesions sized 1 cm or less but in 84% of those with cancers of this size. These

Table 24.2 Neural net scores of Biofield device in relation to histopathology

Neural net index	Normal	Hyperplasia	Atypia	DCIS	Invasive carcinoma
Number	162	72	41	90	296
Median	0.43	0.46	0.48	0.48	0.515
Range	0.41–0.45	0.43–0.47	0.45–0.51	0.47–0.5	0.50–0.53

From Cuzick et al.[11]

results have to be regarded as preliminary but suggest the possibility of a screening test for malignancy in premenopausal women at increased risk, such as those with prior ductal carcinoma in situ (DCIS) or a family history of breast cancer.

TREATMENT OF THE PRIMARY TUMOUR

Complete excision of the primary tumour remains the cornerstone of surgical treatment for early breast cancer. Although this can be achieved with an almost invisible scar and imperceptible tissue deficit, nevertheless the procedure can indelibly mark the patient. As more patients are being diagnosed with small mammographically detected cancers confirmed preoperatively by stereotactic core biopsy, so it may be increasingly asked whether intervention with a scalpel is necessary. Until the 1980s the surgeon's knife was an essential instrument in the extirpation of cancer. This changed with the advent of breast conservation when radiotherapists were able to show that less extensive surgery was safe, if backed up with breast irradiation. Even after apparently complete local excision, withholding radiotherapy was associated with an unacceptably high (40%) breast relapse rate, usually in the same quadrant.[12] Attempts to give either external or interstitial treatment to the affected quadrant have met with varying degrees of success but may be associated with development of fibrosis, which diminishes the cosmetic outcome and may lead to problems distinguishing scar tissue from recurrent disease.[13,14]

An alternative approach would be to use interstitial laser filaments to destroy small breast cancers. Ideally the diagnosis would be made by stereotactic core biopsy to confirm that the cancer was of grade I, tubular or mucoid type and axillary imaging would have indicated no metastatic spread. Subsequently another stereotactic needle would be inserted after which a laser filament (0.1–0.6 mm) would be introduced until its tip lay within the tumour. Using the neodymium: yttrium–aluminimum–garnet (Nd:YAG) laser a calculated energy output could then be delivered in order to induce tumour vaporization and surrounded necrosis extending 5 mm beyond the lesion. As a precaution, subsequent stereotactic biopsies could be taken from the margins to confirm complete destruction of both invasive and non-invasive disease.

Developmental work has been carried out by Robinson et al, using a subcutaneous porcine fat model.[15] Using the Nd:YAG laser inserted via a fibreoptic cable, it was found that the time–temperature characteristics of porcine subcutaneous fat were similar to those of the fibrofatty breast tissue of postmenopausal women. When a total energy of less than 2009 joules was administered this resulted in the total tissue necrosis in a volume of 3 cm in diameter, which should be sufficient to destroy mammographically detected cancers up to 1 cm in diameter.

AXILLARY HISTOLOGY

As a result of the inaccuracy of clinical evaluation of the axilla and the importance of nodal status in determining prognosis, axillary clearance has been the gold standard of staging in early breast cancer. Opponents of the procedure have stressed the possibility of shoulder stiffness, lymphoedema and susceptibility to local infection. In addition, it has to be accepted that approximately 50% of those with palpable breast cancers will have a histologically negative axilla and, under these circumstances, it could be argued that the operation was unnecessary. This is not quite true because, with this knowledge, the patient can be better reassured about her prognosis. If a sample rather than a clearance is performed, at least 10 negative nodes must be examined before the axilla can be regarded as being negative with 95% confidence.

Attempts have been made to determine preoperatively the axillary nodal status, using lymphoscintigraphy and colour Doppler. These techniques were very dependent on the skill of the operator and have not gained general acceptance. An alternative approach was used in patients with melanoma, whereby a radioactive isotope was injected at the site of the lesion with the intention of identifying the first lymph node to which drainage occurred (sentinel node).[16] This technique was then applied to breast cancer patients by Krag et al who showed that sentinel nodes could be identified in this way.[17]

Recently, Veronesi et al reported the results of subdermal injection of technetium-99m (^{99m}Tc) labelled human serum albumin over breast cancers in 163 sequential cases who underwent sentinel node biopsy and subsequent axillary clearance.[18] Scintigraphic images were taken after 10, 30 and 180 minutes. A skin marker was placed over the radioactive node which was re-identified peroperatively with a hand-held γ-ray detector probe, after which the node was excised. In three cases no sentinel node was found, but of the others nodal metastases were found in 81 and no tumour in 79. Of the latter group, four patients (5%) were found to have nodal involvement in the axillary clearance specimen.

In 107 cases a frozen section was performed on the sentinel node and in all the 32 positive cases the diagnosis was confirmed at final histology. Of the 75 with negative frozen section diagnosis of the sentinel node, microfoci of malignant cells were found after full histological examination in 18 (24%). The final agreement between histology of the axillary clearance and the sentinel node biopsy was 89/107 (83%). Taking only those 45 patients with cancers less than 1.5 cm in diameter, there was 100% agreement for both sentinel negative (23) and positive (22) cases.

If this work can be confirmed it should provide a rational basis for intraoperative assessment of the axilla, particularly in women with small tumours so that sentinel node-negative cases can be spared a clearance. In addition, those cases with larger tumours who will receive primary radiotherapy could have the sentinel node biopsy performed to determine the need for axillary surgery should the tumour shrink sufficiently to enable breast conservation therapy.

RADIOTHERAPY

Even after histologically confirmed complete excision of small breast cancers, if radiotherapy is not given there is a breast relapse rate of between 20% and 40%. However, in the Milan series comparing quadrantectomy and axillary clearance with and without radiotherapy, breast relapse occurred in 16% of those aged 55 or under but only 3% of women aged over 55 years.[19] Hence it may be possible to avoid radiotherapy in selected older women, particularly in those with ER-positive tumours which have been excised. This may need to be followed by long-term anti-oestrogen therapy.

Rather than whole breast irradiation, quadrant treatment may be used, but, particularly if brachytherapy is contemplated, both dosage and fractionation need to be determined by prospective trials because apparently adequate radiation dosages may lead to totally inadequate local control.[14] Experience with interstitial caesium, given as four fractions lasting about 6 hours to a total dose of 45 Gy has been more encouraging, but such techniques are very labour-intensive and may need to be restricted to older patients who would benefit from having their entire surgical and radiotherapy treatment given during a 5-day hospital stay.

ADJUVANT THERAPY

In absolute terms, more women with breast cancer have been given tamoxifen than any other type of adjuvant therapy and as such it has been responsible for preventing more relapses and deaths from the disease than other endocrine or cytotoxic interventions. Despite this enviable curriculum vitae, tamoxifen remains under suspicion as a potentially genotoxic agent. In a long-term carcinogenicity study, tamoxifen was administered to Wistar rats for 2 years at a dosage of 5–35 mg/kg daily (6–40 times the human dose).[20] Of those given 5 mg per day, hepatocellular carcinomas were found in 10%, compared with 67% of those given 20 mg per day and 67% of those who received 35 mg per day. Interestingly, the mortality rate was lower in those given 5 mg/kg per day than in controls because the latter group developed more fatal pituitary tumours in females and chronic renal disease in males.

Whatever the explanation for these findings and lack of observed hepatocellular cancers in women taking tamoxifen, there is pressure to investigate newer anti-oestrogens such as toremifine or selective oestrogen response modifiers (SERMs) such as raloxifene. The latter agent binds strongly to oestrogen receptors but has minimal oestrogen agonist effect and as such does not induce endometrial proliferation.[21] If raloxifene, or another SERM, can be shown to be equally effective as an adjuvant agent in women with breast cancer, without increased subjective toxicity, tamoxifen may be deposed as the leading endocrine therapy.

The workhorse of adjuvant cytotoxic treatment has been the CMF (cyclophosphamide, methotrexate, 5-fluorouracil) regimen, but although now of proven efficacy the impact on survival is fairly modest. Attempts are being made to improve the effect with anthracyclines, at standard or escalated dosages, with or without growth factor support, but no clear-cut advantages have emerged.[22] As taxol (paclitaxel) has been shown to be effective in anthracycline-resistant advanced breast cancer,[23] albeit with severe toxicity, it is likely that a bold medical oncologist will conduct a trial of its use in high-risk women with early disease. Before all oncologists rush to the yew tree for a breast cancer adjuvant therapy, the cost–benefit implications of such an approach need to be clearly defined. Uncritical acceptance or a desire to use fashionable new therapies may lead to a bankrupting of scarce resources.

SYNOPSIS

- Newer SERMs such as toremifine may replace tamoxifen in the next round of prevention trials.
- Measurement of electrical potentials over suspicious areas may enable the earlier detection of breast cancers and recurrence after breast conservation therapy.
- Instead of surgical excision, interstitial laser filaments may be of use in achieving limited destruction of small screen-detected cancers.
- Determination of sentinel node histology may identify those women with negative nodes who can be spared axillary clearance.
- Whole breast irradiation may be selectively avoided in some patients with early breast cancer with either a boost to the tumour site or sometimes no radiotherapy.
- Better selection of adjuvant therapies will spare some patients from unnecessary chemotherapy, and those who require endocrine therapy while identifying those who will benefit from more intensive treatment.

REFERENCES

1. Cauley JA, Lucas FL, Kuller LH et al. Bone mineral density and risk of breast cancer in older women. The Study of Osteoporotic Fractures. *JAMA* 1996; **276:** 1404–8.
2. Zhang Y, Kiel DP, Kreger BE et al. Bone mass and the risk of breast cancer among postmenopausal women. *N Engl J Med* 1997; **336:** 611–17.
3. Fentiman IS, Zaad S, Chaudary MA et al. Tamoxifen protects against steroid induced bone loss. *Eur J Cancer* 1992; **28:** 684–5.
4. Valavaara R, Pyrhönen S, Heckkinen M et al. Toremifine, a new antioestrogenic compound for treatment of advanced breast cancer. *Eur J Cancer* 1988; **24:** 785–90.
5. Saarto T, Blomqvist C, Ehnholm C et al. Anti-atherogenic effects of adjuvant antioestrogens: a randomised trial comparing the effects of tamoxifen and toremifine on plasma lipid levels in postmenopausal women with node-positive breast cancer. *J Clin Oncol* 1996; **14:** 429–33.
6. Hard GC, Iatropoulos MJ, Jordan K et al. Major difference in the hepatocarcinogenicity and DNA adduct forming ability between toremifine

and tamoxifen in female Crl:CD(BR) rats. *Cancer Res* 1993; **53:** 4534–41.

7. Pyrhönen S, Valavaara R, Modig H et al. Comparison of toremifine and tamoxifen in postmenopausal patients with advanced breast cancer: a randomized double-blind, the 'Nordic' phase III study. *Br J Cancer* 1997; **76:** 270–7.

8. Fentiman IS, Taylor-Papadimitriou J. Cultured human breast cancer cells lose selectivity in direct intercellular communication. *Nature* 1977; **269:** 156–8.

9. Loewenstein WR. Junctional intercellular communication and the control of growth. *Biochim Biopys Acta* 1979; **560:** 1–65.

10. Weiss BA, Ganepola GA, Freeman HP et al. Surface electric potentials as a new modality in the diagnosis of breast lesions. *Breast Dis* 1994; **7:** 91–8.

11. Cuzick J, Holland R, Barth V et al. Electro-potential measurements as a new modality for breast cancer diagnosis: results from a prospective multicentre trial. *Eur J Cancer* 1998; in press.

12. Fisher B, Anderson S, Fisher ER et al. Significance of ipsilateral breast tumour recurrence after lumpectomy. *Lancet* 1991; **338:** 327–31.

13. Magee B, Swindell R, Harris M, Banerjee SS. Prognostic factors for breast recurrence after conservative breast surgery and radiotherapy: results from a randomised trial. *Radiother Oncol* 1996; **39:** 223–7.

14. Fentiman IS, Poole C, Tong D et al. Inadequacy of iridium implant as sole radiation treatment for operable breast cancer. *Eur J Cancer* 1996; **32A:** 608–11.

15. Robinson DS, Parel J-M, Denham DB et al. Stereotactic uses beyond core biopsy: model development for minimally invasive treatment of breast cancer through interstitial laser hyperthermia. *Am Surg* 1996; **60:** 117–18.

16. Van der Veen H, Hoekstra OS, Paul MA et al. Gamma-probe-guided sentinel node biopsy to select patients with melanoma for lymphadenectomy. *Breast J Surg* 1994; **81:** 1769–70.

17. Krag DN, Weaver DL, Alex JC, Fairbank JT. Surgical resection and radiolocalization of the sentinel lymph node in breast cancer using a gamma probe. *Surg Oncol* 1993; **2:** 335–9.

18. Veronesi U, Paganelli G, Galimberti V et al. Sentinel node biopsy to avoid axillary dissection in node negative breast cancer with clinically negative lymph nodes. *Lancet* 1997; **349:** 1864–7.

19. Veronesi U, Luini A, Del Vecchio M et al. Radiotherapy after breast-preserving surgery in women with localized cancer of the breast. *N Engl J Med* 1993; **328:** 1587–91.

20. Greaves P, Goonetilleke R, Nunn G et al. Two-year carcinogenicity study of tamoxifen in Alderley Park Wistar-derived rats. *Cancer Res* 1993; **53:** 3919–24.

21. Black LJ, Sato M, Rowley ER et al. Raloxifene prevents bone loss and reduces serum cholesterol without causing uterine hypertrophy in ovariectomised rats. *J Clin Invest* 1994; **93:** 63–9.

22. Hudis C. New approaches to adjuvant chemotherapy for breast cancer. *Pharmacotherapy* 1996; **16:** 885–93.

23. Seidman A, Reichman B, Crown J et al. Paclitaxel as second and subsequent therapy for metastatic breast cancer: activity independent of prior anthracycline response. *J Clin Oncol* 1995; **13:** 1152–9.

Index